KETO DIET 50

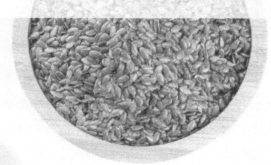

THE COMPLETE KETOGENIC BIBLE FOR PEOPLE OVER 50. BEGINNERS GUIDE TO START LIVING A HAPPY & HEALTHY LIFE, LOSING WEIGHT FAST AND NATURALLY

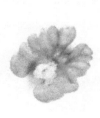

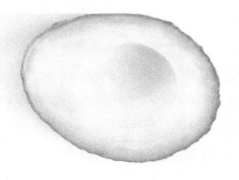

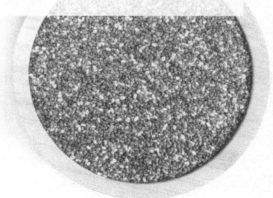

Jillian Collins

KETO AFTER 50

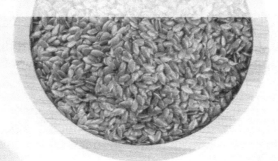

EASY GUIDE TO KETO DIET FOR SENIORS. DISCOVER HOW TO ENGAGE FAT-BURNING HORMONES FOR WEIGHT LOSS NATURALLY, INCREASE LONGEVITY, RESET METABOLISM TO FEEL CONFIDENT AGAIN (KETO RECIPES)

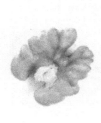
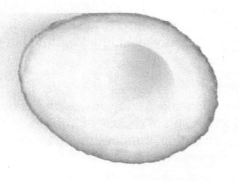
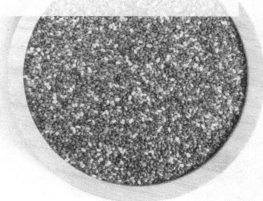

Jillian Collins

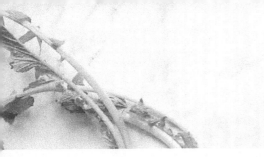
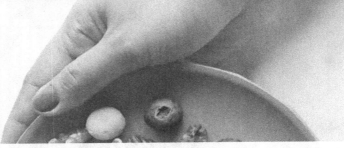

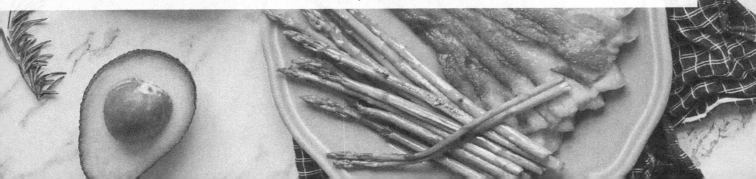

TABLE OF CONTENTS

INTRODUCTION

Are you over 50 and looking for a weight loss solution that works for you and enables you to eat as much as you desire?

If yes, you are in the right place.

This book was written after numerous consultations with people who reached middle age and began to experience weight gain and other related problems.

I am a Nutritionist with a degree in food science, and I am happy to have been able to help many women and men to achieve their goals. This book is intended to give you a full understanding of how a Ketogenic style can improve your physical and mental state without having to disrupt your habits. You must know that after the age of 50, the body for both women and men begins to undergo various changes, and this is why after the age of 50, a specific diet is necessary. This complete guide has been specifically designed to help men and women over 50 understand why a general ketogenic diet is not adequate but must be adapted and modified.

I am passionate about this way of keeping fit because it is not a classic restrictive diet but allows people to adapt gradually. I live a Ketogenic lifestyle, and although I'm 53 and mother of two boys, I can eat ice cream without feeling guilty and wear the clothes I wore at 30. I also involved my husband, who thought it was not easy, but today he feels invigorated and organizes barbecues with friends every week.

You can achieve this all by a one-of-a-kind diet that can help you burn away excess body fat, take your health and body to a new level, and restore your youth after the age of 50. So why is the Ketogenic diet a miracle for us? Let's start from the beginning. The ketogenic diet is a high-fat, medium protein, and low carb diet. The breakdown of a ketogenic diet is:

Fat: 70 to 90 percent of calories

Protein: 15 to 25 percent of calories

Carbs: 5 to 10 percent of calories

These macro-nutrient compositions make the Keto diet a perfect solution to burn fats in the body. The portion of fats is much more than the standard amount that people are used to consuming. This is where the keto diet gets intimidating as we have been told that fats are bad for health; this is not true. Bad fats are those that are harmful to health, whereas good fats are essential for absorbing vital minerals and nutrients.

Typically, the human body's natural behavior is sugar (glucose), which results from carbohydrate intake through foods. The glucose is then used as fuel by the body to perform its activities. However, glucose is not the most effective and efficient energy source for the body as it brings many serious health issues like coronary diseases, hypertension, diabetes, and obesity (to name a few). Sugar supply doesn't remain consistent in the blood, and that's why we face spikes of energy and become hungry again after eating recently. We also become tired after eating a high-carb meal and often plop down on the couch to take a nap. Glucose from carbs is the first choice of fuel by the body, but when it isn't used and burned through exercises, it is converted into fats, and we gain weight. When our body needs sugar for energy, it doesn't burn the converted in fat, and instead, it sends signals to the brain that provoke us to eat high sugar foods like chips, cookies, etc.

To break the diet routine of consuming more carbs/sugar and become more obese, the body burns off fats through a high-fat keto diet. It means that you are burning fats that have led you to gain weight. The keto diet brings the body into a ketosis state, which is a metabolic state where the body starts processing fats for fuel when carb reserves are depleted. Ketosis transforms fats into ketones that act as a source of energy, and ultimately, as fats keep burning, our weight sheds as well. The change in the body's natural behavior for fuel doesn't let you experience cravings or make you feel hungry, which are annoying side effects of other diets. You will become healthy, fitter, and sharper.

THANK YOU

I hope you'll enjoy these book; is part of the larger labor of love, which led me to create this project. I've put a lot of time, effort, and commitment into providing you with the only guide you'll need to understand how to approach the Ketogenic Diet, start a new lifestyle, and feel happy and Healthy again. All I ask in return is that if you love this book, please leave me an honest review.

I will read all with attention.

Thank you.

CHAPTER 1 - WHAT IS KETO DIET?

As you'd probably already know, the ketogenic diet is a low-carb diet where you eliminate or minimize carbohydrates' consumption. Proteins and fats replace the extra carbs while you cut back on pastries and sugar.

HOW DOES IT WORK?

See, when you consume less than 50 grams of carbs per day, your body starts to run out of blood sugar (which is used as fuel to provide your body quick energy). Once there are no sugar reserves left, your body will start to utilize fat and protein for energy. This entire process is known as ketosis, and this is exactly what helps you lose weight.

Compared to other diets, keto has a better chance of helping you lose weight more quickly. The diet is also incredibly popular as you're not encouraged to starve yourself. It would help if you worked towards a more high-fat and protein diet, which isn't as difficult as counting calories.

IS KETO GOING ALRIGHT FOR PEOPLE WITH DIABETES?

Now you're probably wondering, what do I do if I have diabetes? For starters, visit your physician. Talking to your physician is important regardless of what kind of diet you choose. However, note that keto diets generally do work well to improve insulin sensitivity.

For better results, seek a doctor's help if you have diabetes. Keto diets can have a drastic impact on your body and overall lifestyle; hence, it's always better to seek professional guidance.

How the Body Changes When You're Over 50

This isn't going to be fun to read, but once you hit your 50s, you're likely to experience some changes in your body. The most common include:

· Weight Gain

According to the Centers for Disease Control and Prevention (CDC), men and women are likely to gain one to two pounds each year as they transition from adulthood to middle age. This doesn't get any better for women as they hit menopause. While the gain in belly fat isn't directly linked to menopause, hormonal changes may cause you to put on a few pounds, depending on the lifestyle and environmental changes.

- Metabolism Slows Down

You've probably heard a lot about your metabolism changing as you grow older. That's probably why you can't chow down junk food as you used to when you were in your teens. So, what is metabolism, and how does it affect your body?

In simple terms, metabolism is how quickly your body processes or converts food and liquids into energy. As you grow older, metabolism slows down, and the body starts to convert those extra calories into fat. This is probably why you should skip those convenience meals and start to eat healthier.

WHY SHOULD YOU SWITCH TO KETO?

Once you start to hit 50, you likely don't indulge in strenuous activities anymore, so your body will need fewer calories to function. This is when you should start eliminating added sugars from your diet. Also, most packaged meals or meals provided in the hospital for the elderly are processed and contain empty calories, including mashed potatoes, bread, pasta, and puddings. These foods not only taste bland, but they also lack nutrition to keep your body strong and healthy.

Plus, a low-carb diet that is rich in healthy vegetables and meat will prove to be far better for people suffering from insulin insensitivity and your overall health. Hence, start reading food labels more often and opt for healthier options. A recent study from the Hebrew University of Jerusalem has indicated how eating a diet rich in healthy fats can help you lose weight in the long-term.

MACRONUTRIENTS AND KETO
MACRONUTRIENTS

The food you consume provides nutrition to the body. Various types of nutrients are present in the food. They are broadly classified into macronutrients and micronutrients. Macronutrients are those nutrients required in significant quantities in the food to provide necessary energy and raw material to build different body parts. These are:

- Carbohydrates

11

- Proteins

- Fats

CARBOHYDRATES

Carbohydrates are important energy sources of the body. In a Keto diet plan, you have to cut on your carbs to eliminate this energy source and compel your body to spend the already present food stores in your body. These food stores are present as fat in your body. Once your body turns to these fat deposits in the body for energy, you start to lose weight.

Carbohydrates should not constitute more than 5–10% of your daily caloric intake.

Carbohydrates are present in a variety of foods. You should make sure that the small quota of carbohydrates you can consume comes from healthy carbohydrate sources like the low-carb vegetables and fruits, e.g., broccoli, lemon, and tomatoes.

PROTEINS

Proteins are really important because they provide subunits, which are building blocks of the body. They produce various hormones, muscles, enzymes, and other working machinery of the body. They provide energy to the body as well.

No more than 20–25% of your daily caloric intake should come from proteins. As a rule of thumb, a healthy person should consume about 0.5–0.7 grams of proteins per pound of total body weight.

Many people make a mistake in a keto diet consuming much more protein than they should. This not only puts additional strain on their kidneys but is also very unhealthy for the digestive system.

Eat a good variety of proteins from various sources like tofu, fish, chicken, and other white meat sources, including seeds, nuts, eggs, and dairy (though you shouldn't fill your diet with cheese). Red meat like beef can be enjoyed less frequently. We also suggest you avoid processed meats, which are typically laden with artificial preservatives.

Processed meat refers to meat that's modified through a series of processes, which might include salting, smoking, canning, and, most importantly, treated with preservatives. Such variants typically include sausages, jerky, and salami. As these meats are not even considered healthy for normal diets, we suggest limiting your portions to only once or twice a week.

FATS

In keto, fats serve as the mainstay of your diet. It seems counterintuitive to consume what you want to eliminate from your body, but that is exactly how this strategy works. But before you go about loading your body with all types of fats, keep the following things in your mind:

1.   You have to cut on carbs before this high-fat diet can be of any benefit to the body.

2.   Fats should take up about 70—75% of your daily caloric intake.

3.   Fats are of various types, and you have to be aware of the kind of fats you should consume.

Dietary fats can be divided into two kinds: healthy and harmful. Unsaturated fats belong to the healthier group, whereas saturated and trans-unsaturated fats belong to the unhealthier category. Aside from the differences in their health effects, these fats essentially differ in terms of chemical structure and bonding.

·   Saturated Fats

Saturated fats drive up cholesterol levels and contain harmful LDL cholesterol that can clog arteries anywhere in the body, especially the heart, and increase the risk of cardiovascular diseases. A diet high in saturated fat has an increased chance of reducing the risks of heart diseases. These fats are mainly contained in animal origin (except fish, which contains a small part). They are also present in plant-based foods, such as coconut oil. However, coconut oil contains medium-chain fatty acids, which are saturated fats different from animal origin, and therefore considered a healthy food.

Saturated fats are mostly contained in:

·   Whole milk dairy products, including milk and cheese

·   Butter

·   Skin-on chicken

·   Red meat such as pork, lamb, and beef

While there's no doubt that these foods are keto-friendly, they should not be consumed in large quantities, regardless of what diet you follow. It's also worth noting that some saturated fats are rated better in the health department than others. For instance, milk is healthier than consuming red meat. We suggest you limit butter and pork derived from animal fat as they overall tend to be unhealthy.

·   Unsaturated Fats

These 'good fats' contain healthy cholesterol. Unsaturated fats can most commonly be found in nuts, veggies, and fish. These fats keep your heart healthy and are a good substitution for saturated fats.

Unsaturated fats can be divided into:

Trans Fats: Trans fats, or trans-fatty acids, are a particular form of unsaturated fat. These unhealthy fats are manufactured through a partial hydrogenation food process. Moreover, some studies differentiate the health risks of those obtained industrially or transformed by cooking, from those naturally present in food (for example, vaccenic acid); the latter would be harmless or even beneficial to health.

The industrial foods that contain these hydrogenated fats are mainly: fried foods (especially French fries), margarine, microwave popcorn, brioche, sweet snacks, and pretzels.

While these foods may taste good, they're an unhealthy kind of fat and should be avoided.

Trans fats are known to increase unhealthy cholesterol levels in the blood, thus increasing the risks of cardiovascular disease. The WHO (World Health Organization) has the aim of global elimination of industrially-produced trans fats from food supplies by 2023.

CALCULATING YOUR DAILY CALORIC INTAKE

Many people think that calculating your calories while you are on a keto diet is not very important, but it is always good to watch how many calories you consume a day. It would help if you calculated how much calories you get to consume every day by the idea of how much weight you want to lose.

If your body needs 2,000 calories a day, but you consume only 1,400, your body is in a caloric deficit, so it will have to tap into your body's fat reserves, and this will result in a loss of weight. There are various calculators available online that can be used to calculate your daily caloric intake taking into account your objectives, age, height, activity level, and other factors.

In general, if you want to lose weight, you need to subtract around 600 calories from your daily caloric needs. So less than 1,000–1,200 calories if you are a woman and less than 1,400–1,600 calories if you are a man.

HAVING A MEAL PLAN

When you have a complete meal plan laid out in front of you, you are in a better position to have an idea as to what your diet would look like in the days to come. If you have to spontaneously decide what you will prepare to eat every time you are in the kitchen, your chances of getting off the rails become pretty high.

You can start by first calculating how many calories you are going to consume a day.

The next step would be to decide which macronutrients will have to be incorporated and in what proportion for your body to reach that goal. Remember that the rule of thumb is 75, 20, 5: for fats, proteins, and carbs, respectively.

CHAPTER 2 - KETO DIET FOR 50 AND ABOVE

Some part of aging involves a level of decrease by how we can work, yet it doesn't need to be disabling and segregating. It is a sad reality for some seniors and older people in our general public. The high-carb prepared eating routine frequently recommended for individuals of this age bunch isn't helping, either. Instead of seeing getting older as deplorable, we can bolster better mental and physical wellbeing at any age through an increasingly legitimate eating regimen. Furthermore, there are numerous focal points of following a ketogenic diet for old grown-ups in all actuality.

BENEFITS OF FOLLOWING A KETOGENIC DIET

Here is a part of the ways being in ketosis and eating well ketogenic foods can address concerns frequently looked by seniors today:

INSULIN OPPOSITION

Many residents in our public are overweight and managing diabetes. It is not funny at all, as diabetes can prompt things like vision misfortune, kidney infection.

BONE HEALTH

Osteoporosis, in which diminished bone thickness makes bones delicate and weak, is one of the most well-known conditions seen in older people. It is because the parts with the most noteworthy places of osteoporosis will, in general, have the most elevated rate of daily utilization. What's much better is to concentrate on a keto diet low in poisons, which meddle with ingestion, and is wealthy in all micronutrients instead of over-burden on a particular macronutrient (calcium).

INFLAMMATION

For some individuals, aging incorporates more agony from wounds that occurred at a younger age or joint issues like joint pain. Being in ketosis can help lessen the creation of substances considered cytokines that advance irritation, which can help with these kinds of conditions.

SUPPLEMENT INSUFFICIENCIES

Older adults will, in general, have higher inadequacies in effective supplements like iron deficiency and nutrient b12 lack, which can prompt neurological conditions like dementia, mind mist, and weariness.

FATS

Insufficiency can prompt issues with discernment, skin, vision, and nutrient lacks.

VITAMINE D

Insufficiency causes intellectual hindrance in older adults, increment the danger of coronary illness, and even increase the chance of malignant growth.

The top-notch sources of creature protein on the ketogenic diet can, without much of a stretch record, be fantastic sources of these effective supplements.

KETO IN CONTROLLING BLOOD SUGAR

As we've talked about, there is an association between inadequate glucose and cerebrum-related conditions like Alzheimer's sickness, dementia, and Parkinson's Disease. A few factors that may add to Alzheimer's infection incorporate:

- An abundance admission of carbohydrates, mainly from fructose, which is radically decreased in the ketogenic keto diet
- An absence of keto dietary fats and cholesterol, which are bottomless and sound on the ketogenic keto diet
- Oxidative pressure, which being in ketosis ensures against

Utilizing a ketogenic keto diet to assist control with blooding sugar and improve sustenance may help enhance insulin reaction as well as secure against memory issues that regularly happened with age.

SIGNIFICANCE OF KETO FOR AGING

Keto nourishments convey a large amount of sustenance per calorie. It is significant because the basal metabolic rate (the ratio of calories required every day to endure) is less for seniors. Yet, they despise everything that needs an equal amount of supplements from more youthful individuals.

An individual aged 65+ will have a lot harder time living on lousy nourishments than a high schooler or 20-something whose body is as yet flexible. It makes it much increasingly vital for seniors to eat nourishments that are wellbeing supporting and infection battling. It can indeed mean the distinction between appreciating the brilliant years without limit or spending them in torment and misery.

Subsequently, seniors need to eat a progressively ideal eating routine by keeping away from "void calories" from sugars or nourishments wealthy in enemies of supplements, for example, entire grains, and expanding their amount of supplement rich in fats and proteins.

Likewise, a significant part of the nourishment picked by older individuals (or given in an emergency clinic or clinical settings) will, in general, be vigorously prepared and extremely poor in supplements, for example, white bread, pasta, prunes, pureed potatoes, and puddings.

The high-carb keto diet so broadly pushed by the legislature isn't best for supporting our senior residents and their long-term wellbeing. An eating regimen low in carbohydrates and wealthy in animal and plant fats is obviously better for advancing better insulin affectability, fewer occurrences of subjective decay, and generally speaking, better wellbeing. In a Keto Talk web recording with Jimmy Moore, Dr. Adam Nally discusses how he has numerous older patients excelling on a keto diet. In light of the data talked about, this bodes well.

KETOSIS FOR LONGEVITY

Regardless of our age, it's never an impractical notion to improve your odds of feeling and work great for an excellent remainder. It's never the point where it's possible to begin growing, although the sooner we start, the better our odds of maintaining a strategic distance from the ailment. In any event, for the individuals who have spent numerous years not considering their bodies just as they should, ketosis for seniors can fix a part of the harm.

As we talk about ketosis for life span article, we can start making changes that help healthy weight, glucose, resistance, and the sky is the limit from there, the more prominent possibility of having less torment and enduring further down the road. We're all getting older, and demise is, obviously, unavoidable. In any case, what we can control to a degree is the personal satisfaction en route. Individuals are recently living longer, but at the same time, we're getting more broken down by following the standard eating routine of the more significant part. The ketogenic keto diet can assist seniors with improving their well-being, so they can flourish instead of being wiped out or in torment during the later, long periods of life.

CHAPTER 3 - THE SCIENCE BEHIND THE KETO DIET

To bring the body into a ketogenic condition, you need to follow a high-fat diet and small carbohydrates without any grains, or almost any. The composition will be roughly 80% fat and 20% protein. That will be the rule for the very first two days.

When the body absorbs carbs, it induces an insulin surge with the insulin emitted by the pancreas. Common sense assures us that if we then eliminate carbs, the insulin does not hold excess calories as the perfect fat. Now your body has no carbs as an energy source, so your body should look for a new source.

If you decide to remove extra weight, this works well. The body must break down the extra fat and function with it, rather than carbs, as energy.

That particular condition is known as 'Ketosis.' This state, in which you want the body to be in, can make great sense in case you want to lose excess fat while keeping muscle.

Let's move on now to the portion of the diet and how to prepare it. With every pound of lean mass, you would need to ingest no less than one gram of protein. It will aid with strengthening and restoring muscle tissue during exercises. That means 65% protein and 30% fat.

Effectively, if you weigh 150 pounds, that means 150 g of protein a day. If you multiply it four times (number of calories equivalent to 600 calories in a gram of protein), any of the calories will come from fat. If the caloric maintenance is 3,000, you need to consume about 500, less that might imply that one day if you require 2,500 calories, about 1,900 calories should come from the fats!

To fuel the body, you have to consume fats, which will also burn up excess fat! That is the diet plan rule; you've got to consume fats! The downside of taking healthy fats and the keto diet is that you're not going to be thirsty. Fat processing of food is slow, operating to the benefit and making you feel satisfied.

You're going to be working on Monday—Friday, and then on the other days, you're going to have a 'carb-up.' When this process begins when the last exercise is on Friday, post-training, you need to take a liquid carbohydrate with your whey shake. This will help to produce an insulin surge, allowing us to provide the carbohydrates that the body urgently requires for restoring muscle mass and for glycogen stores to expand and refill.

Consume whatever you like during this specific process (carb-up): pizzas, crisps, spaghetti, and ice cream. Somehow, this will be beneficial for you because it can refresh the body for the week ahead and provide the food that your body requires.

Switch your focus on to the no-carb and high-fat average protein diet program as Sunday starts. Holding the body in Ketosis and losing fat is the optimal remedy, by muscle.

An additional benefit of Ketosis is when you enter the ketosis state and burn the fat, the body will deplete from carbohydrates. Packing up with carbs can make you appear as full as before (but even fewer body fat!), perfect for holiday activities if you visit the seaside or parties!

Let us recap on the diet schedule now.

Get in ketosis state by removing carbs and taking moderate/low protein and high fat.

Take some fiber to keep the pipes as clear as ever; you should realize what I mean.

If the ketosis protein consumption has been collected, the lean mass per pound will be no less than that of one gram of protein.

So it is! It does require determination not to eat carbs during the week because certain products contain carbs; however, note that you would be greatly rewarded for the devotion.

You must not live on end days in Ketosis condition because it is dangerous and will wind up with yourself turning to make use of protein as a source of food that is a no-no.

Ketogenic diet systems are structured primarily to trigger a ketosis condition within the body. If the volume of glucose in the body is low, the whole body turns to fat as a source of energy replacement.

The body has main sources of fuel, one of which is:

GLUCOSE

Free fatty acids (FFA) and, to a lesser degree, ketones from FFA Fat by-products are kept in the triglyceride type. Typically, they are split into long-chain fatty acids and glycerol. The removal of glycerol from the triglyceride molecule enables the three free fatty acid (FFA) molecules to be used as energy to introduce the bloodstream.

The glycerol molecule goes into the liver, where three molecules of it combine to create one molecule of sugar. Additionally, when the body consumes fat, it creates glucose as a by-product. Its glucose may be used to power different regions of the brain and body parts that can't operate on FFA molecules.

However, though glucose on its triglycerides will travel through the blood, cholesterol takes a carrier to go through the bloodstream. In a carrier known as LDL or low-density lipoprotein, cholesterol and triglycerides are packed. Thus, the larger the LDL particles, the greater the number of triglycerides it has.

The general process of energy-burning of fat deposits produces co2, oxygen, and ketone-known components. The liver produces ketones out of the free essential fatty acids. Right now, they consist of two classes of atoms joined by a purposeful carbonyl unit.

The body cannot store ketones, and therefore they should be used or excreted at times. The body often excretes them as acetone through the breath and as acetoacetate through the urine.

The ketones may be used as a source of energy for body cells. The subconscious will use ketones to generate between 70—75 percent of the energy requirement.

As for alcoholic drinks, ketones take priority over carbohydrates as food resources. That means that they should be consumed first when filled with the bloodstream before glucose can be used as a fuel.

CHAPTER 4 - THE MAIN FEATURES OF THE KETOGENIC DIET

LOSING WEIGHT

For most people, this is the foremost benefit of switching to keto! Their previous diet method may have stalled for them, or they were noticing weight creeping back on. With keto, studies have shown that people have been able to follow this diet and relay fewer hunger pangs and suppressed appetite while losing weight at the same time! You are minimizing your carbohydrate intake, which means fewer blood sugar spikes. Often, those fluctuations in blood sugar levels make you feel more hungry and prone to snacking in between meals. Instead, by guiding the body towards ketosis, you are eating a more fulfilling diet of fat and protein and harnessing energy from ketone molecules instead of glucose. Studies show that low-carb diets effectively reduce visceral fat (the fat you commonly see around the abdomen that increases as you become obese). This reduces your risk of obesity and improves your health in the long-term.

REDUCE THE RISK OF TYPE 2 DIABETES

The problem with carbohydrates is how unstable they make blood sugar levels. This can be very dangerous for people who have diabetes or are pre-diabetic because of unstable blood sugar levels or family history. Keto is a great option because of the minimal intake of carbohydrates it requires. Instead, you are harnessing most of your calories from fat or protein, which will not cause blood sugar spikes and, ultimately, pressure the pancreas to secrete insulin. Many studies have found that diabetes patients who followed the keto diet lost more weight and ultimately reduced their fasting glucose levels. This is monumental news for patients who have unstable blood sugar levels or are hoping to avoid or reduce their diabetes medication intake.

IMPROVE CARDIOVASCULAR RISK SYMPTOMS TO OVERALL LOWER YOUR CHANCES OF HAVING HEART DISEASE

Most people assume that following a keto diet that is so high in fat content has to increase your risk of coronary heart disease or heart attack, but the research proves otherwise! Research shows that switching to keto can lower your blood pressure, increase your HDL good cholesterol, and reduce your triglyceride fatty acid levels. That's because the fats you are consuming on keto are healthy and high-quality fats, so they reverse many unhealthy symptoms of heart disease. They boost your "good" HDL cholesterol levels and decrease your "bad" LDL cholesterol levels. It also decreases the level of triglyceride fatty acids in the bloodstream. A high level of these can lead to stroke, heart attack, or premature death. And what are the high levels of fatty acids linked to?

LOW CONSUMPTION OF CARBOHYDRATES

With the keto diet, you are drastically cutting your carbohydrates intake to improve fatty acid levels and improve other risk factors. A 2018 study on the keto diet found that it can improve 22 out of 26 risk factors for cardiovascular heart disease! These factors can be very important to some people, especially those who have a history of heart disease in their family.

INCREASES THE BODY'S ENERGY LEVELS

Let's briefly compare the difference between the glucose molecules synthesized from a high carbohydrate intake versus ketones produced on the keto diet. The liver makes ketones and use fat molecules you already stored. This makes them much more energy-rich and a lasting fuel source compared to glucose, a simple sugar molecule. These ketones can physically and mentally give you a burst of energy, allowing you to have greater focus, clarity, and attention to detail.

DECREASES INFLAMMATION IN THE BODY

Inflammation on its own is a natural response by the body's immune system, but when it becomes uncontrollable, it can lead to an array of health problems, some severe, and some minor. The health concerns include acne, autoimmune conditions, arthritis, psoriasis, irritable bowel syndrome, and even acne and eczema. Often, removing sugars and carbohydrates from your diet can help patients of these diseases avoid flare-ups— and the delightful news is keto does just that! A 2008 research study found that keto decreased a blood marker linked to high inflammation in the body by nearly 40%. This is glorious news for people who may suffer from inflammatory disease and want to change their diet to see improvement.

INCREASES YOUR MENTAL FUNCTIONING LEVEL

As we mentioned earlier, the energy-rich ketones can boost the body's physical and mental alertness levels. Research has shown that keto is a much better energy source for the brain than simple sugar glucose molecules are. With nearly 75% of your diet coming from healthy fats, the brain's neural cells and mitochondria have a better energy source to function at the highest level. Some studies have tested patients on the keto diet and found they had higher cognitive functioning, better memory recall, and less memory loss. The keto diet can even decrease the occurrence of migraines, which can be very detrimental to patients.

THE CALORIE AND NUTRIENT BALANCE

Do you know why else the Ketogenic Diet is good for you, specifically, as someone who just hit 50 years old? You should keep in mind that as a person advances in age, their calorie needs to decrease. For example, instead of 2,000 calories per day, you'll need only 1,800 calories per day. Why is that? Well, when we start to get old, our physical activity significantly decreases. Hence, we don't need as much energy in our system. However, that doesn't mean our nutrient needs also go down. We still need the same amount of vitamins and minerals.

The Ketogenic Diet manages to hit a balance between these two needs. You get high nutrition for every calorie you get—which means that you'll maintain a decent amount of weight without feeling less energetic for day to day activities.

HEART DISEASES

Keto diets help women over 50 to shed those extra pounds. Reducing any amount of weight greatly reduces the chances of a heart attack or any other heart complications. Through the carefully selected diet routine, you are not only losing weight and enjoying delicious meals, but you are significantly boosting your heart's health and reviving yourself from the otherwise dull state that you may have been in before.

DIABETES CONTROL

Needless to say, the careful selection of ingredients, when cooked together, provide rich nutrients, free from any processed or harmful contents such as sugar. Add to that the fact that keto automatically controls your insulin levels. The result is a glucose level that is always under control, and continued control would lead to a day where you will say goodbye to the medications you might be taking for diabetes.

CHAPTER 5 - WHAT TO EAT AND AVOID

I've had people complain about the difficulty of switching their grocery list to one that's Ketogenic-friendly. The fact is that food is expensive, and most of the food you have in your fridge is probably packed full of carbohydrates. It is why if you're committing to a Ketogenic Diet, you need to do a clean sweep. That's right, everything that's packed with carbohydrates should be identified and set aside to make sure that you are not overeating.

WHAT TO EAT ON THE KETO DIET

FATS AND OILS

Because fats will be included as part of all your meals, we recommend that you choose the highest quality ingredients that you can afford. Some of your best choices for fat are:

- Ghee or Clarified butter

- Avocado

- Coconut Oil

- Red Palm Oil

- Butter

- Coconut Butter

- Peanut Butter

- Chicken Fat

- Beef Tallow

- Non-hydrogenated Lard

- Macadamias and other nuts

- Egg Yolks

- Fish rich in Omega-3 Fatty Acids like salmon, mackerel, trout, tuna, and shellfish

PROTEIN

Those on a keto diet will generally keep fat intake high, carbohydrate intake low, and protein intake at a moderate level. Some on the keto diet for weight loss have better success with higher protein and lower fat intake.

- Fresh meat: beef, veal, lamb, chicken, duck, pheasant, pork, etc.

- Deli meats: bacon, sausage, ham (make sure to watch out for added sugar and other fillers)

- Eggs: preferably free-range or organic eggs

- Fish: wild-caught salmon, catfish, halibut, trout, tuna, etc.

- Other seafood: lobster, crab, oyster, clams, mussels, etc.

- Peanut Butter: this is a great source of protein, but make sure to choose a brand that contains no added sugar

DAIRY

Compared to other weight-loss diets, the keto diet actually encourages you to choose dairy products that are full fat. Some of the best dairy products that you can choose are:

- Hard and soft cheese: cream cheese, mozzarella, cheddar, etc.

- Cottage cheese

- Heavy whipping cream

- Sour cream

- Full-fat yogurt

VEGETABLES

Overall, vegetables are rich in vitamins and minerals that contribute to a healthy body. However, if you're aiming to avoid carbs, it's best that you limit starchy vegetables such as potatoes, yams, peas, corn, beans, and most legumes. Other vegetables that are high in carbohydrates, such as parsnips and squash, should also be limited. Instead, stick with green leafy vegetables and other low-carb veggies. Choose local or organic varieties if it fits with your budget.

- Spinach
- Lettuce
- Collard greens
- Mustard greens
- Bok choy
- Kale
- Alfalfa sprouts
- Celery
- Tomato
- Broccoli
- Cauliflower

FRUITS

Your choice of fruit on the keto diet is typically restricted to avocado and berries because fruits are high in carbohydrates and sugar.

DRINKS

- Water
- Black coffee
- Herbal tea
- Wine: white wine and dry red wine are OK if they are only consumed occasionally.

OTHERS

- Homemade mayo: if you want to buy mayo from the store, make sure that you watch out for added sugar
- Homemade mustard
- Any type of spices or herbs

- Stevia and other non-nutritive sweeteners such as Swerve

- Ketchup (Sugar-free)

- Dark chocolate/cocoa

FOODS TO AVOID
1. BREAD AND GRAINS

Bread is a staple food in many countries. You have loaves, bagels, tortillas, and the list goes on. However, no matter what form bread takes, they still contain a lot of carbs. The same applies to whole-grain as well because they are made from refined flour. Depending on your daily carb limit, eating a sandwich or bagel can put your way over your daily limit. So if you want to eat bread, it is best to make keto variants at home instead. Grains such as rice, wheat, and oats contain a lot of carbs too. So limit or avoid that as well.

2. FRUITS

Fruits are healthy for you. They are found to make you have a lower risk of heart disease and cancer. However, there are a few that you need to avoid in your keto diet. The problem is that some of those foods contain quite a lot of carbs, such as banana, raisins, dates, mango, and pear. As a general rule, avoid sweet and dried fruits. Berries are an exception because they do not contain as much sugar and are rich in fiber. So you can still eat some of them, around 50 grams. Moderation is key.

3. VEGETABLES

Vegetables are healthy for your body. Most of the keto diet does not care how many vegetables you eat so long as they are low in starch. Vegetables that are high in fiber can aid with weight loss. On the one hand, they make you feel full for longer, so they help suppress your appetite. Another benefit is that your body would burn more calories to break and digest them.

Moreover, they help control blood sugar levels and aid with your bowel movements. But that also means you need to avoid or limit vegetables that are high in starch because they have more carbs than fiber. That includes corn, potato, sweet potato, and beets.

4. PASTA

Pasta is also a staple food in many countries. It is versatile and convenient. As with any other suitable food, pasta is rich in carbs. So when you are on your keto diet, spaghetti, or many different types of pasta are not recommended. You can probably eat a small portion, but that is not suggested. Thankfully, that does not mean you need to give up on it altogether. If you are craving pasta, you can try some other alternatives that are low in carbs such as spiralized veggies or shirataki noodles.

5. CEREAL

Cereal is also a massive offender because sugary breakfast cereals contain a lot of carbs. That also applies to "healthy cereals." Just because they use other words to describe their product does not mean that you should believe them. That also applies to oatmeal, whole-grain cereals, etc. So if you get your cereal when you are doing keto, you are already way over your carb limit, and we haven't even added milk into the equation! Therefore, avoid whole-grain cereal or cereals that we mention here altogether.

CHAPTER 6 - WOMEN AFTER 50 AND KETOGENIC DIET

Getting to the age of 50 means many physical and psychological changes in women, such as menopause, hormonal problems, inflammation, irritability, weak muscles and bones, lethargy, and the list goes on. Some women develop diabetes, Alzheimer's, and cardiovascular issues as well.

WHY A NORMAL KETO DIET IS NOT RECOMMENDED FOR WOMEN AFTER 50

With a regular Keto diet, you cut your carbs down to minimum levels, i.e., less than 15 grams. Cutting down carbs severely and suddenly is bad for you because, due to aging, your metabolism decreases by 25%, and with every passing year, your bones and muscles become weaker and weaker.

We also become more vulnerable to many physiological and psychological diseases, such as cardiovascular disease, obesity, Alzheimer's, or diabetes. Adopting a regular Keto diet plan can result in many side effects, such as:

- Headaches

- Dizziness

- Fatigue

- Brain fog and difficulty focusing

- Lack of motivation and irritability

- Nausea

- Keto flu

INFLAMMATION

These side effects cause many women to pull back and lose hope. It's all because you haven't been told before about the likely side effects that you can suffer if you dive headfirst into the Keto diet. However, by consuming the right amount of fats while eating as much as you desire within the range of the specific foods presented in this book, you will get your desired results.

For this, you need a specific Keto diet plan, which will not only benefit you through weight loss but will also help build muscles, stabilizes your blood sugar levels, and maximize your energy levels. And for all this, the Keto diet for women over 50 is a perfect option for you.

FOR AGING AND MENOPAUSE

For aging women, menopause will bring severe changes and challenges, but the ketogenic diet can help you switch gears effortlessly to continue enjoying a healthy and happy life. Menopause can upset hormonal levels in women, which consequently affects brainpower and cognitive abilities. Furthermore, due to less production of estrogens and progesterone, your sex drive declines, and you suffer from sleep issues and mood problems. Let's have a look at how a ketogenic diet will help to solve these side effects.

ENHANCED COGNITIVE FUNCTIONS

Usually, hormone estrogen ensures the continuous flow of glucose into your brain. But after menopause, the estrogen levels begin to drop dramatically, so does the amount of glucose reaching the brain. As a result, your available brainpower will start to deteriorate. However, by following the keto diet for women after 50, the problem of glucose intake is circumvented. It results in enhanced cognitive functions and brain activity.

HORMONAL BALANCE

Usually, women face significant symptoms of menopause due to hormonal imbalances. The keto diet for women after 50 works by stabilizing these imbalances such as estrogen—this aids in experiencing fewer and bearable menopausal symptoms like hot flashes. The keto diet also balances blood sugar levels and insulin and helps in controlling insulin sensitivity.

INTENSIFIED SEX DRIVE

The keto diet surges the absorption of vitamin D, which is essential for enhancing sex drive. Vitamin D ensures stable levels of testosterone and other sex hormones that could become unstable due to low levels of testosterone.

BETTER SLEEP

Glucose disturbs your blood sugar levels dramatically, which in turn leads to a low quality of sleep. Along with other menopausal symptoms, good sleep becomes a massive problem as you age. The keto diet for women after 50 not only balances blood glucose levels but also stabilizes other hormones like cortisol, melatonin, and serotonin, warranting an improved and better sleep.

REDUCES INFLAMMATION

Menopause can upsurge the inflammation levels by letting potential harmful invaders in our system, which result in uncomfortable and painful symptoms. Keto diet for women after 50 uses the healthy anti-inflammatory fats to reduce inflammation and lower pain in your joints and bones.

FUEL YOUR BRAIN

Are you aware that your brain is composed of 60% fat or more? It infers that it needs a more considerable amount of fat to keep it functioning optimally. In other words, the ketones from the keto diet serve as the energy source that fuels your brain cells.

NUTRIENT DEFICIENCIES

Older women tend to have higher deficiencies in essential nutrients such as an iron deficiency, which leads to brain fog and fatigue; vitamin B12 deficiency, which leads to neurological conditions like dementia; fats deficiency, that can lead to problems with cognition, skin, vision; and vitamin D deficiency that not only causes cognitive impairment in older adults and increase the risk of heart disease but also contribute to the risk of developing cancer. On a keto diet, the high-quality proteins ensure adequate and excellent sources of these critical nutrients.

CONTROLLING BLOOD SUGAR

There is a relationship between low blood sugar levels and brain diseases, such as Alzheimer's disease, Parkinson's disease, or dementia. Some factors contributing to Alzheimer's disease may include:

- Enormous intake of carbohydrates, especially from fructose—which is drastically reduced in the ketogenic diet.

- Lack of nutritional fats and good cholesterol—which are copious and healthy in the keto diet.

·   Keto diet helps to control blood sugar levels and improve nutrition, which in turn not only improves insulin response and resistance but also protects against memory loss—which is often a part of aging.

CHAPTER 7 - KETO FOR MEN AFTER 50

When you reach the age of 50, you will notice many changes in your body. Among the most common symptoms are a loss of muscle, sleeplessness, and finer skin. You don't have to worry about this. Still, you have to pay much more attention than usual to your lifestyle. It is essential to keep fit, do exercise, and have a healthy and correct diet under all macros.

From this point of view, the ketogenic diet offers enormous advantages, as seen in the previous chapters. You can apply it even if you have health problems. Of course, a visit to a nutritionist can help you personalize your diet even more effectively. But this is "something more," the information in this book is more than enough; you just need to study it and apply it diligently.

As said, the functions of our body change according to age. The thing that changes most is our metabolism; it is physiological that it slows down with age. This change is due both to aging and to our lifestyle. Current metabolism is a consequence of our lifestyle in recent years.

A healthy lifestyle, with frequency, and low-abundance meals, with moderate alcohol consumption, will have a faster metabolism than a lifestyle consisting of large meals eaten once a day, alcohol consumption, and insomnia.

The ketogenic diet can help you from this point of view, eliminating carbohydrates and promoting the elimination of fats from our body. Another advantage is its flexibility; in fact, you can play with macros and adapt them to your needs, lifestyle, and progress made, of course.

Start gradually; your body has adapted for years to an unhealthy lifestyle, so do not overdo it overnight. Take your time and slowly reach your goals. There is no need to run; this is a marathon, not a 100-meters race.

At first, you may feel tired, exhausted, without energy. Don't worry; it's a normal thing; it's your body adapting to the new food style. You're taking away its main source of energy, carbohydrates; logically, it has to adapt. It must change the main energy source, it must switch to using fats, but this takes time, two or three days are necessary. The drop-in sugars could decrease your pressure for a couple of days, avoid exercise, and there will be no problems. The resulting benefits will be enormous.

KETO FOR MEN AFTER 50

Men also go through quite a lot of internal and external changes. These include, but are not limited to, physical changes, habitual changes, and so on. While the chemistry inside the body of both remains broadly the same, whether young or old, there are things which men are more likely to develop or lose than women, these include some diseases, ailments, infections, frequent changes, and disorders. The worst news is it happens as soon as you cross 45 years old. That means you are at least five years late already, or that is what you think.

KETO FOR WOMEN VS. MEN

In reality, since women and men have been created differently, our approach to Keto Diet may differ and should be different. These are the biological indifferences that we have no control with. We will be discussing the differences between males and females when it comes to approaching the Keto Diet.

Then, how should men do it or women do it? Here's a thing we need to understand about the Keto Diet. First and foremost is that it is very bio-individual. Even there are different ways to do it among men as well as among women. Just understand that it is individual, and it might take some adjustments as you go throughout the process. But for all men and all women, it's really important to become Keto adaptive first before you start to adjust things; what we mean by that is you need to do Keto strict for the first thirty days or so until you get adapted. Your body is becoming more efficient, and it is adapting to this new fuel source called ketones. It is going to take a while before your body gets adapted. But once you get adapted, there might be some difference in men versus women, as some women tend not to do well in the long-term with intermittent fasting.

So, a lot of people that do Keto do intermittent fasting as well because it puts you in a modified state of ketosis, so you are producing some ketones, but women don't do it in the long-term because of their hormones are different from men and their cycles during that time of the month.

Therefore, what we recommend to all women out there is that if you have become adapted to the Ketogenic Diet is that you should be cycling in and out of ketosis from time to time and specifically try it out adding in healthy carbs, not pizza, French fries or soda, but healthy carbs like fruit, potatoes, sweet potatoes, maybe a little bit of rice the week before your cycle. Adding those carbohydrates during nighttime could help balance those hormones to not experience their side effects from going on Keto long-term. And that is what we've seen helps a lot of clients that are adding those and also they are not as grumpy or angry. This stuff can help out with those symptoms and side effects. Thus, add in carbohydrates the week before your cycle.

Also, for men, it is best recommended that you test your hormones and get your blood work done every couple of months, so you know how your body is changing and adapting; therefore, you know if you need to switch things up or maybe do the target a ketogenic diet for a week or two and see how your body responds and adapts. It would be best if you became your experimentations, so you know what is best for you moving forward.

The truth is, there is a wide variety of people who can benefit from the Ketogenic Diet, whether they are young, old, man, or woman. Still, the Ketogenic Diet has been especially beneficial for women due to their different hormones and conditions.

HOW TO START A KETO DIET WHEN YOU'RE OVER 50?

Once you have decided, the next thing to do is speak to your doctor about it. As discussed, whether or not you're suffering from a medical condition, it's important to speak to your doctor to learn more about the keto diet and if it's right for you. Let's take a look at some steps to take when getting started:

DO YOUR RESEARCH ON KETO-FRIENDLY FOOD

First of all, you need to acquire a list of foods to eat and avoid. Depending on your budget and location, some of those foods may be difficult to find. So you may need to look for food alternatives that are also keto-friendly. Moreover, learn how to spot "hidden carbs" in the food items you purchase. Many foods may claim to be keto-friendly but may contain additional carbs or sugars.

PRACTICE PORTION CONTROL

Just because you're allowed to eat foods rich in fats and proteins doesn't mean you should eat excessive amounts. Although you don't have to count calories every time you eat, you should practice portion control so you don't go overboard. This is where a high-quality food scale comes in handy.

BE PREPARED TO EXPERIENCE SOME SIDE EFFECTS

Although these side effects don't happen to most people, you might be unlucky enough to experience them. One of the most common side effects is a condition known as the "keto flu." You will know that you have this condition if you experience side effects such as headaches, fatigue, irritability, a lack of motivation, brain fog (an inability to focus), sugar cravings, muscle cramps, dizziness, and nausea. However, if you already know what to watch out for, you don't have to worry. Most of these side effects are temporary and will go away. Also, try not to let the side effects discourage you from sticking with the diet.

EXERCISE

This is optional, but you should take care of your muscles at your age as they start to degrade. You will feel better, your health will improve, and your weight will go down faster.

CONSULT A NUTRITION SPECIALIST

This book is a valuable tool to get an idea of a ketogenic diet, the benefits, and how to avoid classic mistakes. It is a complete guide, with which, if studied well, you will certainly be able to set your diet according to your daily needs. However, consulting a doctor is never a bad idea; you can discuss your opinions and give you valuable advice. I recommend consulting your doctor, especially in health problems and cases where you have never been on a diet.

CHAPTER 8 - TIPS FOR SENIORS WHO WANT TO START, WHICH YOU WILL NOT FIND ELSEWHERE

LEARN HOW TO COUNT YOUR MACROS

This is especially important at the beginning of your journey. As time goes on, you will learn how to estimate your meals without using a food scale.

PREPARE YOUR KITCHEN FOR YOUR KETO-FRIENDLY FOODS

Once you've made a choice, it's time to get rid of all the foods in your kitchen that aren't allowed in the keto diet. To do this, check the nutritional labels of all the food items. Of course, there's no need to throw everything away. You can donate foods you don't need to food kitchens and other institutions that give food to the needy.

PURCHASE SOME KETO STRIPS FOR YOURSELF

These are important so you can check your ketone levels and track your progress. You can purchase keto strips in pharmacies and online. For instance, some of the best keto strips available on Amazon are: Perfect Keto Ketone Test Strips, Smackfat Ketone Strips, and One Earth Ketone Strips.

FIND AN ACTIVITY YOU ENJOY

When you have done enough exercise, you will know what activities you like. One way to encourage yourself to exercise more regularly is by making it entertaining than a chore. If possible, stick to your favorite activities, and you can get the most out of your exercises. Keep in mind that the activities you enjoy may not be effective or needed, so you need to find other exercises to compensate for, which you may not enjoy. For instance, if you like jogging, you can work your leg muscles, but your arms are not involved. So, you need to do pushups or other strength training exercises.

CHECK WITH A HEALTHCARE PROVIDER

Your dietitian can tell you whether a keto diet would work. Still, it helps to check in with your healthcare provider to ensure that you do not have any medical condition that prevents you from losing weight, such as hypothyroidism and polycystic ovarian syndrome. It helps to know well in advance whether your body is even capable of losing fat in the first place before you commit and see no result.

HYDRATE PROPERLY

That means drinking enough water or herbal tea and ditch sweetened beverages or other drinks that contain sugar altogether. Making the transition will be difficult for the first few weeks, but your body will thank you for it. There is nothing healthier than good old plain water, and the recommended amount is 2 gallons a day.

SUPPLEMENTS

When you get older, your body starts to lose its ability to absorb certain nutrients, which leads to deficits. For example, vitamin B12 and folate are some of the most common nutrients that people over 50 lack. They have an impact on your mood, energy level, and weight loss rate.

HAVE THE RIGHT MINDSET

Your mindset is one of the most important things you need to change when you've decided to follow the keto lifestyle. Without the right mindset, you might not stick with the diet long enough to enjoy all its benefits. Also, the proper mindset will keep you motivated to keep going no matter what challenges come your way.

GET ENOUGH SLEEP

Getting enough sleep helps your body regulate the hormones within it, so try to aim for 7 to 9 hours of sleep a day. You can get more restful sleep by creating a nighttime routine that involves not looking at a computer, phone, or TV screen for at least 1 hour before going to bed. You can drink warm milk or water to help your body relax or even do 10 to 20 minutes of stretching to get a restful sleep.

KEEP A FOOD LOG

Add the calories and divide them into three to get an average. Now that you know how many takes, you can figure out how much you need to pay on average per day to reach your goals.

CHAPTER 9 - 7-DAYS PLAN DETOX FOR WEIGHT LOSS

DAY ONE

Breakfast: Chorizo Breakfast Bake

Lunch: Sesame Pork Lettuce Wraps

Supper: Avocado Lime Salmon

All out macros: Calories: 1,520 Protein: 110g Fat: 109g Net Carbs: 16g

DAY TWO

Breakfast: Leftover Chorizo Breakfast Bake with 3 Slices Thick-Cut Bacon

Lunch: Spiced Pumpkin Soup

Supper: Leftover Avocado Lime Salmon

All out macros: Calories: 1,570 Fat: 124g Protein: 92g Net Carbs: 16g

DAY THREE

Breakfast: Baked Eggs in Avocado

Lunch: Easy Beef Curry

Supper: Veggies and Rosemary Roasted Chicken

All out macros: Calories: 1,700 Fat: 128.5g Protein: 103g Net Carbs: 22g

DAY FOUR

Breakfast: Lemon Poppy Ricotta Pancakes with 3 Slices Thick-Cut Bacon

Lunch: Leftover Spiced Pumpkin Soup with ½ Medium Avocado

Supper: Leftover Rosemary Roasted Chicken and Veggies

All out macros: Calories: 1,665 Fat: 130g Protein: 95.5g Net Carbs: 23.5g

DAY FIVE

Breakfast: Leftover Lemon Poppy Ricotta Pancakes with 3 Slices Thick-Cut Bacon

Lunch: Leftover Spiced Pumpkin Soup

Supper: Cheesy Sausage Mushroom Skillet with 1 Slice Thick-Cut Bacon

All out macros: Calories: 1,650 Fat: 126g Protein: 100.5g Net Carbs: 22.5g

DAY SIX

Breakfast: Sweet Blueberry Coconut Porridge with 1 Slice Thick-Cut Bacon

Lunch: Leftover Easy Beef Curry

Supper: Leftover Cheesy Sausage Mushroom Skillet

All out macros: Calories: 1,670 Protein: 100g Fat: 112g Net Carbs: 33.5g

DAY SEVEN

Breakfast: Leftover Sweet Blueberry Coconut Porridge

Lunch: Leftover Easy Beef Curry

Supper: Rosemary and Garlic with Lamb Chops

All out macros:Calories: 1,625 Protein: 110.5g Fat: 108g Net Carbs: 27g

CHAPTER 10 - IMPROVE YOUR KETOGENIC DIET WITH FITNESS

Can you remember when the last time you squat was? During physical education at school? Or maybe you tried to do a workout a few months ago, but then you lost your motivation?

Every diet that you respect must be associated with an adequate training regimen; they are two sides of the same coin, both important and necessary sacrifices and motivations.

It only takes a second to decide that it's worth it, 10 minutes for your first workout, and two weeks to feel the difference.

Everyone knows that doing physical activity improves wellbeing, but many are not familiar with all the benefits.

Here are the main benefits you can get when you start exercising:

- Lower risk of chronic diseases

- Mood and mental health improve

- Balanced energy levels during the day and better sleep quality

- Slowing down of aging processes

- Better brain health

- Positive effects on the microbiome

- Guaranteed sex life

MY GENERAL ADVICE IS:

- Cardio (minimum amount of activity): at least 150 minutes of moderate activity during the week. You can replace them with 75 minutes of intense activity or a combination of both.

- Train your strength (highly recommended): exercises involving the main muscle groups two or more days a week.

- For extra benefits: all minimal cardio activity can add 300 minutes (moderate level) or 150 minutes (intense level) per week (or a combination of both).

It may sound challenging, but the good thing is that you can adapt these tips to your schedule. As long as cardio activities are performed for at least 10 minutes, you can divide your active minutes into how many training sessions. Depending on your personal goal, you can choose to start with cardio or strength training.

TYPES OF PHYSICAL ACTIVITIES

What are the most common types of physical activity?

Cardio: any activity that increases your heart rate and makes you breathe faster is considered cardio. Usually refers to activities aimed at improving endurance, such as:

- Moderate level: brisk walking, dancing, jumping, jogging, cycling, swimming, push-ups, etc.

- Intense level: running, fast cycling, fast walking uphill, fast swimming.

Strength training: any activity that uses endurance to increase muscle strength. Using your body weight as resistance has many benefits!

Flexibility and mobility training: exercises to maintain and improve passive (flexibility) and active (mobility) movement.

WHAT TYPE OF PHYSICAL ACTIVITY IS BEST FOR LOSING WEIGHT?

Any exercise that requires high effort (for you) will have similar effects—especially for a beginner. So the truth is that... it doesn't matter! Choose activities that you enjoy and that you can imagine continuing to do for more than a month or two. After all, losing weight depends on the calorie deficit. So be sure also to adjust your diet to get the results you want.

TIPS TO START WORKING OUT

The first step is to reach a level of fitness where you no longer feel you "hate sport." Here's how to do it:

FIND THE INSPIRATION AND SET A GOAL

How many times have you forced yourself to start a training plan to lose 5 kg, and you have not succeeded? Try a different approach and first decide what you want to improve. Think about what you would like to do—whether it's exercising for 30 minutes without stopping or participating in the next marathon, improving your fitness for more energy and being more productive at work, and being able to keep up with your children.

START GRADUALLY AND SET YOUR PROGRESS

Starting gradually means focusing first and foremost on short-term goals.

Focus on one week at a time. Do your scheduled workout for the day. Then do the next one. Challenge yourself to cut 15—50 minutes a day, as often as possible, to do some movement.

Once the first week is over, rethink your workouts and move on to the next level—aim to do one more workout the following week, or even just five minutes more of cardio.

Establishing a training routine and respecting it is more important than the duration and type of training you do. Even a short 7—10-minute workout can give real benefits, especially for beginners on really busy days.

It takes time to see the results. That's why you need a monitoring system that shows you the best day by day and gives you motivation when you don't want to train. Be proud of every minute you record in your training plan!

PREPARE FOR OBSTACLES WITH A PLAN B

Skipping a workout or catching the flu shouldn't distract you from your goal. Each of us often encounters obstacles along our path after the first 2—3 weeks.

The goal is not to be perfect, but to improve over time. It is essential not to give up just as you don't give up school for a bad grade or quit your job when there's a problem.

Here are some possible solutions when you encounter an obstacle:

- Have you planned a workout but suddenly ran out of energy? If you already feel tired in the morning, stop training, and concentrate on what you eat during the rest of this day. If you start feeling too tired in the afternoon, do a short workout to relax and do some movement.

- Are you feeling stressed, or have you lost your motivation? It is normal to feel like this. Skip a day and make sure you get enough sleep.

- Did you miss a couple of days of training and feel guilty? Think about the cause: was it a particularly abundant meal, a difficult day, or a busy schedule? Keep this in mind because it will happen again sooner or later. Get ready to pick up where you left off. Even a setback can lead to new thoughts and renewed motivation.

EXTRA TIPS FOR BEGINNERS
DO A MEDICAL CHECK

It is always a good idea to check with your doctor or physiotherapist before starting a new lifestyle, such as a new training routine—especially if you are over 45 years old, suffer from chronic diseases, or have suffered injuries in the past.

DO NOT EXAGGERATE WITH INTENSITY

No effort, no results? Should you push yourself beyond your limits as a beginner? Yes, but only to maintain consistency in training.

How long does your body take to get used to training?

It depends on how long it has been since you were in shape ... but don't be put off by muscle pain. A common saying goes that "it takes two weeks to feel a change, four weeks to see a change and eight weeks to see the others."

Make an effort to be more active, but don't train if you feel pain. The real battle is in your head, and it's all about getting through the first few months. Once you've got used to it and learned how to do the exercises, it's time to push yourself even further to overcome your limits.

CARE FOR THE SHAPE

Avoid injuries and get better results by learning from the most common mistakes. In the beginning, you may feel confused by all the tips you need to keep in mind to take care of the exercises' shape. Focus on improving only one exercise at a time, not altogether. Don't force yourself. Do what you can by taking care of the shape and be patient; strength and endurance go hand in hand with constancy!

WORKOUT TO DO AT HOME AND TRAINING PLANS

There are many workouts that you can do at home and without the need for tools:

- Abdominals: 3 exercises to do at home

- Perfect for the morning: 7-minute energizing workout

- Abdominals: 4 core workouts to do at home

- Strongback: 6 exercises to strengthen it

- Mobility exercises for knees and wrists

- 10-minutes full body intense training

CHAPTER 11 - HEALTH TIPS FOR PEOPLE AFTER 50

Nobody told you that life was going to be this way! But don't worry. There's still plenty of time to make amendments and take care of your health. Here are a couple of tips that will allow you to lead a healthier life in your fifties:

START BUILDING ON IMMUNITY

Every day, our body is exposed to free radicals and toxins from the environment. The added stress of work and family problems doesn't make it any easier for us. To combat this, you must start consuming healthy veggies that contain plenty of antioxidants and build a healthier immune system.

This helps ward off unwanted illnesses and diseases, allowing you to maintain good health.

Adding more healthy veggies to your keto diet will help you obtain various minerals, vitamins, and antioxidants.

CONSIDER QUITTING SMOKING

It's never too late to try to quit smoking, even if you are in your fifties. Once a smoker begins to quit, the body quickly starts to heal the previous damages caused by smoking.

Once you start quitting, you'll notice how you'll be able to breathe easier while acquiring a better sense of smell and taste. Over a period of time, eliminating the habit of smoking can greatly reduce the risks of high blood pressure, strokes, and heart attack. Please note how these diseases are much more common among people in the fifties and above than in younger people.

Not to mention, quitting smoking will help you stay more active and enjoy better health with your friends and family.

STAY SOCIAL

We've already mentioned this, but it's worth pondering on again and again. Aging can be a daunting process, and trying to get through it all on your own isn't particularly helpful. We recommend you to stay in touch with friends and family or become a part of a local community club or network. Some older people find it comforting to get an emotional support animal.

Being surrounded by people you love will give you a sense of belonging and will improve your mood. It'll also keep your mind and memory sharp as you engage in different conversations.

HEALTH SCREENINGS YOU SHOULD GET AFTER YOUR FIFTIES

Your fifties are considered the prime years of your life. Don't let the joy of these years be robbed away from you because of poor health. Getting simple tests done can go a long way in identifying any potential health problems that you may have. Here is a list of health screenings you should get done:

CHECK YOUR BLOOD PRESSURE

Your blood pressure is a reliable indicator of your heart health. In simple words, blood pressure is a measure of how fast blood travels through the artery walls. Very high or even very low blood pressure can be a sign of an underlying problem. Once you reach your 40s, you should have your blood pressure checked more often.

EKG

The EKG reveals your heart health and activity. Short for electrocardiogram, the EKG helps identify problems in the heart. The process works by highlighting any rhythm problems that may be in the heart, such as poor heart muscles, improper blood flow, or any other form of abnormality. Getting an EKG is also a predictive measure for understanding the chances of a heart attack. Since people starting their fifties are at greater risk of getting a heart attack, you should get yourself checked more often.

MAMMOGRAM

Mammograms help rule out the risks of breast cancer. Women who enter their fifties should ideally get a mammogram after every ten years. However, if you have a family history, it is advisable that you get one much earlier to rule out cancer possibilities.

BLOOD SUGAR LEVELS

If you're somebody who used to grab a fast food meal every once in a while before you switched to keto, then you should definitely check your blood sugar levels more carefully. Blood sugar levels indicate whether or not you have diabetes. And you know how the saying goes, "prevention is better than cure." It's best to clear these possibilities out of the way sooner than later.

CHECK FOR OSTEOPOROSIS

Unfortunately, as you grow older, you also become susceptible to a number of bone diseases. Osteoporosis is a bone-related condition in which bones begin to lose mass, becoming frail and weak. Owing to this, seniors become more prone to fractures. This can make even the smallest of falls detrimental to your health.

ANNUAL PHYSICAL EXAM

Your insurance must be providing coverage for your annual physical exam. So, there's no reason why you should not take advantage of it. This checkup helps identify the state of your health. You'll probably be surprised by how much doctors can tell from a single blood test.

PROSTATE SCREENING EXAM

Once men hit their fifties, they should be screened for prostate cancer (similar to how women should get a mammogram and pap smear). Getting a screening done becomes especially important if cancer runs in your family.

EYE EXAM

As you start to aging, you'll notice how your eyesight will start to deteriorate. It's quite likely that vision is not as sharp as it used to be. Ideally, you should have gotten your first eye exam during your 40s, but it isn't too late. Get one as soon as possible to prevent symptoms from escalating.

BE WARY OF ANY WEIRD MOLES

While skin cancer can become a problem at any age, older adults should pay closer attention to any moles or unusual skin tags in their bodies. While most cancers can be easily treated, melanoma can be particularly quite dangerous. If you have noticed any recent moles in your body that have changed in color, size, or shape, make sure to visit the dermatologist.

CHECK YOUR CHOLESTEROL LEVELS

We've talked about this plenty of times, but it's worth mentioning again. High cholesterol levels can be dangerous to your health and can be an indicator of many diseases. Things become more complicated for conditions that don't show particular symptoms. Your total cholesterol levels should be below 200 mg per deciliter just to be on the safe side. Your doctor will take a simple blood test and will give you a couple of guidelines with the results. In case there is something to be worried about, you should make serious dietary and lifestyle changes. Within the first few weeks, just about everyone who follows this program experiences a rapid and significant weight loss. I've had readers tell me they've lost about 14 pounds in 14 days. These outcomes vary from person to person. If you have much extra weight to lose, it's likely to come off quicker. Some of the weight loss will be water weight, and it will feel right that the scale is going down fast. It may get you motivated to continue.

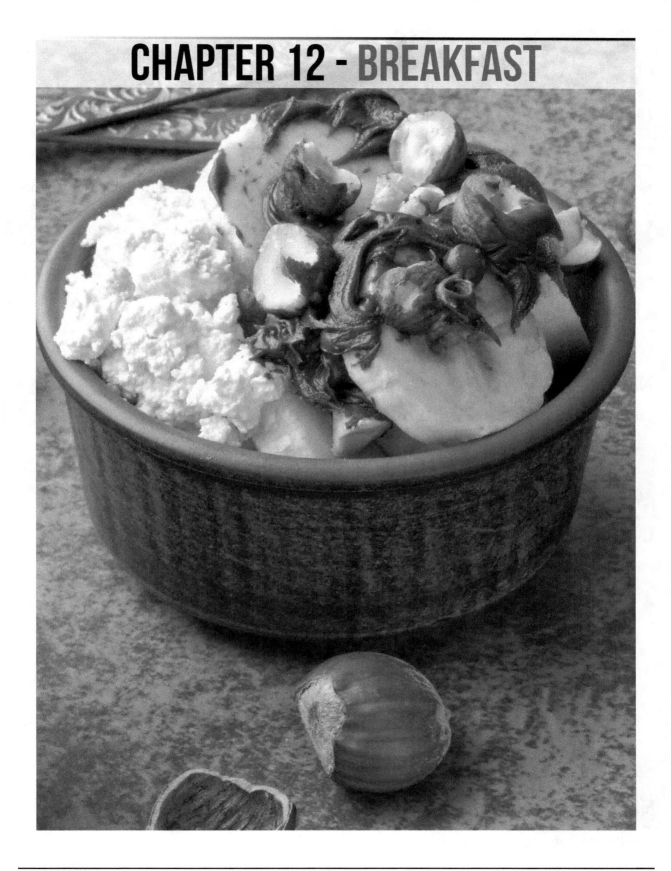

1. BLUEBERRY NUTTY OATMEAL

COOKING: 6-8H　　PREPARATION: 10'　　SERVINGS: 6

INGREDIENTS

- » 1 tablespoon of coconut oil (melted)
- » ½ cup of chopped pecans
- » ½ cup of sliced almonds
- » 1 avocado (diced)
- » 1 cup of coconut milk
- » 1 cup of coconut (shredded)
- » 2 cups of water
- » 2 ounces (57 g) of protein powder
- » ¼ cup of granulated erythritol
- » 1 teaspoon of ground cinnamon
- » ¼ teaspoon of ground nutmeg
- » ½ cup of blueberries (for garnish)

DIRECTIONS

1. Coat the insert of a slow cooker with melted coconut oil.
2. Put all ingredients except for the blueberries in the slow cooker, and stir until thoroughly mixed.
3. Cook covered on low heat for about 6 to 8 hours.
4. Divide the oatmeal among six serving bowls and garnish with the blueberries before serving. TIP: To add more flavors to this oatmeal, serve topped with a dollop of plain Greek yogurt.

NUTRITION:

Calories: 372, Fat: 33.2g, Carbs: 3.9g, Protein: 14.3g

2. KETO GOAT CHEESE SALMON FAT BOMBS

COOKING: 0'　　PREPARATION: 10'　　SERVINGS: 12

INGREDIENTS

- » ½ cup of butter (at room temperature)
- » ½ cup of goat cheese (at room temperature)
- » 2 ounces (57 g) of smoked salmon
- » 2 teaspoons of freshly squeezed lemon juice
- » Pinch of freshly ground black pepper

DIRECTIONS

1. Line a baking sheet with parchment paper. Set aside.
2. Make the fat bombs: Mix the butter, goat cheese, smoked salmon, pepper, and lemon juice in a bowl. Stir well to incorporate.
3. Scoop tbsp.-sized mounds of the mixture onto the parchment-lined baking sheet.
4. Transfer the fat bombs to the fridge for 2 to 3 hours until firm but not completely solid.
5. Remove from the fridge and let chill at room temperature for 8 minutes before serving.
6. TIP: Store the fat bombs in a sealed airtight container in the fridge for up to 1 week.

NUTRITION:

Calories: 196, Fat: 18.2g, Carbs: 0g, Protein: 8.1g

3. FRIED PORK RIND CRUSTED SALMON CAKES

COOKING: 25'　　　**PREPARATION: 15'**　　　**SERVINGS: 5**

INGREDIENTS

- » SALMON CAKES:
- » 6 ounces (170 g) of canned Alaska wild salmon, drained
- » 1 egg (lightly beaten)
- » 2 tablespoons of pork rinds (crushed)
- » 3 tablespoons of mayonnaise (divided)
- » Pink Himalayan salt (to taste)
- » Freshly ground black pepper (to taste)
- » MAYO DIPPING SAUCE:
- » 1 tablespoon of ghee
- » ½ tablespoon of Dijon mustard

NUTRITION:

Calories: 382.9, Fat: 31.3g, Carbs: 1.1g, Protein: 24.2g

DIRECTIONS

1. Mix the salmon, beaten egg, pork rinds, 1½ tablespoons of mayo, salt, and pepper in a large bowl until well combined.
2. Make the salmon cakes: on a lightly floured surface, scoop out 2 tablespoons of the salmon mixture and form a patty with your palm, about ½ inch thick. Repeat with the remaining salmon mixture.
3. Melt the ghee in a large skillet over medium-high heat.
4. Fry the patties for about 6 minutes until golden brown on both sides, flipping once.
5. Remove from the heat to a plate lined with paper towels. Set aside.
6. Combine the remaining mayo and mustard in a small bowl. Stir well.
7. Serve the salmon cakes with the mayo dipping sauce on the side.
8. TIP: If you don't have a large skillet that fits all the patties, you can cook them in batches.

4. CRAB SALAD STUFFED AVOCADOS

COOKING: 20　　　**PREPARATION: 0**　　　**SERVINGS: 2**

INGREDIENTS

CRAB SALAD:
- » ½ cup of cream cheese
- » 4½ ounces (128 g) of Dungeness crab meat
- » ¼ cup of chopped (peeled English cucumber)
- » ¼ cup of chopped red bell pepper
- » 1 teaspoon of chopped cilantro
- » ½ scallion (chopped)
- » Pinch of sea salt and freshly ground black pepper (to taste)

STUFFED AVOCADOS:
- » 1 avocado (peeled, halved lengthwise and pitted)
- » ½ teaspoon of freshly squeezed lemon juice

1. Make the crab salad: place the cream cheese, crab meat, cucumber, red pepper, cilantro, scallion, salt, and pepper in a medium bowl. Mix well until blended. Set aside.
2. Rub the cut parts of the avocado with fresh lemon juice.
3. Using a spoon, stuff each avocado halve with the crab salad. Serve immediately, or cover it with plastic wrap and refrigerate until ready to serve.
4. TIP: The crab salad can be made ahead and refrigerated until you want to stuff the avocado halves.

NUTRITION:

Calories: 378, Fat: 31.2g, Carbs: 5.1g, Protein: 19.2g

5. ARTICHOKE CAPONATA WITH GRILLED SALMON FILLETS

COOKING: 20'   **PREPARATION: 15'**   **SERVINGS: 4**

INGREDIENTS

- ¼ cup of olive oil (divided)
- 2 celery stalks (chopped)
- 1 tablespoon of garlic (minced)
- 1 onion (chopped)
- ½ cup of marinated artichoke hearts (chopped)
- 2 tomatoes (chopped)
- 2 tablespoons of dry white wine
- ¼ cup of apple cider vinegar
- 2 tablespoons of chopped pecans
- ¼ cup of pitted green olives (chopped)
- 4 (4-ounce/113g) of salmon fillets
- Freshly ground black pepper (to taste)
- 2 tablespoons of chopped fresh basil (for garnish)

DIRECTIONS

1. Make the caponata: heat 3 tablespoons of olive oil in a nonstick skillet over medium heat until shimmering.

2. Add the celery, garlic, and onion to the skillet and sauté for 4 minutes or until the onion is translucent.

3. Add the artichoke hearts, tomatoes, dry white wine, vinegar, pecans, and olives to the skillet.

4. Sauté to mix well and bring to a boil.

5. Turn down the heat to low and simmer for 6 minutes or until the liquid reduces by one third. Set the skillet aside.

6. Preheat the grill to medium-high heat.

7. On a clean work surface, brush the salmon fillets with olive oil, and sprinkle the salt and pepper to season.

8. Arrange the salmon on the preheated grill grates and grill for 8 minutes or until cooked through.

9. Flip the salmon halfway through.

10. Transfer the salmon to four plates, and pour the caponata over each salmon and serve with basil on top.

11. TIP: To make it a complete meal, you can serve it with roasted green beans and spicy chicken stew.

NUTRITION:

Calories: 340.9, Fat: 25.3g, Carbs: 4.1g, Protein: 24.g

CHAPTER 10 - LUNCH

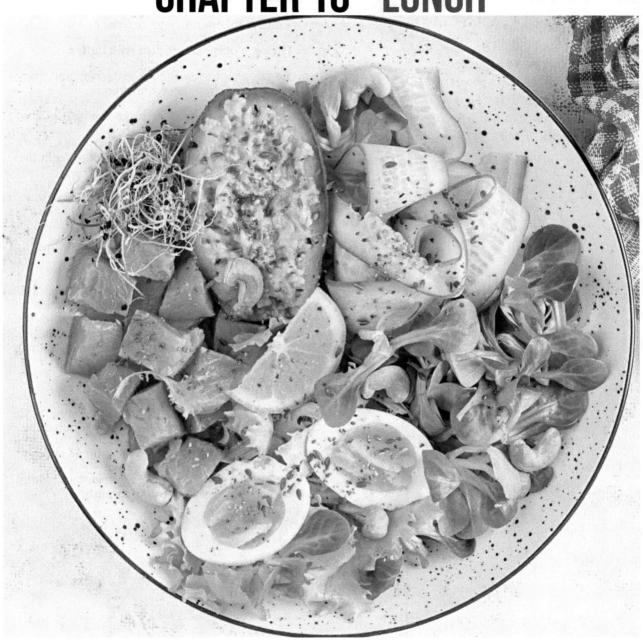

6. ROASTED LEMON CHICKEN SANDWICH

COOKING: 1H 30'   **PREPARATION: 15'**   **SERVINGS: 12**

INGREDIENTS

- » 1 kg. of whole chicken
- » 5 tablespoons of butter
- » 1 lemon (cut into wedges)
- » 1 tablespoon of garlic powder
- » Salt and pepper to taste
- » 2 tablespoons of mayonnaise
- » Keto-friendly bread

DIRECTIONS

1. Preheat the oven to 350 degrees F.

2. Grease a deep baking dish with butter.

3. Ensure that the chicken is patted dry and that the gizzards have been removed.

4. Combine the butter, garlic powder, salt, and pepper.

5. Rub the entire chicken with it, including in the cavity.

6. Place the lemon and onion inside the chicken and place the chicken in the prepared baking dish.

7. Bake for about 1½ hours, depending on the size of the chicken.

8. Baste the chicken often with the drippings. If the drippings begin to dry, add water. The chicken is done when a thermometer inserts it into the thickest part of the thigh, reads 165 degrees F, or when the clear juices run when the thickest part of the thigh is pierced.

9. Allow the chicken to cool before slicing.

10. To assemble the sandwich, shred some of the breast meat and mix with the mayonnaise.

11. Place the mixture between the 2 bread slices.

12. TIP: To save the chicken, refrigerated for up to 5 days or freeze for up to 1 month.

NUTRITION

Calories: 214, Fat: 11.8g, Carbs: 1.6g, Protein: 24.4g

7. KETO-FRIENDLY SKILLET PEPPERONI PIZZA

COOKING: 6'   PREPARATION: 10'   SERVINGS: 4

INGREDIENTS

FOR CRUST

» ½ cup of almond flour
» ½ teaspoon of baking powder
» 8 large egg whites (whisked into stiff peaks)
» Salt and pepper to taste

TOPPINGS

» 3 tablespoons of unsweetened tomato sauce
» ½ cup of shredded cheddar cheese
» ½ cup of pepperoni

DIRECTIONS

1. Gently incorporate the almond flour into the egg whites. Ensure that no lumps remain.

2. Stir in the remaining crust ingredients.

3. Heat a nonstick skillet over medium heat. Spray with nonstick spray.

4. Pour the batter into the heated skillet to cover the bottom of the skillet.

5. Cover the skillet with a lid and cook the pizza crust to cook for about 4 minutes or until bubbles that appear on the top.

6. Flip the dough and add the toppings, starting with the tomato sauce and ending with the pepperoni.

7. Cook the pizza for 2 more minutes.

8. Allow the pizza to cool slightly before serving.

9. TIP: It can be stored in the refrigerator for up to 5 days and frozen for up to 1 month.

NUTRITION

Calories: 175, Fat: 12g , Carbs: 1.9g, Protein: 14.3g.

8. CHEESY CHICKEN CAULIFLOWER

COOKING: 10'   PREPARATION: 5'   SERVINGS:4

INGREDIENTS

» 2 cups of cauliflower florets (chopped)
» ½ cup of red bell pepper (chopped)
» 1 cup of roasted chicken, shredded (Lunch Recipes: Roasted Lemon Chicken Sandwich)
» ¼ cup of shredded cheddar cheese
» 1 tablespoon of butter
» 1 tablespoon of sour cream
» Salt and pepper (to taste)

DIRECTIONS

1. Stir fry the cauliflower and peppers in the butter over medium heat until the veggies are tender.

2. Add the chicken and cook until the chicken is warmed through.

3. Add the remaining ingredients and stir until the cheese is melted.

4. Serve warm.

NUTRITION

Calories: 144, Fat: 8.5g , Carbs: 4g , Protein: 13.2g.

9. LEMON BAKED SALMON

COOKING: 30' **PREPARATION: 10'** **SERVINGS: 4**

INGREDIENTS

» 1 lb. of salmon
» 1 tablespoon of olive oil
» Salt and pepper to taste
» 1 tablespoon of butter
» 1 lemon (thinly sliced)
» 1 tablespoon of lemon juice

DIRECTIONS

1. Preheat your oven to 400 degrees F.

2. Grease a baking dish with the olive oil and place the salmon skin-side down.

3. Season the salmon with salt and pepper then top with the lemon slices.

4. Slice half the butter and place over the salmon.

5. Bake for 20 minutes or until the salmon flakes easily.

6. Melt the remaining butter in a saucepan. When it starts to bubble, remove from heat and allow to cool before adding the lemon juice.

7. Drizzle the lemon butter over the salmon and serve warm.

NUTRITION

Calories: 211, Fat: 13.5g, Carbs: 1.5g, Protein: 22.2g

10. BAKED SALMON

COOKING: 10' **PREPARATION: 10'** **SERVINGS: 4**

INGREDIENTS

» Cooking spray
» 3 cloves of garlic (minced)
» ¼ cup of butter
» 1 teaspoon of lemon zest
» 2 tablespoons of lemon juice
» 4 salmon of fillets
» Salt and pepper to taste
» 2 tablespoons of parsley (chopped)

DIRECTIONS

1. Preheat your oven to 425 degrees F.

2. Grease the pan with cooking spray.

3. In a bowl, mix the garlic, butter, and lemon zest and lemon juice.

4. Sprinkle salt and pepper on salmon fillets.

5. Drizzle with the lemon butter sauce.

6. Bake in the oven for 12 minutes.

7. Garnish with parsley before serving.

NUTRITION

Calories: 345, Total Fat: 22.7g, Saturated Fat: 8.9g, Cholesterol: 109mg, Sodium: 163mg, Carb: 1.2g, Dietary Fiber: 0.2g, Total Sugars: 0.2g, Protein: 34.9g, Potassium: 718mg

11. BUTTERED COD

COOKING: 5'   **PREPARATION: 5'**   **SERVINGS: 4**

INGREDIENTS

- » 1 ½ lb. of cod fillets (sliced)
- » 6 tablespoons of butter (sliced)
- » ¼ teaspoon of garlic powder
- » ¾ teaspoon of ground paprika
- » Salt and pepper to taste
- » Lemon slices
- » Chopped parsley

DIRECTIONS

1. Mix the garlic powder, paprika, salt, and pepper in a bowl.
2. Season codpieces with seasoning mixture.
3. Add 2 tablespoons of butter in a pan over medium heat.
4. Let half of the butter melt.
5. Add the cod and cook for 2 minutes per side.
6. Top with the remaining slices of butter.
7. Cook for 3 to 4 minutes.
8. Garnish with parsley and lemon slices before serving.

NUTRITION

Calories: 295, Total Fat: 19g, Saturated Fat: 11g, Cholesterol: 128mg, Sodium: 236mg, Carb: 1.5g, Dietary Fiber: 0.7g, Total Sugars: 0.3g, Protein: 30.7g, Potassium: 102mg

12. TUNA SALAD

COOKING: 0'   **PREPARATION: 15'**   **SERVINGS: 2**

INGREDIENTS

- » 1 cup of tuna flakes
- » 3 tablespoons of mayonnaise
- » 1 teaspoon of onion flakes
- » Salt and pepper to taste
- » 3 cups of romaine lettuce

DIRECTIONS

1. 1. Mix the tuna flakes, mayonnaise, onion flakes, salt, and pepper in a bowl.
2. 2. Serve with lettuce.

NUTRITION

Calories: 130, Total Fat: 7.8g, Saturated Fat: 1.1g, Cholesterol: 13mg, Sodium: 206mg, Total Carbohydrate: 8.5g, Dietary Fiber: 0.6g, Total Sugars: 2.6g, Protein: 8.2g, Potassium: 132mg

13. KETO FROSTY

COOKING: 0' **PREPARATION: 45'** **SERVINGS: 5**

INGREDIENTS

- » 1 ½ cups of heavy whipping cream
- » 2 tablespoons of cocoa powder (unsweetened)
- » 3 tablespoons of swerve
- » 1 teaspoon of pure vanilla extract
- » Salt to taste

DIRECTIONS

1. In a bowl, combine all the ingredients.
2. Use a hand mixer and beat until you see stiff peaks forming.
3. Place the mixture in a Ziploc bag.
4. Freeze for 35 minutes.
5. Serve in bowls or dishes.

NUTRITION

Calories: 164 , Total Fat: 17g, Saturated Fat: 10.6g, Cholesterol: 62mg, Sodium: 56mg, Carb: 2.9g, Dietary Fiber: 0.8g, Total Sugars: 0.2g, Protein: 1.4g, Potassium: 103mg

14. COCONUT CRACK BARS

COOKING: 3' **PREPARATION: 2'** **SERVINGS: 20**

INGREDIENTS

- » 3 cups of coconut flakes (unsweetened)
- » 1 cup of coconut oil
- » ¼ cup of maple syrup

DIRECTIONS

1. Line a baking sheet with parchment paper.
2. Put coconut in a bowl.
3. Add the oil and syrup.
4. Mix well.
5. Pour the mixture into the pan.
6. Refrigerate until firm.
7. Slice into bars before serving.

NUTRITION

Calories: 147 , Total Fat: 14.9g, Saturated Fat: 13g, Cholesterol: 0mg, Sodium: 3mg, Carb: 4.5g, Dietary Fiber: 1.1g, Total Sugars: 3.1g, Protein: 0.4g, Potassium: 51mg

15. STRAWBERRY ICE CREAM

COOKING: 0'   **PREPARATION: 1H 20'**   **SERVINGS: 4**

INGREDIENTS

- » 6 slices bacon
- » 1 avocado
- » 2 Persian cucumbers
- » 2 medium carrots
- » 4 oz. cream cheese

DIRECTIONS

1. Warm-up oven to 400F. Line a baking sheet. Place bacon halves in an even layer and bake, 11 to 13 minutes.

2. Meanwhile, slice cucumbers, avocado, and carrots into parts roughly the width of the bacon.

3. Spread an even layer of cream cheese in the cooled down bacon. Divide vegetables evenly and place it on one end. Roll up vegetables tightly. Garnish and serve.

NUTRITION

Carbohydrates: 11g, Protein: 28g, Fat: 30g

16. TROUT AND CHILI NUTS

COOKING: 0'   **PREPARATION: 10'**   **SERVINGS: 3**

INGREDIENTS

- » 1.5kg of rainbow trout
- » 300gr of shelled walnuts
- » 1 bunch of parsley
- » 9 cloves of garlic
- » 7 tablespoons of olive oil
- » 2 fresh hot peppers
- » The juice of 2 lemons
- » Halls

DIRECTIONS

1. Clean and dry the trout, then place them in a baking tray.

2. Chop the walnuts, parsley, and chili peppers then mash the garlic cloves.

3. Mix the ingredients by adding olive oil, lemon juice, and a pinch of salt.

4. Stuff the trout with some of the sauce and use the rest to cover the fish.

5. Bake at 180° for 30/40 minutes.

6. Serve the trout hot or cold.

INGREDIENTS

Calories: 226 , Fat: 5g , Dietary Fiber: 2g, Carbs: 7g, Protein: 8g

17. FIVE GREENS SMOOTHIE

COOKING: 25'   **PREPARATION: 10'**   **SERVINGS: 3**

INGREDIENTS

- » 6 kale leaves (chopped)
- » 3 stalks celery (chopped)
- » 1 ripe avocado (skinned, pitted, sliced)
- » 1 cup of ice cubes
- » 2 cups of spinach (chopped)
- » 1 large cucumber (peeled and chopped)
- » Chia seeds to garnish

DIRECTIONS

1. In a blender, add the kale, celery, avocado, and ice cubes, and blend for 45 seconds.

2. Add the spinach and cucumber, and process for another 45 seconds until smooth.

3. Pour the smoothie into glasses, garnish with chia seeds, and serve the drink immediately.

NUTRITION

Calories: 124, Fat: 7.8g, Carbs: 2.9g, Protein: 3.2g

CHAPTER 11 - SNAKS

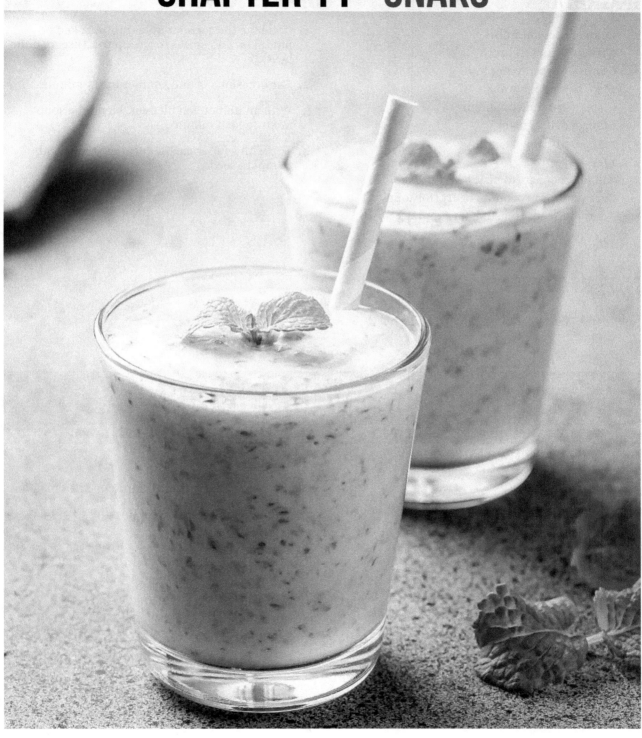

18. QUICK PUMPKIN SOUP

COOKING: 20'　　　**PREPARATION: 10'**　　　**SERVINGS: 4-6**

INGREDIENTS

- » 1 cup of coconut milk
- » 2 cups of chicken broth
- » 6 cups of baked pumpkin
- » 1 tsp. of garlic powder
- » 1 tsp. of ground cinnamon
- » 1 tsp. of dried ginger
- » 1 tsp. of nutmeg
- » 1 tsp. of paprika
- » Salt and pepper (to taste)
- » Sour cream or coconut yogurt (for topping)
- » Pumpkin seeds (toasted, for topping)

DIRECTIONS

1. Combine the coconut milk, broth, baked pumpkin, and spices in a soup pan (use medium heat).
2. Stir occasionally and simmer for 15 minutes.
3. With an immersion blender, blend the soup mixture for 1 minute.
4. Top with sour cream or coconut yogurt and pumpkin seeds

NUTRITION

Calories: 123, Fat: 9.8g, Carbs: 8.1g, Protein: 3.1g

19. FRESH AVOCADO SOUP

COOKING: 10'　　　**PREPARATION: 5'**　　　**SERVINGS: 2**

INGREDIENTS

- » 1 ripe avocado
- » 2 romaine lettuce leaves (washed and chopped)
- » 1 cup of coconut milk (chilled)
- » 1 tbsp. of lime juice
- » 20 fresh mint leaves
- » Salt (to taste)

DIRECTIONS

1. Mix all your ingredients thoroughly in a blender.
2. Chill in the fridge for 5–10 minutes.

NUTRITION

Calories: 280, Fat: 26g, Carbs: 12g, Protein: 4g

20. CREAMY GARLIC CHICKEN

COOKING: 15'　　　**PREPARATION: 5'**　　　**SERVINGS: 4**

INGREDIENTS

- » 4 chicken of breasts (finely sliced)
- » 1 tsp. of garlic powder
- » 1 tsp. of paprika
- » 2 tbsp. of butter
- » 1 tsp. of salt
- » 1 cup of heavy cream
- » ½ cup of sun-dried tomatoes
- » 2 cloves of garlic (minced)
- » 1 cup of spinach (chopped)

DIRECTIONS

1. Blend the paprika, garlic powder, and salt and sprinkle over both sides of the chicken.
2. Melt the butter in a frying pan (choose medium heat).
3. Add the chicken breast and fry for 5 minutes each side. Set aside.
4. Add the heavy cream, sun-dried tomatoes, and garlic to the pan and whisk well to combine.
5. Cook for 2 minutes.
6. Add spinach and sauté for an additional 3 minutes. Return the chicken to the pan and cover with the sauce.

NUTRITION

Calories: 280, Fat: 26g, Carbohydrates: 12g, Protein: 4g

21. SHRIMP SCAMPI WITH GARLIC

COOKING: 10'　　　**PREPARATION: 5'**　　　**SERVINGS: 4**

INGREDIENTS

- » 1 pound of shrimp
- » 3 tbs. of olive oil
- » 1 bulb of shallot (sliced)
- » 4 cloves of garlic (minced)
- » ½ cup of pinot grigio
- » 4 tbsp. of salted butter
- » 1 tbsp. of lemon juice
- » ½ tsp. of sea salt
- » ¼ tsp. of black pepper
- » ¼ tsp. of red pepper flakes
- » ¼ cup of parsley (chopped)

DIRECTIONS

1. Pour the olive oil into the heated frying pan.
2. Add the garlic and shallots and fry for about 2 minutes.
3. Combine the Pinot Grigio, salted butter, and lemon juice.
4. Pour this mixture into the pan and cook for 5 minutes.
5. Put the parsley, black pepper, red pepper flakes, and sea salt into the pan and whisk well.
6. Add the shrimp and fry until they are pink (about 3 minutes).

NUTRITION

Calories: 344, Fat: 7g, Carbohydrates: 7g, Protein: 32g

22. CHINESE PORK BOWL

COOKING: 15' **PREPARATION: 5'** **SERVINGS: 4**

INGREDIENTS

- » 1¼ pounds of pork belly (cut into bite-size pieces)
- » 2 tbsp. of tamari soy sauce
- » 1 tbsp. of rice vinegar
- » 2 cloves of garlic (smashed)
- » 3 oz. of butter
- » 1 pound of Brussels sprouts (rinsed, trimmed, halved, or quartered)
- » ½ leek (chopped)
- » Salt and ground black pepper (to taste)

DIRECTIONS

1. Fry the pork over medium-high heat until it is starting to turn golden brown.
2. Combine the garlic cloves, butter, and Brussels sprouts.
3. Add to the pan, whisk well and cook until the sprouts turn golden brown.
4. Stir the soy sauce and rice vinegar together and pour the sauce into the pan.
5. Sprinkle with salt and pepper.
6. Top with chopped leek

NUTRITION

Calories: 993 Fat: 97g Carbs: 7g Protein: 19g

23. CHICKEN PAN WITH VEGGIES AND PESTO

COOKING: 20' **PREPARATION: 10'** **SERVINGS: 4**

INGREDIENTS

- » 2 tbsp. of olive oil
- » 1 pound of chicken thighs (skinless, boneless, sliced into strips)
- » ¾ cup of oil-packed sun-dried tomatoes (chopped)
- » 1 pound of asparagus ends
- » ¼ cup of basil pesto
- » 1 cup of cherry tomatoes (red and yellow, halved)
- » Salt (to taste)

DIRECTIONS

1. Heat olive oil in a frying pan over medium-high heat.
2. Put salt on the chicken slices and then put it into a skillet, add the sun-dried tomatoes and fry for 5–10 minutes.
3. Remove the chicken slices and season with salt.
4. Add asparagus to the skillet.
5. Cook for additional 5–10 minutes.
6. Place the chicken back in the skillet, pour in the pesto, and whisk.
7. Fry for 1–2 minutes. Remove from the heat.
8. Add the halved cherry tomatoes and pesto. Stir well and serve.

NUTRITION

Calories: 423 Fat: 32g Carbohydrates: 12g Protein: 2g

24. CABBAGE SOUP WITH BEEF

COOKING: 20'　　　**PREPARATION: 15'**　　　**SERVINGS:4**

INGREDIENTS

- » 2 tbsp. of olive oil
- » 1 medium onion (chopped)
- » 1 pound of fillet steak (cut into pieces)
- » ½ stalk celery (chopped)
- » 1 carrot (peeled and diced)
- » ½ head small green cabbage (cut into pieces)
- » 2 cloves of garlic (minced)
- » 4 cups of beef broth
- » 2 tbsp. of fresh parsley (chopped)
- » 1 tsp. of dried thyme
- » 1 tsp. of dried rosemary
- » 1 tsp. of garlic powder
- » Salt and black pepper (to taste)

DIRECTIONS

1. Heat oil in a pot (use medium heat).
2. Add the beef and cook until it is browned.
3. Put the onion into the pot and boil for 3–4 minutes.
4. Add the celery and carrot.
5. Stir well and cook for about 3–4 minutes.
6. Add the cabbage and boil until it starts softening.
7. Add garlic and simmer for about 1 minute.
8. Pour the broth into the pot.
9. Add the parsley and garlic powder.
10. Mix thoroughly and reduce heat to medium-low.
11. Cook for 10–15 minutes.

NUTRITION

Calories: 177 Fat: 11g Carbs: 4g Protein:12g

25. CAULIFLOWER RICE SOUP WITH CHICKEN

COOKING: 1H   PREPARATION: 10'   SERVINGS: 5

INGREDIENTS

- » 2½ pounds of chicken breasts (boneless and skinless)
- » 8 tbsp. of butter
- » ¼ cup of celery (chopped)
- » ½ cup of onion (chopped)
- » 4 cloves of garlic (minced)
- » 2 12-ounce of packages steamed cauliflower rice
- » 1 tbsp. of parsley (chopped)
- » 2 tsp. of poultry seasoning
- » ½ cup. of carrot (grated)
- » ¾ tsp. of rosemary
- » 1 tsp. of salt
- » ¾ tsp. of pepper
- » 4 ounces of cream cheese
- » 4¾ cup of chicken broth

DIRECTIONS

1. Put shredded chicken breasts into a saucepan and pour in the chicken broth.
2. Add salt and pepper. Cook for 1 hour.
3. In another pot, melt the butter.
4. Add the onion, garlic, and celery.
5. Sauté until the mix is translucent.
6. Add the riced cauliflower, rosemary, and carrot.
7. Mix and cook for 7 minutes.
8. Add the chicken breasts and broth to the cauliflower mix.
9. Put the lid on & simmer for 15 minutes.

NUTRITION

Calories: 415 Fat: 30g Carbs: 6g Protein: 27g

CHAPTER 11 - DINNER

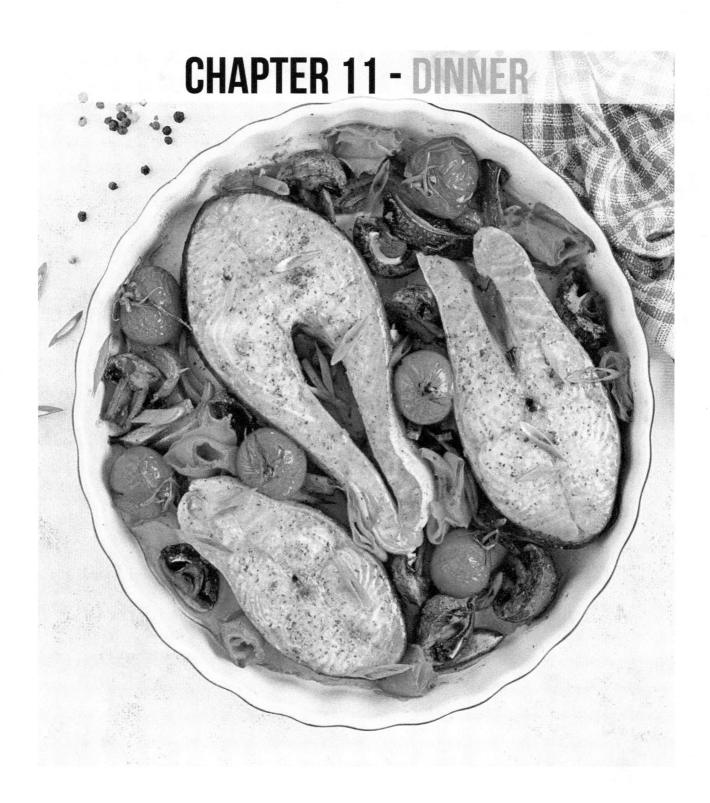

26. CHIPS

INGREDIENTS

- » Oil spray (make sure its avocado)

What you need for the coating:
- » 1 tablespoon of paprika
- » ½ of a tablespoon of cayenne pepper for a little bit of a kick
- » ½ of a tablespoon of onion powder
- » ¼ of a cup of nutritional yeast
- » ½ tablespoon of garlic powder

What you need for the chip:
- » A bag of pork rinds (take note that whatever bag you choose will change the nutrition information at the end of the recipe)

DIRECTIONS

1. Add the coating ingredients to a spice grinder and blend until everything becomes smooth.

2. Spray your pork rinds with oil as it will make the coating stick better.

3. Transfer the rinds to a plastic bag and pour the toppings in before you begin to shake it.

NUTRITION

Calories: 97, Fat: 2.7g, Carbs: 2g, Fiber: 1g, Protein: 14g

27. PICKLE

INGREDIENTS

- » 1 can of tuna (go for a version that is light flaked)
- » ¼ cup of mayo (it needs to be sugar-free if you can get it and a light version)
- » 1 tablespoon of dill
- » 5 or 6 pickles depending on what you need

DIRECTIONS

1. Cut your pickles in half so that they are lengthwise.

2. Seed your pickles.

3. Drain the tuna and then mix the dill, mayo, and tuna in a bowl before mixing.

4. Spoon the tuna mixture onto the pickle. It will only take you five minutes.

5. You can get up to four servings from this.

NUTRITION

Calories: 47.1 Fiber: 1.4g Protein: 6.01g Carbs: 3.6g Fat: 0.6g

28. PINWHEEL DELIGHT

COOKING: 5'   PREPARATION: 5'   SERVINGS: 20

INGREDIENTS

» 1 block of cream cheese (8 ounces)
» 10 slices of salami (genoa) and pepperoni
» 4 tablespoons of pickles (make sure they are finely diced)

DIRECTIONS

1. Have your cream cheese brought to room temperature.

2. Whip the cream cheese until it becomes fluffy.

3. Spread your cream cheese in a rectangle that is a quarter-inch thick. Make sure to use an appropriate sized plastic wrap.

4. Put pickles on top of cream cheese

5. Place the salami over the cream cheese in layers that are overlapping so that each cream cheese layer is covered.

6. Place another layer of the wrap over the layer of salami and press down. Be gentle.

7. Flip your whole rectangle over so that the bottom cream cheese layer is now facing the top instead.

8. Peel back your plastic wrap off very carefully from the top cream cheese layer.

9. You should begin rolling this into a log shape, slowly removing the bottom layer of your plastic wrap as you go along.

10. Place the pinwheel in a tight plastic wrap.

11. Place in the fridge overnight or if you can't wait at least four hours.

12. Slice, whatever thick you want it.

NUTRITION

Calories: 47 Fat: 4.2g Carbs: 0.8g Protein: 1g

29. ZESTY OLIVES

COOKING: 5' **PREPARATION: 5'** **SERVINGS: 6**

INGREDIENTS

- » ¼ cup of oil (make sure that it is extra virgin olive oil)
- » ¼ teaspoon of pepper flakes (red and crushed)
- » 1 thinly sliced garlic clove
- » 1 tablespoon of lemon juice
- » 1 strip of zest from a lemon
- » 1 cup of olives
- » 2 sprigs of thyme (make sure it's fresh)
- » 1 tablespoon of orange juice
- » 1 strip of zest from an orange

DIRECTIONS

1. Get a saucepan.
2. Heat your oil over medium-high heat.
3. Add zest, thyme, garlic, and zest in and cook it.
4. Be sure that you stir occasionally.
5. Cook for a few minutes, and you will notice that the garlic is golden.
6. You will then need to stir in the olives and cook them as well.
7. Stir them as they cook but only cook for two minutes. You want them to be warmed.
8. Turn off your heat.
9. Stir in your juice.
10. Place in a dish.

NUTRITION

Calories: 180 Fat: 20g Carbs: 2g

30. DEVILED EGGS KETO STYLE!

COOKING: 5' **PREPARATION: 5'** **SERVINGS: 20**

INGREDIENTS

- » 10 large eggs (hardboiled)
- » 1 avocado (make sure it is ripe)
- » 1 lemon (you will need to juice this)
- » 1 tablespoon of mustard (use Dijon)
- » Paprika (use smoked)

DIRECTIONS

1. Slice your eggs in half and take out the yolks.
2. Combine your yolks, avocado, and lemon juice in a bowl and stir thoroughly.
3. Spoon the mixture into the egg halves.
4. Sprinkle the top with paprika.

NUTRITION

Calories: 50 Fat: 4g Fiber: 1gCarbs: 1g Protein: 3g

---

31. CUCUMBER

INGREDIENTS

» 1 cup of cucumbers (make sure they are sliced)
» 10 olives (Kalamata olives. Use large ones)

DIRECTIONS

1. Mix them in a bowl, and there you go!

NUTRITION

Calories: 71 Fat: 4.8g Fiber: 2.3g Carbs: 5g Protein: 1.29g

32. NUTTY YOGURT

INGREDIENTS

» 2 ounces of yogurt (use whole milk Greek yogurt)
» ½ teaspoon of cinnamon
» 1 tablespoon of walnuts (chopped)

DIRECTIONS

1. Place the yogurt in a dish.
2. Add the walnuts.
3. Add the cinnamon.

NUTRITION

Calories: 160 Fiber: 0.5g Fat: 12.5g Protein: 8g Carbs: 6g

33. CREAMY BOAT

COOKING: 0'   **PREPARATION: 5'**   **SERVINGS: 4**

INGREDIENTS

» 2 stalks of celery
» 2 tablespoons of cream cheese

DIRECTIONS

1. Clean the celery and cut it into pieces.

2. Place the pieces on a plate before adding cream cheese to them.

3. Repeat this process if necessary.

NUTRITION

Calories: 113 Fat: 10.1g Fiber: 1.3g Carbs: 4g Protein: 2.3g

CHAPTER 15 - DESSERTS

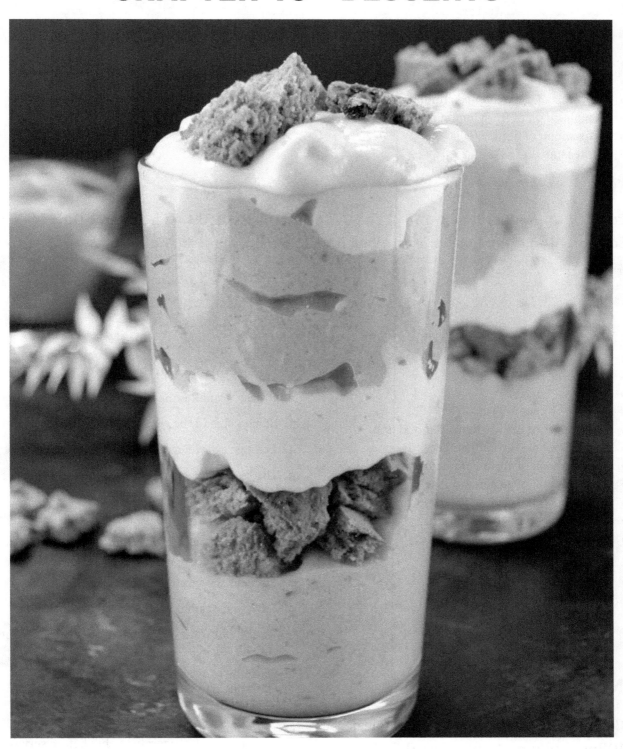

34. RASPBERRY MOUSSE

COOKING: 10'   **PREPARATION: 10'**   **SERVINGS: 4**

INGREDIENTS

- » 2 ½ cups of fresh raspberries
- » 1/3 cups of granulated erythritol
- » 1/3 cups of unsweetened almond milk
- » 1 tablespoon of fresh lemon juice
- » 1 teaspoon of liquid stevia
- » ¼ teaspoon of salt

DIRECTIONS

1. In a food processor, add all the listed ingredients and pulse until smooth.

2. Transfer the mixture into serving glasses and refrigerate to chill before serving.

NUTRITION

Calories: 44 Net Carbs: 4.3 g Total Fat: 0.8 g Saturated Fat: 0.1 g Cholesterol: 0mg

Sodium: 164mg Total Carbs: 9.4g Fiber: 5.1g Sugar: 3.5g Protein: 1g

35. EGG CUSTARD

COOKING: 55'   **PREPARATION: 15'**   **SERVINGS: 8**

INGREDIENTS

- » 5 organic eggs
- » Salt (as required)
- » ½ cup of yacon syrup
- » 20 ounces of unsweetened almond milk
- » ¼ teaspoon of ground ginger
- » ¼ teaspoon of ground cinnamon
- » ¼ teaspoon of ground nutmeg
- » ¼ teaspoon of ground cardamom
- » 1/8 teaspoon of ground cloves
- » 1/8 teaspoon of ground allspice

DIRECTIONS

1. Preheat your oven to 325°F.

2. Grease 8 small ramekins.

3. In a bowl, add the eggs and salt and beat well.

4. Arrange a sieve over a medium bowl.

5. Through a sieve, strain the egg mixture into a bowl.

6. Add the Yacon syrup in eggs and stir to combine.

7. Add the almond milk and spices and beat until well combined.

8. Transfer the mixture into prepared ramekins.

9. Now, place ramekins in a large baking dish.

10. Add hot water in the baking dish about 2-inch high around the ramekins.

11. Place the baking dish in the oven and bake for about 30−40 minutes or until a toothpick inserted in the center comes out clean.

12. Remove ramekins from the oven and set aside to cool. Refrigerate to chill before serving.

NUTRITION

Calories: 77 Fat: 3.8g Carbs: 6g Cholesterol: 102mg Sodium: 116mg Fiber: 0.5g Sugar: 3.7g Protein: 3.8g

36. MOCHA ICE CREAM

COOKING: 15'   **PREPARATION: 15'**   **SERVINGS: 2**

INGREDIENTS

- » 1 cup of unsweetened coconut milk
- » ¼ cup of heavy cream
- » 2 tablespoons of granulated erythritol
- » 15 drops of liquid stevia
- » 2 tablespoons of cacao powder
- » 1 tablespoon of instant coffee
- » ¼ teaspoon of xanthan gum

NUTRITION

Calories: 246 Carbs: 6.2g Fat: 23.1g

Cholesterol: 21mg Sodium: 52mg Fiber: 2g

Sugar: 3g Protein: 2.8g

DIRECTIONS

1. In a container, add the ingredients (except xanthan gum) and with an immersion blender, blend until well combined.

2. Slowly, add the xanthan gum and blend until a slightly thicker mixture is formed.

3. Transfer the mixture into ice cream maker and process according to manufacturer's instructions.

4. Now, transfer the ice cream into an airtight container and freeze for at least 4–5 hours before serving.

37. COTTAGE CHEESE PUDDING

COOKING: 45   **PREPARATION: 10'**   **SERVINGS: 6**

INGREDIENTS

PUDDING
- » 1 cup of cottage cheese
- » ¾ cup of heavy cream
- » 3 organic eggs
- » ¾ cup of water
- » ½ cups of granulated erythritol
- » 1 teaspoon of organic vanilla extract

TOPPING
- » 1/3 cup of heavy whipping cream
- » 1/3 cup of fresh raspberries

DIRECTIONS

1. Preheat your oven to 350°F.

2. Grease 6 (6-ounce) ramekins.

3. Add all the ingredients (except cinnamon) and pulse in a blender until smooth.

4. Transfer the mixture into prepared ramekins evenly.

5. Now, place ramekins in a large baking dish.

6. Add hot water in the baking dish, about 1-inch up sides of the ramekins.

7. Bake for about 35 minutes.

8. Serve warm with the topping o heavy whipping cream and raspberries.

NUTRITION

Calories: 226 Fat: 19.6g Carbs: 3.7g Protein: 9g

38. VANILLA CRÈME BRÛLÉE

COOKING: 1H 20'   **PREPARATION: 20'**   **SERVINGS: 4**

INGREDIENTS

» 2 cups of heavy cream
» 1 vanilla bean (halved with seeds scraped out)
» 4 organic egg yolks
» 1/3 teaspoon of stevia powder
» 1 teaspoon of organic vanilla extract
» Pinch of salt
» 4 tablespoon of granulated erythritol

DIRECTIONS

1. Preheat your oven to 350°F.

2. In a pan, add heavy cream over medium heat and cook until heated.

3. Stir in the vanilla bean seeds and bring to a gentle boil.

4. Reduce the heat to very low and cook, covered for about 20 minutes.

5. Meanwhile, in a bowl, add the remaining ingredients (except erythritol) and beat until thick and pale mixture forms.

6. Remove the heavy cream from heat and through a fine-mesh strainer, strain into a heat-proof bowl.

7. Slowly, add the cream in egg yolk mixture beating continuously until well combined.

8. Divide the mixture into 4 ramekins evenly.

9. Arrange the ramekins into a large baking dish.

10. In the baking dish, add hot water about half of the ramekins.

11. Bake for about 30–35 minutes.

12. Remove the pan from the oven and then let it cool slightly.

13. Refrigerate the ramekins for at least 4 hours.

14. Just before serving, sprinkle the ramekins with erythritol evenly.

15. Holding a kitchen torch about 4–5-inches from the top, caramelize the erythritol for about 2 minutes.

16. Set aside for 5 minutes before serving.

NUTRITION

Calories: 264 Fat: 26.7g Carbs: 2.4g Protein: 3.9g

39. LEMON SOUFFLÉ

INGREDIENTS

- » 2 large organic eggs (whites and yolks separated)
- » ¼ cups of granulated erythritol (divided)
- » 1 cup of ricotta cheese
- » 1 tablespoon of fresh lemon juice
- » 2 teaspoons of lemon zest (grated)
- » 1 teaspoon of poppy seeds
- » 1 teaspoon of organic vanilla extract

DIRECTIONS

1. Preheat your oven to 375°F.

2. Grease 4 ramekins.

3. Add egg whites and beat in a clean glass bowl until it has a foam-like texture.

4. Add 2 tablespoons of erythritol and beat the mixture until it is stiff.

5. In another bowl, add ricotta cheese, egg yolks, and the remaining erythritol until it is mixed thoroughly.

6. Put the lemon juice and lemon zest in the bowl and mix well.

7. Add the poppy seeds and vanilla extract and mix again.

8. Add the whipped egg whites into the ricotta mixture and gently stir.

9. Place the mixture into prepared ramekins evenly.

10. Bake for about 20 minutes.

11. Remove from the oven and serve immediately.

NUTRITION

Calories: 130 Fat: 7.7g Carbs: 4g Protein: 10.4g

40. CREAM CAKE

COOKING: 1H 5'   PREPARATION: 15'   SERVINGS: 12

INGREDIENTS

- » 2 cups of almond flour
- » 2 teaspoons of organic baking powder
- » ½ cup of butter (chopped)
- » 2 ounces of cream cheese (softened)
- » 1 cup of sour cream
- » 1 cups of granulated erythritol
- » 1 teaspoon of organic vanilla extract
- » 4 large organic eggs
- » 1 tablespoon of powdered erythritol

DIRECTIONS

1. Preheat your oven to 350°F.

2. Generously, grease a 9-inch Bundt pan.

3. Add almond flour and baking powder in a large bowl and mix well. Set aside.

4. In a microwave-safe bowl, add butter and cream cheese and microwave for about 30 seconds.

5. Remove from microwave and stir well.

6. Add sour cream, erythritol, and vanilla extract and mix until well combined.

7. Add the cream mixture into the bowl of the flour mixture and mix until well combined.

8. Add eggs and mix until well combined.

9. Transfer the mixture into the prepared pan evenly.

10. Bake for about 50 minutes or until a toothpick inserted in the center comes out clean.

11. Remove from the oven and put onto a wire rack to cool for about 10 minutes.

12. Carefully, invert the cake onto a wire rack to cool completely.

13. Just before serving, dust the cake with powdered erythritol.

14. Cut into 12 equal-sized slices and serve.

NUTRITION

Calories: 258 Fat: 24.3g Carbs: 5.5g
Protein: 7.2g

CHAPTER 17 - 30 DAYS MEAL PLAN

DAYS	BREAKFAST	LUNCH/DINNER	SNACKS
1	Blueberry Nutty Oatmeal	Baked Salmon	Pickle
2	Crab Salad Stuffed Avocados	Buttered Cod	Deviled Eggs Keto Style!
3	Keto Goat Cheese Salmon Fat Bomb	Shrimp Scampi with Garlic	Nutty Yogurt
4	Fried Pork Rind Crusted Salmon Cakes	Roasted Lemon Chicken Sandwich	Chips
5	Bacon Hash	Cabbage Soup with Beef	Pinwheel Delight
6	Bagels with Cheese	Baked Salmon	Zesty olives
7	Baked Apples	Buttered Cod	Strawberry Rhubarb Custard
8	Crab Salad Stuffed Avocados	Chinese Pork Bowl	Creme Brulee
9	Banana Pancakes	Roasted Lemon Chicken Sandwich	Pickle
10	Fried Pork Rind Crusted Salmon Cakes	Shrimp Scampi with Garlic	Vanilla Frozen Yogurt

11	Brunch BLT Wrap	Quick Pumpkin Soup	Ice Cream
12	Keto Goat Cheese Salmon Fat Bomb	Roasted Lemon Chicken Sandwich	Nutty Yogurt
13	Coconut Porridge Keto	Chinese Pork Bowl	Mocha Mousse
14	Crab Salad Stuffed Avocados	Baked Salmon	Zesty olives
15	Creamy Basil, Baked Sausage	Cabbage Soup with Beef	Creme Brulee
16	Almond, Coconut, Egg Wraps	Baked Salmon	Pickle
17	Fried Pork Rind Crusted Salmon Cakes	Buttered Cod	Chocolate Muffins
18	Bacon and Cheese Frittata	Quick Pumpkin Soup	Deviled Eggs Keto Style!
19	Blueberry Nutty Oatmeal	Roasted Lemon Chicken Sandwich	Chips
20	Bacon Hash	Trout and Chili Nuts	Mocha Mousse
21	Bagels with Cheese	Buttered Cod	Pinwheel Delight
22	Keto Goat Cheese Salmon Fat Bomb	Chinese Pork Bowl	Creme Brulee

23	Baked Eggs In The Avocado	Baked Salmon	Nutty Yogurt
24	Fried Pork Rind Crusted Salmon Cakes	Shrimp Scampi with Garlic	Chocolate Muffins
25	Keto Goat Cheese Salmon Fat Bomb	Quick Pumpkin Soup	Pickle
26	Blueberry Nutty Oatmeal	Roasted Lemon Chicken Sandwich	Vanilla Frozen Yogurt
27	Cheesy Bacon and Egg Cups	Cabbage Soup with Beef	Deviled Eggs Keto Style!
28	Blueberry Nutty Oatmeal	Buttered Cod	Chocolate Avocado Ice Cream
29	Fried Pork Rind Crusted Salmon Cakes	Tuna Salad	Chips
30	Crab Salad Stuffed Avocados	Fresh Avocado Soup	Pickle

CONCLUSION

Your dedication to improve your health and lose weight is phenomenal since you have been able to reach the end of this guidebook. While it is hard to lose weight, if you can maintain the guidelines you have learned in this guidebook and stay motivated, your life will change in ways that you cannot imagine. You are on the right path in getting both mental and physical health. Even though adjusting to eating a healthy diet after being accustomed to eating a lot of convenience foods is a challenge; you will feel the difference in energy levels that you will experience. You will look good and be safe from many of the common nutrition-related diseases and conditions, and besides of all that, your quality of life will improve significantly.

We are all different; thus, you should take time to really understand what a weight loss program involves and try out the program gradually. If you nosedive into a weight loss program is not advisable since it may not be for you. No regiment works perfectly for everyone; thus, you should select a plan and modify it in a way that suits you. There are many weight loss programs with mind-blowing results, but they may be too hard to follow or just unsafe to practice.

Your workout intensity, the duration, and your resting period are all factors that should be considered. It works best when it is a constant in your daily activities, and as it is not a permanent change of your physical and psychological condition.

To get the maximum weight loss experience, you should listen to your body. It means that you should pay attention to how it responds to your diet and fasting regiment because the body system determines the time for you to eat, time for you to exercise and even how many calories you take in. Thus you will be in full control of your weight loss once you are in control of your diet and fasting program.

You should know that even though the ketogenic diet is about carbohydrate restriction, it doesn't excessively restrict them. You should make sure you eat enough. If you avoid food with calories too much, you will be moody, and it can even stop your weight loss process. You should also vary your food choices so that you make sure that you are getting the nutrients that your body needs to maintain a good healthy lifestyle.

Getting all the nutrients that you require from a ketogenic diet is possible. Unfortunately for some, this is not possible. If you do not feel okay, you should go and see a doctor to determine if you have any nutritional deficiencies. He/she will be able to recommend supplements for you from that information.

For health reasons, weight loss should be a slow process. Losing 2 pounds a day is okay, but anything more than that is too much. Engage in your day-to-day occupations while fasting as this is a time-flying route. Good luck with your keto diet journey!

THANK YOU

Finally, if you enjoyed this book, then I'd like to ask you for a favor, would you be kind enough to leave a review for this book on Amazon? It'd be greatly appreciated!

It would be crucial to help me with this project that I care about a lot. I believe that regardless of the book and the mission that matters. Everybody deserves a healthier and more just life. Maybe people are not aware of it.

Maybe we can help.

With Love,

Jillian Collins

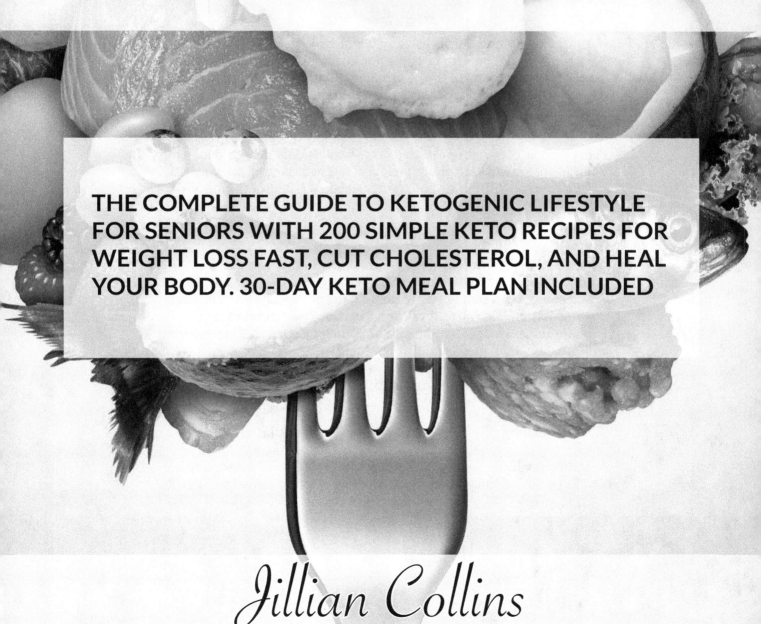

KETO DIET COOKBOOK AFTER 50

THE COMPLETE GUIDE TO KETOGENIC LIFESTYLE FOR SENIORS WITH 200 SIMPLE KETO RECIPES FOR WEIGHT LOSS FAST, CUT CHOLESTEROL, AND HEAL YOUR BODY. 30-DAY KETO MEAL PLAN INCLUDED

Jillian Collins

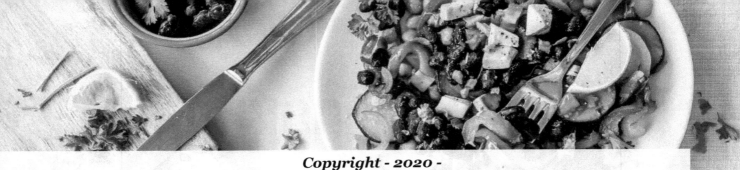

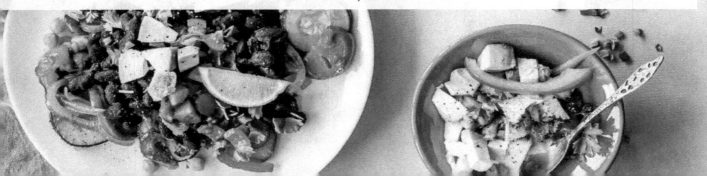

TABLE OF CONTENTS

INTRODUCTION

All of us gradually get older. It is a sure fact of our life. But even though we are aging all the time, we do not need to be old, not yet anyway. Because believe me, it is possible to be active and vibrant at fifty and beyond if you make some smart choices and take care of yourself. Deciding to follow the keto way of life is the smartest choice that anyone could ever make when choosing the right and suitable diet at this age. The keto diet isn't just good for weight loss, although that is probably its most important and noticeable feature. It gives so much more to our body while helping you lose and then maintain our weight.

When the keto diet helps you lose weight, it also reduces your risk of cardiovascular disease. When you lose weight and decrease the amount of fat and cholesterol in the body, there will be less to accumulate in the arteries, and the blood will naturally flow better with less restriction.

Being overweight can cause high blood pressure. Losing weight plus being in a healthy weight will ease the strain on your heart. If the blood pressure is not pumping too high, it will not cause weak arteries' weak spots. If there are no soft spots, then there is no place for plaque to collect.

For you, who are over 50 and want to be better and healthier, adopting the keto way of life will help eliminate your kidneys' problems and improve their function. Kidney stones and gout are caused mainly by the elevation of certain urine chemicals that help create uric acid, which we eliminate in the bathroom. When ketones begin to rise, the acid in urine will briefly increase as your body begins to eliminate all waste products from the metabolized fats. However, the level will decrease and remain lower than before as long as you are on the keto diet.

The best overall advantage of the keto lifestyle is that it will lower your overall weight, positively affecting your entire body. Losing weight will mean freedom from the effects of obesity, which can help eliminate metabolic syndrome and type 2 diabetes. The condition known as metabolic syndrome happens when the body becomes resistant to insulin, and the insulin your body produces is no recognized by the cells in your body. That causes the body to store your excess blood sugar as fat in your body, especially around the stomach area. When we begin the keto diet and enter Ketosis, the body will be forced to use these fat stores for energy, and the body's production of insulin will be returned to normal. The number of proteins in the diet will help our muscles keep their strength and tone and not begin to wither as so often happens in older women.

The keto diet will result in increased brain function and the ability to focus. The brain typically uses sugar to fuel its processes, but the consumption of sugar has its problems. The mind can easily switch to using ketones for fuel and energy. Always remember that ketones are the by-product of Ketosis that makes you burn fat.

Inflammation is a part of life, especially for people over the age of fifty. There is the right kind of inflammation, such as when white blood cells rush to a particular body area to kill an infection. Most older people are plagued by the wrong forms of inflammation, which make your joints swell and cause early morning stiffness. Losing weight will help to eliminate inflammation in the body.

This ultimate guide can give you full knowledge regarding the Keto Diet and answer the questions that keep you from sailing to your new healthy Keto-lifestyle. Trust me; you don't want to miss this opportunity! Full-packed of Keto knowledge and, of course, the highlights to this is giving you simple, fast, and easy-to-follow Keto recipes, and 30 days meal plan for men and women exclusively made separately, that will complete your Keto-journey!

Following the keto diet will mean that you will eat less food, but it will be more filling and more nutritious. When you eat fats and proteins instead of carbs, you will feel fuller much longer with less food. Lowering your caloric will keep your weight loss, and less weight will make you healthier. It will also slash your risk of developing certain diseases and will minimize the effects of others. These are the life improvements that the keto lifestyle has to offer you.

I hope you'll enjoy these book; is part of the larger labor of love, which led me to create this project. I've put a lot of time, effort, and commitment into providing you with the only guide you'll need to understand how to approach the Ketogenic Diet, start a new lifestyle, and feel happy and Healthy again. All I ask in return is that if you love this book, please leave me an honest review.

I will read all with attention.

Thank you.

CHAPTER 1. UNDERSTANDING KETO OVER 50

Now comes the exciting part. I am sure you have been wondering how a Keto diet will help you, a person who is 50 years or more in age, and why is it so important, right? Do not worry as I shall provide you with an answer that satisfies both questions.

IS THE KETOGENIC DIET HEALTHY AFTER 50?

As we grow in age, the body's natural fat-burning ability reduces. When that happens, our body stops receiving a healthy dose of nutrients correctly; therefore, we will develop diseases and ailments. With the keto diet, we are pushing the body into Ketosis and bypassing the need to worry about our body's ability to burn fat. Once in Ketosis, our body will now burn fat forcefully for survival.

Once more, our system will now start to regain strength. An even better aspect that follows is our insulin level because it drops. If you are diagnosed with type 2 diabetes and others, the drop-in insulin might even reverse the effects and eliminate the diseases from your body altogether.

It is also essential to highlight that as we get older, we start losing more than just the ability to burn fat. During this phase of our life, once we hit around 50 years of age, we come across various obstacles, some chronic in nature, which transpire only because our body can no longer function at rates like it did when we were young. Ketogenic diets help us regain that edge and feel energized from within.

There are hundreds of thousands of stories, all pointing out how this revolutionary diet is especially helpful for older adults and the elderly. Therefore, it is a no-brainer for people above 50 who have spent ages trying to search for a healthy lifestyle choice of diet. With such a high success rate, there is no harm in trying, right?

Keto has been producing results that have attracted the top minds of every people who benefit from it for a fairly long time. Considering the unique nature of this lifestyle of eating, the results have been somewhat encouraging.

GETTING INTO KETOSIS

With a further understanding of ketones and how they work, you may now be wondering how to get into Ketosis yourself. While it is a pretty straightforward process, it can seem a bit confusing at first. Below, you will find methods to help you get into Ketosis and how to stay there.

RESTRICT CARBOHYDRATES

It may seem obvious, as it the golden rule of the ketogenic diet, but carbohydrates can be tricky. When people first begin this diet, they typically only focus on their net carbs. If you want to lose weight faster, you will want to focus and limit your carbohydrates. You will generally want to stay below 20g of net carbs and 35g total carbs in an entire day.

RESTRICT PROTEIN

As you begin the ketogenic diet, you will find that many of the recipes include meat. It is beneficial to our diet. But some old folks don't realize that there is such a thing called too much protein. If you eat too much protein in a day, this can lower your body's ketones levels. If you are looking to lose weight on the ketogenic diet, you will want to keep your protein levels to .6g and .8g of protein per lean body mass. You can calculate this number using an online calculator.

DRINK WATER

Drinking enough water is going to be vital while following the ketogenic diet. Not only will drinking enough water to keep everything in your body flowing, but it will also help you with several symptoms caused by starting your new diet. I suggest that you drink about a gallon of water per day. It will help regulate your bodily functions and decrease your hunger levels.

INTERMITTENT FASTING

Fasting is an excellent tool if you are looking to boost your ketone levels. If you have never tried it before, there is a level for just about any person. Through fasting, you will stop snacking and get better results through your diet.

EXERCISE

When you exercise, it will help you get better results when paired with the proper nutrients through the ketogenic diet. I suggest adding anywhere from twenty to thirty minutes of exercise per day for mac results. Whether this is picking some weights up or taking a short walk, a small amount of exercise will be able to help you regulate your blood sugar levels and promote even further weight loss.

SIGNS THAT YOU ARE INTO KETOSIS

As you practice the ketogenic diet further, you will tell you are in Ketosis through the signs and symptoms you will experience. Remember that you will now be providing your body with a new fuel source; it will take a little bit of time to adapt your body to this change. Below, you will find the most common signs that you are into Ketosis:

BAD BREATH

I know, a great introduction to the ketogenic diet, but bad breath is one of the most reported symptoms for individuals who have reached full Ketosis. But don't worry, it is a very common side effect for individuals who follow a low-carb diet. Some have described the scent as a "fruit" smell.

Elevated ketone levels in your body cause this scent. The scent is the acetone that exits your body through breath and urine. And while this symptom is less than ideal for your friends and family, it is a great sign that you are following your diet correctly! To solve this issue, you will want to brush your teeth a few times a day or find a sugar-free gum to chew on.

INCREASED KETONES IN BLOOD, URINE, OR BREATH

As mentioned earlier, you will want to find a method of testing ketones in your body. One of the best ways to do this is to test your blood ketone levels using a meter. When you do this, the meter will be able to measure the amount of BHB in your blood, one of the primary ketones that will be present in your bloodstream. If you are in true Ketosis, your blood ketones should be anywhere from .5-3.0 mmol/L.

WEIGHT LOSS

When you first begin the ketogenic diet, weight loss can happen almost immediately. Some have reported that weight loss has even occurred in the first week! After the initial drop in weight, you should expect to lose body fat consistently. It will be up to you to stick to the diet to keep the weight loss up!

DECREASED APPETITE

Another common symptom of the ketogenic diet is appetite suppression. Many people have reported that they aren't as hungry as they used to be while following this diet. It could potentially be due to the increased protein intake and alterations to the hunger hormones through Ketosis. Either way, a decreased appetite means increased weight loss. It is a win-win situation for anyone following the ketogenic diet.

INCREASED ENERGY

When your body enters Ketosis, you will probably experience a new energy boost that you didn't even know you had in you! Of course, increased energy and focus are a long-term effect of the diet. When you first start, you will most likely experience symptoms such as tiredness and brain fog. Fret not, as this is to be expected as your body adapts to a new fuel source.

The good news is that once you are in Ketosis, your brain will start burning these ketones instead of glucose. It is a very potent fuel for your brain, which is why followers of this diet have reported improved brain function and clarity.

FATIGUE

As mentioned earlier, more than likely, you will experience some fatigue if you are just getting started on the ketogenic diet. On top of fatigue, you may feel overall weak, which is a pretty common side effect of the ketogenic diet. As you probably realize, the switch to running on ketones isn't going to happen overnight. Instead, you should expect these symptoms to subside anywhere from seven to thirty days. To help combat the fatigue, consider taking an electrolyte supplement.

DIGESTIVE ISSUES

Another common symptom of starting this diet is experiencing digestive issues. When you make such a drastic change to your diet, it involves changing the types of foods you eat daily. When this happens, digestive issues like diarrhea and constipation are to be expected. While these symptoms will subside, you may want to note which foods you feel are causing these issues. While you adjust to the new Keto diet, these symptoms should subside.

INSOMNIA

Insomnia is another short-term symptom you may experience when you first make the switch due to the lack of carbs, though it is still misunderstood as to why this happens. But many people who follow the ketogenic diet long term have reported that they sleep better once they have adapted to their new diet. Maybe it seems hard at first, if you can push through the bad, the grass is greener on the other side!

CHAPTER 2. FOODS TO AVOID

Because the diet is a keto, that means you need to avoid high-carbs food. Some of the food you avoid is even healthy, but it just contains too many carbs. Here is a list of typical food you should limit or avoid altogether.

BREAD AND GRAINS

No matter what form bread takes, they still pack a lot of carbs. The same applies to whole grain as well because they are made from refined flour. So, if you want to eat bread, it is best to make keto variants at home instead.

Grains such as rice, wheat, and oats pack a lot of carbs as well. So, limit or avoid that as well.

FRUITS

Fruits are healthy for you. The problem is that some of those foods pack quite a lot of carbs such as banana, raisins, dates, mango, and pear. As a general rule, avoid sweet and dried fruits.

VEGETABLES

Vegetables are just as healthy for your body. For one, they make you feel full for longer, so they help suppress your appetite. But that also means you need to avoid or limit vegetables high in starch because they have more carbs than fiber. That includes corn, potato, sweet potato, and beets.

PASTA

As with any other convenient food, pasta is rich in carbs. So, spaghetti or any different types of pasta are not recommended when you are on your keto diet.

CEREAL

Cereal is also a considerable offender because sugary breakfast cereals pack a lot of carbs. That also applies to "healthy cereals." Just because they use other words to describe their product does not mean that you should believe them. That also applies to oatmeal, whole-grain cereals, etc.

BEER

In reality, you can drink most alcoholic beverages in moderation without fear. Beer is an exception to this rule because it packs a lot of carbs. Carbs in beers or other liquid are considered liquid carbs, and they are even more dangerous than substantial carbs.

SWEETENED YOGURT

Yogurt is very healthy because it is tasty and does not have that many carbs. The problem comes when you consume yogurt variants rich in carbs such as fruit-flavored, low-fat, sweetened, or nonfat yogurt. A single serving of sweetened yogurt contains as many carbs as a single serving of dessert.

JUICE

Fruit juices are perhaps the worst beverage you can put into your system when you are on a keto diet. Another problem is that the brain does not process liquid carbs the same way as stable carbs. Substantial carbs can help suppress appetite, but liquid carbs will only put your need into overdrive.

LOW-FAT AND FAT-FREE SALAD DRESSINGS

If you have to buy salads, keep in mind that commercial sauces pack more carbs than you think, especially the fat-free and low-fat variants.

BEANS AND LEGUMES

These are also very nutritious as they are rich in fiber. However, they are also rich in carbs. You may enjoy a small amount of them when you are on your keto diet, but don't exceed your carb limit.

SUGAR

We mean sugar in any form, including honey. Foods that contain lots of sugar, such as cookies, candies, and cake, are forbidden on a keto diet or any other form of diet that is designed to lose weight. When you are on a keto diet, you need to keep in mind that your diet consists of food rich in fiber and nutritious. So, sugar is out of the question.

CHIPS AND CRACKERS

These two are some of the most popular snacks. Some people do not realize that one packet of chips contains several servings and should not be all eaten in one go. The carbs can add up very quickly if you do not watch what you eat.

MILK

Milk also contains a lot of carbs on its own. Therefore, avoid it if you can even though milk is a good source of many nutrients such as calcium, potassium, and other B vitamins.

GLUTEN-FREE BAKED GOODS

Gluten-free diets are trendy nowadays, but what many people don't seem to realize is that they pack quite a lot of carbs. That includes gluten-free bread, muffins, and other baked products. In reality, they contain even more carbs than their glutenous variant.

CHAPTER 3. KETO SHOPPING LIST

People complain about the difficulty of switching their shopping list to one that's Ketogenic-friendly. The fact is that food is expensive — and most of the food you have in your fridge is probably packed full of carbohydrates. If you're committing to a Ketogenic Diet, you need to do a clean sweep. That's right — everything that's packed with carbohydrates should be identified and set aside. You can donate them to a charity before going out and buying your new Keto-friendly shopping list.

SEAFOOD

Seafood means fish like sardines, mackerel, and wild salmon. Go for shrimp, tuna, mussels, and crab into your diet. The secret is omega-3 fatty acids, which are credited for lots of health benefits. You want to add food rich in omega-3 fatty acids in your diet.

LOW-CARB VEGETABLES

Not all vegetables are right for you when it comes to the Ketogenic Diet. The vegetable choices should be limited to those with low carbohydrate counts. Pack up your cart with items like spinach, eggplant, arugula, broccoli, and cauliflower. You can also put in bell peppers, cabbage, celery, kale, Brussels sprouts, mushrooms, zucchini, and fennel.

These vegetables also contain loads of fiber, which makes digestion easier. Of course, there's also the presence of vitamins, minerals, antioxidants, and various other nutrients that you need for day to day life.

FRUITS LOW IN SUGAR

During an episode of sugar-craving, it's usually a good idea to pick low-sugar fruit items. Just make sure to stock up on avocado, blackberries, raspberries, strawberries, blueberries, lime, lemon, and coconut. Also, note that tomatoes are fruits too, so feel free to make side dishes or dips with tomatoes' loads! Avocadoes are incredibly popular for those practicing the Ketogenic Diet because they contain LOTS of the right kind of fat.

MEAT AND EGGS

While some diets will tell you to skip the meat, the Ketogenic Diet encourages its consumption. Meat is packed with protein that will feed your muscles and give you a consistent energy source throughout the day. It's a slow but sure burn when you eat protein instead of carbohydrates, which are burned faster and therefore stored faster if you don't use them immediately.

But what kind of meat should you be eating? There's chicken, beef, pork, venison, turkey, and lamb. Keep in mind that quality plays a huge role here — you should be eating grass-fed organic beef or organic poultry if you want to make the most out of this food variety.

NUTS AND SEEDS

Nuts and seeds you should add in your cart include chia seeds, brazil nuts, macadamia nuts, flaxseed, walnuts, hemp seeds, pecans, sesame seeds, almonds, hazelnut, and pumpkin seeds. They also contain lots of protein and very little sugar, so they're great if you have the appetite. They're the ideal snack because they're quick, easy, and will keep you full. They're high in calories, though, which is why lots of people steer clear of them.

DAIRY PRODUCTS

OK — some people in their 50s already have a hard time processing dairy products, but you can happily add many of these to your diet for those who don't. Make sure to consume sufficient amounts of cheese, plain Greek yogurt, cream butter, and cottage cheese. These dairy products are packed with calcium, protein, and a healthy kind of fat.

OILS

Nope, we're not talking about essentials oils but rather MCT oil, coconut oil, avocado oil, nut oils, and even extra-virgin olive oil. You can start using those for your frying needs to create healthier food options. The beauty of these oils is that they add flavor to the food, making sure you don't get bored quickly with the recipes. Try picking up different types of Keto-friendly oils to add some variety to your cooking.

COFFEE AND TEA

Instead, beverages would be limited to unsweetened tea or unsweetened coffee to keep sugar consumption low. Opt for organic coffee and tea products to make the most out of these powerful antioxidants.

DARK CHOCOLATE

Yes — chocolate is still on the menu, but it is limited to just dark chocolate. Technically, this means eating chocolate that is 70 percent cacao, which would make the taste a bit bitter.

SUGAR SUBSTITUTES

In a while, the part of this book's recipe, you might be surprised at some of the ingredients required in the list. Because while sweeteners are an essential part of food preparation, you can't just use any sugar in your recipe. Remember: the regular sugar is pure carbohydrate. Even if you're not eating carbohydrates, if you're dumping lots of sugar in your food — you're not following the Ketogenic Diet principles.

So, what do you do? You find sugar substitutes. You can get rid of the old sugar and use any of these as a good substitute.

Stevia. Perhaps the most familiar one in this list. It's a natural sweetener derived from plants and contains very few calories. Typically, the ratio is 200 grams of sugar per 1 teaspoon of powdered stevia.

Sucralose. It contains zero calories and zero carbohydrates. It's an artificial sweetener and does not metabolize — hence the complete lack of carbohydrates.

Erythritol. It's a naturally occurring compound that interacts with the tongue's sweet taste receptors. Hence, it mimics the taste of sugar without actually being sugar. It does contain calories, but only about 5% of the calories you'll find in the regular sugar.

Xylitol. It still contains calories; the calories are just 3 per gram. It's a sweetener that's good for diabetic patients because it doesn't raise the body's sugar levels.

WHAT ABOUT CONDIMENTS?

Condiments are still on the table, but they won't be as tasty as you're used to. Your options include mustard, olive oil mayonnaise, oil-based salad dressings, and unsweetened ketchup. Of all these condiments, ketchup is the one with the most sugar, so make a point of looking for one with reduced sugar content.

WHAT ABOUT SNACKS?

The good news is that there are packed snacks for those who don't have the time to make it themselves. Sugarless nut butter, dried seaweeds, nuts, and sugar-free jerky are all available in stores.

Once you've figured this out, you can quickly make calculations in your head about the carbohydrate content of what you're eating based on the labels. You will find that this can be easily adjusted to your eating habits so that you always know what you're consuming, even if you're not following a set recipe.

CHAPTER 4. BREAKFAST

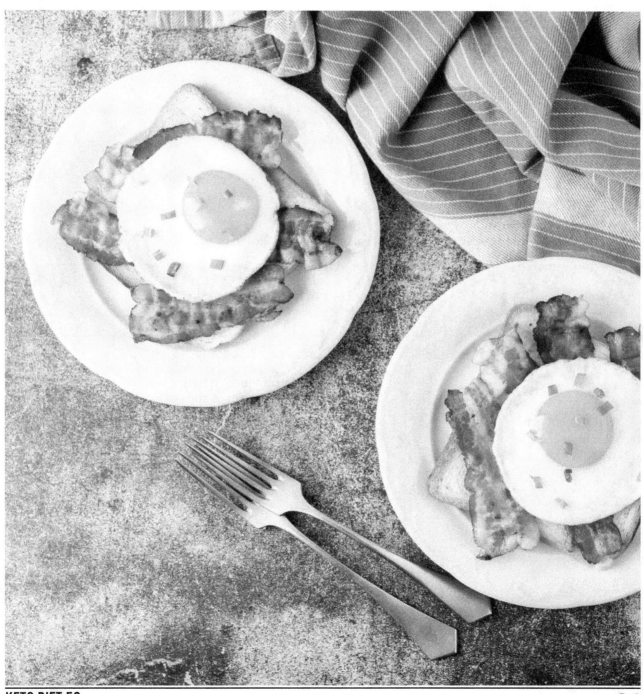

1. BACON & AVOCADO OMELET

COOKING: 5' **PREPARATION: 5'** **SERVINGS: 1**

INGREDIENTS

» **1 slice of crispy bacon**
» **2 organic eggs**
» **.5cup grated parmesan cheese**
» **2 tbsp. Ghee**
» **1 Avocado**

DIRECTIONS

1. Cook the bacon and set aside. Mix the eggs and parmesan cheese. Warm a skillet and add the ghee to melt. Mix in the eggs then cook within 30 seconds. Flip and cook again within 30 seconds. Serve with the crunched bacon bits and sliced avocado.

NUTRITION:

Carbohydrates: 3.3 grams Protein: 30 grams Fats: 63 grams Calories: 719

2. BACON & CHEESE FRITTATA

COOKING: 5' **PREPARATION: 5'** **SERVINGS: 6**

INGREDIENTS

» 1 cup Heavy cream
» 6 eggs
» 5 slices of bacon
» 2 green onions
» 4oz. Cheddar cheese

DIRECTIONS

1. Warm the oven temperature to reach 350 F.
2. Whisk the eggs and seasonings. Put in the pie pan. Bake 30-35 minutes. Cooldown and serve.

NUTRITION:

Protein: 13 grams Carbohydrates: 2 grams Fats: 29 grams Calories: 320

3. BACON & EGG BREAKFAST MUFFINS

COOKING: 30' **PREPARATION: 15'** **SERVINGS: 12**

INGREDIENTS

- » 8 eggs
- » 8 slices of bacon
- » .66 cup Green onion

DIRECTIONS

1. Warm the oven at 350° Fahrenheit. Grease the muffins.
2. Fry the bacon in medium setting until it's crispy, chopped. Mix with the eggs and green onions. Put to muffin thin and bake within 20 to 25 minutes. Cool and serve.

NUTRITION:

Carbohydrates: 0.4 grams Protein: 5.6 grams Fats: 4.9 gramsCalories: 69

4. BACON HASH

COOKING: 10' **PREPARATION: 10'** **SERVINGS: 5**

INGREDIENTS

- » **1 small green pepper**
- » **2 Jalapenos**
- » **1 onion**
- » **4 eggs**
- » **6 slices of bacon**

DIRECTIONS

1. Chop the bacon into chunks. Set aside. Slice the onions and peppers. Dice the jalapenos.
2. Warm-up a skillet and fry the veggies. Once browned, combine the fixings and cook until crispy. Serve with the eggs.

NUTRITION:

Carbohydrates: 9 grams Protein: 23 grams Fats: 24 grams Calories: 366

5. BAGELS WITH CHEESE

COOKING: 15'   **PREPARATION: 10'**   **SERVINGS: 6**

INGREDIENTS

- » 2.5 cups mozzarella cheese
- » 1 tsp. Baking powder
- » 3oz. Cream cheese
- » 1.5 cups Almond flour
- » 2 eggs

DIRECTIONS

1. Shred the mozzarella and combine with the flour, baking powder, and cream cheese. Microwave within one minute. Mix.
2. Cool and put the eggs. Break into six parts and shape into round bagels.
3. Bake within 12 to 15 minutes. Serve.

NUTRITION:

Carbohydrates: 8 grams Protein: 19 grams Fats: 31 grams Calories: 374

6. BAKED APPLES

COOKING: 1 H   **PREPARATION: 10'**   **SERVINGS: 4**

INGREDIENTS

- » 4 tsp. Keto-friendly sweetener
- » .75 tsp. cinnamon
- » .25 cup chopped pecans
- » 4 Granny Smith apples

DIRECTIONS

1. Set the oven temperature at 375° Fahrenheit. Mix the sweetener, cinnamon, and pecans. Core the apple and put the stuffing. Add enough water into the baking dish apple. Bake within 45 minutes to 1 hour. Serve.

NUTRITION:

Carbohydrates: 16 grams Protein: 6.8 grams Fats: 19.9 grams Calories: 175

7. BAKED EGGS IN THE AVOCADO

COOKING: 10'   **PREPARATION: 20'**   **SERVINGS: 1**

INGREDIENTS

» Half avocado
» 1 egg
» 1 tbsp. Olive oil
» .5 cup shredded cheddar cheese

DIRECTIONS

1. Heat the oven to reach 425° Fahrenheit.
2. Remove the avocado flesh. Drizzle with oil and put the eggs.
3. Sprinkle with cheese and bake within 15 to 16 minutes. Serve.

NUTRITION:

Carbohydrates: 0.4 grams Protein: 5.6 grams Fats: 4.9 gramsCalories: 69

8. BANANA PANCAKES

COOKING: 10'   **PREPARATION: 15'**   **SERVINGS: 3**

INGREDIENTS

» Butter
» 2 bananas
» 4 eggs
» 1 tsp. Cinnamon
» 5 tsp. Baking powder

DIRECTIONS

1. Mix the fixings. Cook the pancakes 1-2 minutes per side. Serve.

NUTRITION:

Carbohydrates: 6.8 grams Fats: 7 grams Calories: 157

9. BREAKFAST SKILLET

COOKING: 15'   **PREPARATION: 10'**   **SERVINGS: 2**

INGREDIENTS

- » .75-1lb. organic ground turkey
- » 6 organic eggs
- » 1 cup Keto-friendly salsa

DIRECTIONS

1. Grease the skillet, then put the turkey and simmer. Fold in the salsa and simmer within two to three minutes. Put the eggs to the top of the turkey base. Cook within seven minutes. Serve.

NUTRITION:

Carbohydrates: 7.1 grams Protein: 65.2 grams Fats: 32 grams Calories: 556

10. BRUNCH BLT WRAP

COOKING: 15'   **PREPARATION: 5'**   **SERVINGS: 1**

INGREDIENTS

- » 4 bacon slices
- » 2 Romaine lettuce leaves
- » .25 cup tomatoes
- » 2 tsp. Mayo
- » Pepper

DIRECTIONS

1. Cook the bacon until crispy in a skillet. Spread mayonnaise on one side of the lettuce.
2. Add the bacon and tomato. Roll it up and serve.

NUTRITION:

Carbohydrates: 2 grams Protein: 8 grams Fats: 24 grams Calories: 256

11. CHEESY BACON & EGG CUPS

COOKING: 20' **PREPARATION: 10'** **SERVINGS: 6**

INGREDIENTS

- » 6 bacon slices
- » 6 large eggs
- » .25 cup Cheese
- » 1 spinach
- » Pepper

DIRECTIONS

1. Set the oven setting to 400° Fahrenheit. Cook the bacon in medium-heat. Grease muffin tins. Put the slice of bacon. Mix the eggs and combine with the spinach. Add the batter to tins and sprinkle with cheese. Put salt and pepper. Bake within 15 minutes. Serve.

NUTRITION:

Carbohydrates: 1 gram Protein: 8 grams Fats: 7 grams Calories: 101

12. COCONUT KETO PORRIDGE

COOKING: 10' **PREPARATION: 15'** **SERVINGS: 1**

INGREDIENTS

- » 4tsp. Coconut cream
- » 1 pinch ground psyllium husk powder
- » 1 tbsp. Coconut flour
- » 1 Flaxseed egg
- » 1 oz. coconut butter

DIRECTIONS

1. Toss all of the fixings in a small pan, cook on low heat. Serve.

NUTRITION:

Carbohydrates: 5.4 grams Protein: 10.1 grams Fats: 22.8 grams Calories: 401

13. CREAM CHEESE EGGS

COOKING: 5'　　　**PREPARATION: 5'**　　　**SERVINGS: 1**

INGREDIENTS

- » 1 tbsp. butter
- » 2 eggs
- » 2 tbsp. Soft cream cheese with chives

DIRECTIONS

1. Warm-up a skillet and melt the butter. Whisk the eggs with the cream cheese.
2. Cook until done. Serve.

NUTRITION:

Carbohydrates: 3 grams Protein: 15 grams Fats: 31 grams Calories: 341

14. CREAMY BASIL BAKED SAUSAGE

COOKING: 5'　　　**PREPARATION: 5'**　　　**SERVINGS: 12**

INGREDIENTS

- » 3 lb. Italian sausage
- » 8 oz. Cream cheese
- » .25 cup Heavy cream
- » .25 cup Basil pesto
- » 8 oz. Mozzarella

DIRECTIONS

Set the oven at 400° Fahrenheit.
Put the sausage to the dish and bake within 30 minutes. Combine the heavy cream, pesto, and cream cheese. Pour the sauce over the casserole and top it off with the cheese.
Bake within 10 minutes. Serve.

NUTRITION:

Carbohydrates: 4 grams Protein: 23 grams Fats: 23 grams Calories: 316

15. ALMOND COCONUT EGG WRAPS

COOKING: 5'   **PREPARATION: 5'**   **SERVINGS: 4**

INGREDIENTS

» 5 organic eggs
» 1 tbsp. coconut flour
» .25 tsp. Sea Salt
» 2 tbsp. Almond meal

DIRECTIONS

1. Blend the fixings in a blender. Warm-up a skillet, medium-high. Put two tablespoons of batter then cook within 3 minutes. Flip to cook for another 3 minutes. Serve.

NUTRITION:

Carbohydrates: 3 grams Protein: 8 grams Fats: 8 grams Calories: 111

16. BANANA WAFFLES

COOKING: 30'   **PREPARATION: 30'**   **SERVINGS: 4**

INGREDIENTS

» 4 eggs
» 1 banana
» ¾ cup coconut milk
» ¾cup almond flour
» Salt
» 1tbsp. ground psyllium husk powder
» ½tsp. vanilla extract
» 1 tsp. baking powder
» 1 tsp. ground cinnamon
» Butter

DIRECTIONS

1. Mash the banana then put all the fixing and whisk. Fry the waffles in a pan. Serve!

NUTRITION:

Carbohydrates: 4g Fat: 13g Protein: 5g Calories: 155

17. KETO CINNAMON COFFEE

COOKING: 5' **PREPARATION: 5'** **SERVINGS: 1**

INGREDIENTS

» 2tbsp. ground coffee
» 1/3 cup heavy whipping cream
» 1tsp. ground cinnamon
» 2 cups of water

DIRECTIONS

1. Start by mixing the cinnamon with the ground coffee. Pour in hot water, whip the cream until stiff peaks. Serve with cinnamon.

NUTRITION:

Net Carbs: 1g Fiber: 1g Fat: 14g Protein: 1g Calories: 136

18. KETO WAFFLES AND BLUEBERRIES

COOKING: 10-15' **PREPARATION: 15'** **SERVINGS: 8**

INGREDIENTS

» 8 eggs
» 5 oz. melted butter
» 1 tsp. vanilla extract
» 2 tsp. baking powder
» 1/3 cup coconut flour
» Topping:
» 3 oz. butter
» 1 oz. blueberries

DIRECTIONS

1. Mix the butter and eggs, put in the remaining items except topping.
2. Cook the batter in medium heat. Serve with blueberries plus batter.

NUTRITION:

Net Carbs: 3g Fiber: 5g Fat: 56g Protein: 14g Calories: 575

19. BAKED AVOCADO EGGS

COOKING: 30' **PREPARATION: 30'** **SERVINGS: 4**

INGREDIENTS

» avocados
» 4 eggs
» ½ cup bacon bits
» 2 tbsp. chives
» 1 sprig basil
» 1 cherry tomato
» Salt
» pepper
» Shredded cheddar cheese

DIRECTIONS

1. Warm-up the oven to 400 degrees Fahrenheit
2. Remove the avocado seed. Break eggs onto the center hole of the avocado. Put salt and pepper.
3. Top with bacon bits and bake within 15 minutes. Serve!

NUTRITION:

Calories: 271 Fat: 21g Fiber: 5g Protein: 13g Carbohydrates: 7g

20. MUSHROOM OMELET

COOKING: 5' **PREPARATION: 15'** **SERVINGS: 1**

INGREDIENTS

» 3 eggs
» 1 oz. cheese
» 1 oz. butter
» ¼ yellow onion
» 4 large mushrooms
» vegetables
» Salt
» pepper

DIRECTIONS

1. Beat the eggs, put some salt and pepper.
2. Cook the mushroom and onion. Put the egg mixture into the pan and cook on medium heat.
3. Put the cheese on top of the still-raw portion of the egg.
4. Pry the edges of the omelet and fold it in half. Serve.

NUTRITION:

Carbohydrates: 5g Fiber: 1g Fat: 44g Protein: 26g Calories: 520

21. CHOCOLATE SEA SALT SMOOTHIE

COOKING: 15'   **PREPARATION: 15'**   **SERVINGS: 2**

INGREDIENTS

- » 1 avocado
- » 2 cups almond milk
- » 1 tbsp. tahini
- » ¼ cup of cocoa powder
- » 1 scoop Keto chocolate base

DIRECTIONS

1. Combine all the fixing in a high-speed blender. Add ice and serve!

NUTRITION:

Calories: 235 Fat: 20g Carbohydrates: 11.25 Protein: 5.5g

22. ZUCCHINI LASAGNA

COOKING: 1 H 20'   **PREPARATION: 20'**   **SERVINGS: 9**

INGREDIENTS

- » 3 cups raw macadamia nuts
- » Ricotta
- » 2 tbsp. nutritional yeast
- » 2 tsp. dried oregano
- » 1 tsp. sea salt
- » 1/2 cup water
- » 1/4 cup vegan parmesan cheese
- » 1/2 cup fresh basil, chopped
- » 1 lemon juice
- » Black pepper
- » 1 28-oz marinara sauce
- » 3 medium zucchini squash with a mandolin

DIRECTIONS

1. Warm-up the oven to 375 degrees Fahrenheit
2. Process the macadamia nut in a processor. Add the remaining fixing.
3. Put 1 cup of marinara sauce in a baking dish.
4. Create the lasagna layers using thinly sliced zucchini
5. Scoop ricotta mixture on the zucchini and spread, layer up to the top.
6. Sprinkle parmesan cheese on the topmost layer.
7. Cover with foil and bake within 45 minutes. Remove the foil and bake within 15 minutes.
8. Cool and serve.

NUTRITION:

Calories: 338 Fat: 34g Carbohydrates: 10g Protein: 4.7g

23. VEGAN KETO SCRAMBLE

COOKING: 10-15'   PREPARATION: 15'   SERVINGS: 1

INGREDIENTS

- » 14 oz. firm tofu
- » 3 tbsp. avocado oil
- » 2 tbsp. yellow onion
- » 1.5 tbsp. Nutritional yeast
- » ½ tsp. Turmeric
- » ½ tsp. Garlic powder
- » ½ tsp. salt
- » 1 cup baby spinach
- » 3 grape tomatoes
- » 3 oz. vegan cheddar cheese

DIRECTIONS

1. Sauté the chopped onion until it caramelizes.
2. Crumble the tofu on the skillet. Grease avocado oil onto the mixture with the dry seasonings. Stir.
3. Fold the baby spinach, cheese, and diced tomato. Cook for a few more minutes. Serve.

NUTRITION:

Calories: 212 Fat: 17.5g Net Carbohydrates: 4.74g Protein: 10g

24. BAVARIAN CREAM WITH VANILLA AND HAZELNUTS

COOKING: 0'   PREPARATION: 15'   SERVINGS: 3

INGREDIENTS

- » 54g Mascarpone
- » 7g Soy lecithin
- » 2g Hazelnuts
- » 8g Fruit mousse

DIRECTIONS

1. Prepare the mousse by mixing the mascarpone at room temperature sweetened with one or two drops of liquid saccharin and flavored with a pinch of vanillin. Add the lecithin, blending the mixture well. Put the Bavarian cream in a dessert bowl and decorate with the fruit puree and chopped hazelnuts. Chill and serve.

NUTRITION:

Calories: 318 Carbs: 17g Fat: 25g Protein: 6g

25. VANILLA MOUSSE

COOKING: 0'   **PREPARATION: 15'**   **SERVINGS: 5**

INGREDIENTS

- » 30g Mascarpone
- » 70g Cream
- » 4g Butter
- » 3g Rusk rich in fiber
- » 40g Cheese

DIRECTIONS

1. Prepare the mousse with mascarpone and butter. Sweeten with liquid saccharin and sprinkle with a little decaffeinated coffee in granules. Serve the cheese separately with the buttered rusk and the hot drink prepared with the cream and barley coffee sweetened with saccharin.

NUTRITION:

Calories: 100 Carbs: 11g Fat: 6g Protein: 2g

26. BLUEBERRY BAVARIAN

COOKING: 0'   **PREPARATION: 15'**   **SERVINGS: 3**

INGREDIENTS

- » 40g Mascarpone
- » 5g Soy lecithin
- » 10g Hazelnuts
- » 10g Blueberries

DIRECTIONS

1. Prepare the mousse by mixing the mascarpone at room temperature sweetened with one or two drops of liquid saccharin and flavored with a pinch of vanillin. Add the lecithin, blending the mixture well. Put the Bavarian cream in a dessert bowl and decorate with the chopped blueberries and hazelnuts. Chill and serve.

NUTRITION:

Calories: 150 Carbs: 26g Fat: 2g Protein: 7g

27. STRAWBERRY BAVARIAN

COOKING: 15'   **PREPARATION: 0'**   **SERVINGS: 5**

INGREDIENTS

» 40g Mascarpone
» 4g Butter
» 10g Brazilian nuts
» 10g Strawberries

DIRECTIONS

1. Prepare the Bavarian by mixing the mascarpone at room temperature and the butter. Sweeten to taste and put in a cup then chill. Weigh and roughly break the walnuts and garnish with strawberries before serving.

NUTRITION:

Calories: 153 Carbs: 24g Fat: 6g Protein: 2g

28. ALMOND MOUSSE

COOKING: 0'   **PREPARATION: 15'**   **SERVINGS: 2**

INGREDIENTS

» 1 small green pepper
» 2 Jalapenos
» 1 onion
» 4 eggs
» 6 slices of bacon

DIRECTIONS

1. Prepare the mousse with mascarpone, 1 or 2 drops of saccharin, almond flavoring, and softened butter at room temperature. Serve the cheese aside with a cup of green tea sweetened with saccharin.

NUTRITION:

Calories: 566 Carbs: 53g Fat: 36g Protein: 8g

29. NOUGAT

COOKING: 15'　　**PREPARATION: 15'**　　**SERVINGS: 4**

INGREDIENTS

- » 105g Whole milk
- » 2g Bitter cocoa powder
- » 18g Soy lecithin
- » 10g Sweet almonds
- » 16g Butter
- » 5g Hazelnuts
- » 5g Pistachios

DIRECTIONS

1. Crush the hazelnuts, pistachios, and almonds coarsely and mix them with the butter softened at room temperature. Add the lecithin to the mixture and shape the nougat. Chill. Serve with hot cocoa milk.

NUTRITION:

Calories: 70 Carbs: 3g Fat: 0g Protein: 0g

30. CHOCOLATE CREPES

COOKING: 10'　　**PREPARATION: 15'**　　**SERVINGS: 4**

INGREDIENTS

- » 36g Whole egg
- » 5g Dark chocolate
- » 34g Mascarpone
- » 17g Butter

DIRECTIONS

1. Beat the egg. Cook the crepes in a non-stick pan. Prepare the filling by mixing mascarpone and butter at room temperature, sweetening with one or two drops of liquid saccharin. Melt the dark chocolate in a bain-marie and mix it with the mascarpone cream. Stuff the crepes and serve with a cup of decaffeinated tea without sugar.

NUTRITION:

Calories: 150 Carbs: 19g Fat: 8g Protein: 2g

31. RUSK WITH WALNUT CREAM

COOKING: 10'   **PREPARATION: 15'**   **SERVINGS: 1**

INGREDIENTS

- » 17g Spreadable cream with walnuts
- » 10g Butter
- » 4g Rusk rich in fiber
- » 67g Cream with 35% fat

DIRECTIONS

1. Prepare the hot drink by heating the cream and adding soluble decaffeinated coffee. Sweeten with liquid saccharin. Spread the buttered biscuit with the walnut cream.

NUTRITION:

Calories: 39 Carbs: 7g Fat: 1g Protein: 1g

32. BAVARIAN COFFEE WITH HAZELNUTS

COOKING: 10'   **PREPARATION: 15'**   **SERVINGS: 1**

INGREDIENTS

- » 67g Mascarpone
- » 11g Hazelnuts

DIRECTIONS

1. Prepare the hot drink by heating the water. Weigh the hazelnuts and pass them to the mixer then add them by mixing with the mascarpone held for a few moments at room temperature. Add the remaining part of soluble decaffeinated coffee. Sweeten with saccharin.

NUTRITION:

Calories: 20 Carbs: 3g Fat: 1g Protein: 0g

33. STRAWBERRY BUTTER BAVARIAN

COOKING: 0'   **PREPARATION: 15'**   **SERVINGS: 1**

INGREDIENTS

» 1 slice of crispy bacon
» 2 organic eggs
» .5cup grated parmesan cheese
» 2 tbsp. Ghee
» 1 Avocado

DIRECTIONS

1. Soak a piece of gelatin in hot water. Put it in the Bavarian container and add the exact amount of cream. Add the softened butter at room temperature. Sweeten with liquid saccharin and add the vanilla flavor. Chill and serve with strawberries, a small leaf of mint, and the coarsely chopped hazelnuts. Serve the cheese separately with a cup of jasmine tea sweetened with saccharin.

NUTRITION:

Calories: 80 Carbs: 5g Fat: 7g Protein: 0g

34. CHEESE PLATTERS

COOKING: 0'   **PREPARATION: 15'**   **SERVINGS: 1**

INGREDIENTS

» 45g Ricotta cheese
» 35g Cheese
» 22g Hazelnuts
» 30g Mascarpone cheese
» 26g Butter
» Saccharin and orange flavor

DIRECTIONS

1. Weigh the cheeses' exact quantity and serve them on a small wooden cutting board with hazelnuts in the center. Prepare the mascarpone pastry by weighing the precise amount of mascarpone and softened butter at room temperature.

NUTRITION:

Calories: 39 Carbs: 6g Fat: 1g Protein: 2g

35. HAZELNUT BAVARIAN WITH HOT COFFEE DRINK

COOKING: 0' **PREPARATION: 15'** **SERVINGS: 1**

INGREDIENTS

- » 85g Mascarpone cheese
- » 21g Hazelnuts
- » 3g Butter
- » 15g Wild strawberries

DIRECTIONS

1. Prepare the drink by heating 150 ml of water. Add a teaspoon of decaffeinated coffee and saccharin. Prepare the Bavarian by mixing mascarpone, butter, and hazelnuts passed in the mixer at room temperature, sweetening. Garnish with wild strawberries and chill. Serve.

NUTRITION:

Calories: 3 Carbs: 0g Fat: 0g Protein: 0g

36. MUFFINS WITH COFFEE DRINK

COOKING: 5' **PREPARATION: 0'** **SERVINGS: 1**

INGREDIENTS

- » 1 small green pepper
- » 2 Jalapenos
- » 1 onion
- » 4 eggs
- » 6 slices of bacon

DIRECTIONS

1. Prepare the hot coffee drink by mixing the white flour, cream, and American coffee in a mug. Sweeten to taste. Butter the sugar-free muffin. Serve.

NUTRITION:

Calories: 28 Carbs: 4g Fat: 24g Protein: 9g

37. FRENCH TOAST WITH COFFEE DRINK

COOKING: 15'   **PREPARATION: 10'**   **SERVINGS: 1**

INGREDIENTS

- » 24g Cream with 35% fat
- » 14g Whole egg
- » 15g Sweet cheese
- » 12g Low carb bread without crust
- » 11g Butter
- » For the hot drink:
- » 10g White flour
- » 80g Cream with 35% fat

DIRECTIONS

1. In a small bowl, scramble the egg, cream, finely grated cheese in the mixer. Toast the bread in butter, turn it several times and pour the mixture over it. Garnish with chopped fresh parsley. Prepare the hot drink by shaking the white flour with the cream. Add the soluble decaffeinated coffee and saccharin.

NUTRITION:

Calories: 31 Carbs: 6g Fat: 0g Protein: 1g

CHAPTER 5. LUNCH RECIPES

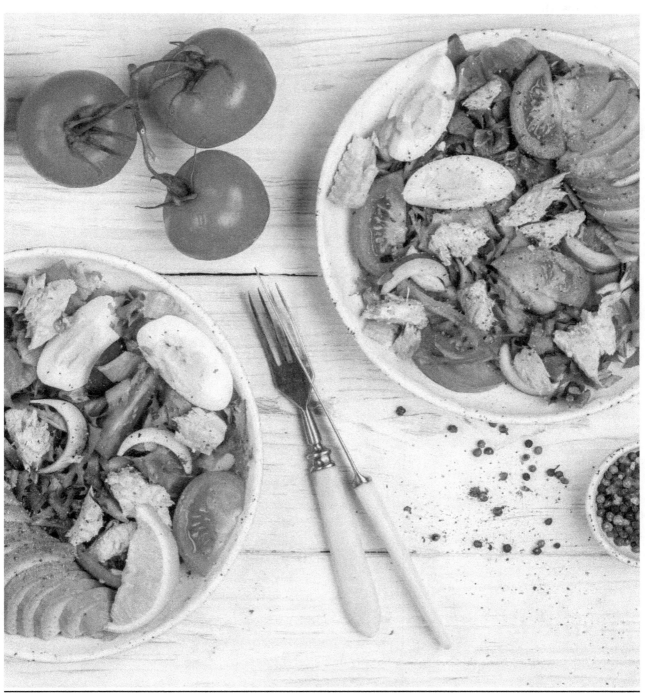

38. TURKEY AND CREAM CHEESE SAUCE

COOKING: 25' **PREPARATION: 15'** **SERVINGS: 5**

INGREDIENTS

- » Two tbsp. butter
- » Two pounds of turkey breast
- » Two cups whipping cream
- » Seven ounces cream cheese
- » One tbsp. tamari soy sauce
- » Pepper
- » Salt
- » 1 & 1/2-ounces capers

DIRECTIONS

1. Warm-up the oven at 170 Celsius, then dissolve half butter in an iron skillet.
2. Rub the breast of turkey with pepper and salt. Fry within five minutes.
3. Bake within ten minutes.
4. Add the drippings of turkey in a pan, cream cheese, and whipping cream. Simmer. Put pepper, soy sauce, and salt. Sauté the small capers in remaining butter.
5. Slice and serve with fried capers and cream cheese sauce.

NUTRITION:

Calories: 810.3 Protein: 47.6g Carbs: 6.9g Fat: 68.6g — Fiber: 0.6g

39. BAKED SALMON AND PESTO

COOKING: 30' **PREPARATION: 15'** **SERVINGS: 4**

INGREDIENTS

- » **For the green sauce:**
- » Four tbsps. green pesto
- » One cup mayonnaise
- » Half cup Greek yogurt
- » Pepper
- » Salt
- » **For the salmon:**
- » Two pounds salmon
- » Four tbsps. green pesto
- » Pepper
- » Salt

DIRECTIONS

1. Put the fillets on a greased baking dish with the skin side down. Add pesto on top. Add pepper and salt.
2. Bake at 200 degrees within thirty minutes.
3. Combine all the listed fixing for the green sauce in a bowl.
4. Serve the baked salmon with green sauce on top.

NUTRITION:

Calories: 1010.2 Protein: 51.6g Carbs: 3.1g Fat: 87.6g Fiber: 0.7g

40. KETO CHICKEN WITH BUTTER AND LEMON

COOKING: 1H 30'   PREPARATION: 15'   SERVINGS: 2

INGREDIENTS

- » Three pounds whole chicken
- » Pepper and salt
- » Two tsp. barbecue seasoning
- » Five ounces butter
- » One lemon
- » Two onions
- » One-fourth cup water
- » One tsp. butter

DIRECTIONS

1. Warm-up oven at 170 degrees. Grease the baking dish.
2. Rub the chicken with pepper, salt, and barbecue seasoning. Put in the baking dish.
3. Arrange lemon wedges and onions surrounding the chicken put slices of butter.
4. Bake within 1 hour and 30 minutes. Slice and serve.

NUTRITION:

Calories: 980.3 Protein: 57.2g Carbs: 0.4g Fat: 81.3g Fiber: 0.1g

41. GARLIC CHICKEN

COOKING: 40'   PREPARATION: 15'   SERVINGS: 4

INGREDIENTS

- » Two ounces butter
- » Two pounds chicken drumsticks
- » Pepper
- » Salt
- » lemon juice
- » Two tbsps. olive oil
- » Seven cloves garlic
- » Half cup parsley

DIRECTIONS

1. Warm-up oven at 250 degrees Celsius.
2. Put the chicken in a baking dish. Add pepper and salt.
3. Add olive oil with lemon juice over the chicken. Sprinkle parsley and garlic on top.
4. Bake within forty minutes. Serve.

NUTRITION:

Calories: 540.3 Protein: 41.3g Carbs: 3.1g Fat: 38.6g Fiber: 1.6g

42. SALMON SKEWERS WRAPPED WITH PROSCIUTTO

COOKING: 4'   **PREPARATION: 15'**   **SERVINGS: 4**

INGREDIENTS

- ¼ cup basil
- One-pound salmon
- One pinch black pepper
- Four ounces prosciutto
- One tbsp. olive oil
- Eight skewers

DIRECTIONS

1. Start by soaking the skewers in a bowl of water.
2. Cut the salmon fillets lengthwise. Thread the salmon using skewers.
3. Coat the skewers in pepper and basil. Wrap the slices of prosciutto around the salmon.
4. Warm-up oil in a grill pan. Grill the skewers within four minutes. Serve.

NUTRITION:

Calories: 670.5 Protein: 27.2g Carbs: 1.2g Fat: 61.6g Fiber: 0.3g

43. BUFFALO DRUMSTICKS AND CHILI AIOLI

COOKING: 40'   **PREPARATION: 15'**   **SERVINGS: 4**

INGREDIENTS

- **For the chili aioli:**
- Half cup mayonnaise
- One tbsp. smoked paprika powder
- One clove garlic
- **For the chicken:**
- Two pounds chicken drumsticks
- Two tbsps. of each:
- White wine vinegar
- Olive oil
- One tbsp. tomato paste
- One tsp. of each:
- Salt
- Paprika powder
- Tabasco

DIRECTIONS

1. Warm-up oven at 200 degrees.
2. Combine the listed marinade fixing. Marinate the chicken drumsticks within ten minutes.
3. Arrange the chicken drumsticks in the tray. Bake within forty minutes.
4. Combine the listed items for the chili aioli in a bowl. Serve.

NUTRITION:

Calories: 567.8 Protein: 41.3g Carbs: 2.2g Fat: 43.2g Fiber: 1.1g

44. SLOW COOKED ROASTED PORK AND CREAMY GRAVY

COOKING: 8H 15'   PREPARATION: 15'   SERVINGS: 6

INGREDIENTS

- » **For the creamy gravy:**
- » Two cups whipping cream
- » Roast juice
- » **For the pork:**
- » Two pounds pork roast
- » Half tbsp. Salt
- » One bay leaf
- » Five black peppercorns
- » Three cups of
- » water
- » Two tsp. thyme
- » Two cloves garlic
- » Two ounces ginger
- » One tbsp. of each:
- » Paprika powder
- » Olive oil
- » One-third tsp. black pepper

DIRECTIONS

1. Warm-up your oven at 100 degrees.
2. Add the meat, salt, water in a baking dish. Put peppercorns, thyme, and bay leaf. Put in the oven within eight hours. Remove. Reserve the juices. Adjust to 200 degrees.
3. Put ginger, garlic, pepper, herbs, and oil. Rub the herb mixture on the meat. Roast the pork within fifteen minutes.
4. Slice the roasted meat. Strain the meat juices in a bowl. Boil for reducing it by half.
5. Add the cream. Simmer within twenty minutes. Serve with creamy gravy.

NUTRITION:

Calories: 586.9 Protein: 27.9g Carbs: 2.6g Fat: 50.3g Fiber: 1.5g

45. BACON-WRAPPED MEATLOAF

COOKING: 1H   PREPARATION: 15'   SERVINGS: 4

INGREDIENTS

- » **For the meatloaf:**
- » Two tbsps. butter
- » One onion
- » Two pounds beef
- » Half cup whipping cream
- » Two ounces cheese
- » One large egg
- » One tbsp. oregano
- » One tsp. Salt
- » Half tsp. black pepper
- » Seven ounces bacon
- » **For the gravy:**
- » 1& 1/2 cup whipping cream
- » Half tbsp. tamari soy sauce

DIRECTIONS

1. Warm-up your oven at 200 degrees Celsius.
2. Dissolve the butter in a pan. Add the onion. Cook within four minutes. Keep aside.
3. Combine onion, ground meat, and the remaining fixing except for the bacon in a large bowl.
4. Make a firm loaf. Use bacon strips for wrapping the loaf.
5. Bake the meatloaf for forty-five minutes.
6. Put the juices from the baking dish and cream, then boil. Simmer within ten minutes. Add the soy sauce. Slice and serve with gravy.

NUTRITION:

Calories: 1020.3 Protein: 46.7g Carbs: 5.6g Fat: 88.9g Fiber: 1.2g

46. LAMB CHOPS AND HERB BUTTER

COOKING: 4' **PREPARATION: 15'** **SERVINGS: 4**

INGREDIENTS

» Eight lamb chops
» One tbsp. each:
» Olive oil
» Butter
» Pepper
» Salt
» For the herb butter:
» Five ounces butter
» One clove garlic
» Half tbsp. garlic powder
» Four tbsps. parsley
» One tsp. lemon juice
» One-third tsp. Salt

DIRECTIONS

1. Season the lamb chops with pepper and salt.
2. Warm-up olive oil and butter in an iron skillet. Add the lamb chops. Fry within four minutes.
3. Mix all the listed items for the herb butter in a bowl. Cool.
4. Serve with herb butter.

NUTRITION:

Calories: 722.3 Protein: 42.3g Carbs: 0.4g Fat: 61.5g Fiber: 0.4g

47. CRISPY CUBAN PORK ROAST

COOKING: 4' **PREPARATION: 15'** **SERVINGS: 6**

INGREDIENTS

» Five pounds pork shoulder
» Four tsp. Salt
» Two tsp. cumin
» One tsp. black pepper
» Two tbsps. oregano
» One red onion
» Four cloves garlic
» orange juice
» lemons juiced
» One-fourth cup of olive oil

DIRECTIONS

1. Rub the pork shoulder with salt in a bowl. Mix all the remaining items of the marinade in a blender.
2. Marinate the meat within eight hours. Cook within forty minutes. Warm-up your oven at 200 degrees. Roast the pork within thirty minutes.
3. Remove the meat juice. Simmer within twenty minutes. Shred the meat.
4. Pour the meat juice. Serve.

NUTRITION:

Calories: 910.3 Protein: 58.3g Carbs: 5.3g Fat: 69.6g — Fiber: 2.2g

48. KETO BARBECUED RIBS

COOKING: 1H 10'   **PREPARATION: 15'**   **SERVINGS: 4**

INGREDIENTS

- » One-fourth cup Dijon mustard
- » Two tbsps. of each:
- » Cider vinegar
- » Butter
- » Salt
- » Three pounds of spare ribs
- » Four tbsps. paprika powder
- » Half tbsp. chili powder
- » 1&1/2 tbsp. garlic powder
- » Two tsp. of each:
- » Onion powder
- » Cumin
- » Two & 1/2 tbsp. black pepper

DIRECTIONS

1. Warm-up a grill for thirty minutes.
2. Mix vinegar and Dijon mustard in a bowl, put the ribs and coat.
3. Mix all the listed spices. Rub the mix all over the ribs. Put aside. Put ribs on an aluminum foil. Add some butter over the ribs. Wrap with foil. Grill within one hour. Remove and slice.
4. Put the reserved spice mix. Grill again within ten minutes. Serve.

NUTRITION:

Calories: 980.3 Protein: 54.3g Carbs: 5.8g Fat: 80.2g Fiber: 4.6g

49. TURKEY BURGERS AND TOMATO BUTTER

COOKING: 15'   **PREPARATION: 15'**   **SERVINGS: 4**

INGREDIENTS

- » **For the chicken** patties:
- » Two pounds of chicken
- » One egg
- » Half onion
- » One tsp. Salt
- » Half tsp. black pepper
- » One a half tsp. thyme
- » Two ounces butter
- » **For the fried cabbage:**
- » Two pounds green
- » cabbage
- » Three ounces butter
- » One tsp. Salt
- » Half tsp. black pepper (ground)
- » **For the tomato butter:**
- » Four ounces butter
- » One tbsp. tomato paste
- » One tsp. red wine vinegar
- » Pepper
- » Salt

DIRECTIONS

1. Warm-up your oven at 100 degrees.
2. Combine the listed items for the patties in a large bowl. Shape the mixture into patties.
3. Fry the chicken patties for five minutes, each side. Keep warm in the oven.
4. Warm-up butter in a pan. Put the cabbage, plus pepper and salt. Fry for five minutes.
5. Whip the items for the tomato butter in a bowl using an electric mixer.
6. Serve with a dollop of tomato butter from the top.

NUTRITION:

Calories: 830.4 Protein: 33.6g Carbs: 6.7g Fat: 71.5g Fiber: 5.1g

50. KETO HAMBURGER

COOKING: 70'   **PREPARATION: 15'**   **SERVINGS: 4**

INGREDIENTS

- » For the burger buns:
- » Two cups almond flour
- » Five tbsps. ground psyllium husk powder
- » Two tsp. baking powder
- » One tsp. Salt
- » 1&1/2 cup water
- » Two tsp. cider vinegar
- » Three egg whites

- » One tbsp. sesame seed
- » For the hamburger:
- » Two pounds beef
- » 1-ounce olive oil
- » Pepper and salt
- » 1&1/2-ounce lettuce
- » One tomato
- » One red onion
- » Half cup mayonnaise
- » Five ounces bacon

DIRECTIONS

1. Mix all the blue cheese dressing items in a bowl. Chill within forty minutes.
2. Combine the chicken with olive oil and spices. Marinate for thirty minutes.
3. Bake in the oven for twenty-five minutes. Toss the chicken wings with parmesan cheese in a bowl.
4. Serve with blue cheese dressing by the side.

NUTRITION:

Calories: 1070.3 Protein: 53.4g Carbs: 6.1g Fat: 85.3g Fiber: 12.3g

51. CHICKEN WINGS AND BLUE CHEESE DRESSING

COOKING: 25'   **PREPARATION: 70'**   **SERVINGS: 4**

INGREDIENTS

- » One-third cup mayonnaise
- » One-fourth cup sour cream
- » Three tsp. lemon juice
- » One-fourth tsp. of each:
- » Salt
- » Garlic powder
- » Half cup whipping cream
- » Three ounces blue cheese

- » **For the chicken wings:**
- » Two pounds chicken wings
- » Two tbsps. olive oil
- » One-fourth tsp. garlic powder
- » One clove garlic
- » One-third tsp. black pepper
- » One tsp. Salt
- » Two ounces parmesan cheese

DIRECTIONS

1. Put the fillets on a greased baking dish with the skin side down. Add pesto on top. Add pepper and salt.
2. Bake at 200 degrees within thirty minutes.
3. Combine all the listed fixing for the green sauce in a bowl.
4. Serve the baked salmon with green sauce on top.

NUTRITION:

Calories: 839.3 Protein: 51.2g Carbs: 2.9g Fat: 67.8g Fiber: 0.2

52. SALMON BURGERS WITH LEMON BUTTER AND MASH

COOKING: 15'   **PREPARATION: 70'**   **SERVINGS: 4**

INGREDIENTS

- » For the salmon burgers:
- » Two pounds salmon
- » One egg
- » Half yellow onion
- » One tsp. Salt
- » Half tsp. black pepper
- » Two ounces butter
- » For the green mash:
- » One-pound broccoli
- » Five ounces of butter
- » Two ounces parmesan cheese
- » Pepper
- » Salt
- » For the lemon butter:
- » Four ounces butter
- » Two tbsps. lemon juice
- » Pepper
- » Salt

DIRECTIONS

1. Warm-up your oven at 100 degrees.
2. Cut the salmon into small pieces. Combine all the burger items with the fish in a blender. Pulse for thirty seconds. Make eight patties.
3. Warm-up butter in an iron skillet. Fry the burgers for five minutes.
4. Boil water, along with some salt in a pot, put the broccoli florets. Cook for three to four minutes. Drain. Add parmesan cheese and butter. Blend the ingredients using an immersion blender. Add pepper and salt.
5. Combine lemon juice with butter, pepper, and salt. Beat using an electric beater.
6. Put a dollop of lemon butter on the top and green mash by the side. Serve.

NUTRITION:

Calories: 1025.3 Protein: 44.5g Carbs: 6.8g Fat: 90.1g Fiber: 3.1g

53. EGG SALAD RECIPE

COOKING: 20'   **PREPARATION: 15'**   **SERVINGS: 6**

INGREDIENTS

- » 3 tbsp. mayonnaise
- » 3 tbsp. Greek yogurt
- » 2 tbsp. red wine vinegar
- » Kosher salt
- » Ground black pepper
- » Eight hard-boiled eggs
- » Eight strips bacon
- » One avocado
- » 1/2 c. crumbled blue cheese
- » 1/2 c. cherry tomatoes
- » 2 tbsp. chives

DIRECTIONS

1. Stir mayonnaise, cream, and the red wine vinegar in a small bowl put pepper and salt.
2. Mix the eggs, bacon, avocado, blue cheese, and cherry tomatoes in a large bowl. Fold in the mayonnaise dressing put salt and pepper. Garnish with the chives and serve.

NUTRITION:

Calories: 200 Carbs: 3g Fat: 18g Protein: 10g

54. TACO STUFFED AVOCADOS

COOKING: 25' **PREPARATION: 10'** **SERVINGS: 8**

INGREDIENTS

- » Four ripe avocados
- » Lime juice
- » 1 tbsp. extra-virgin olive oil
- » One onion
- » 1 lb. ground beef
- » One packet taco seasoning
- » Kosher salt
- » Ground black pepper
- » 2/3 c. Mexican cheese
- » 1/2 c. lettuce
- » 1/2 c. quartered grape tomatoes
- » Sour cream

DIRECTIONS

1. Scoop a bit of avocado flesh. Put. Squeeze lime juice overall avocados.
2. Warm-up oil in a skillet over medium heat. Put onion, and cook within 5 minutes. Put ground beef and taco seasoning. Put salt and pepper, and cook within 6 minutes. Remove and drain.
3. Fill every half of the avocado with beef, then top with reserved avocado, cheese, lettuce, tomato, and a sour dollop cream. Serve.

NUTRITION:

Calories: 324 Carbs: 16g Fat: 24g — Protein: 15g

55. BUFFALO SHRIMP LETTUCE WRAPS

COOKING: 20' **PREPARATION: 15'** **SERVINGS: 4**

INGREDIENTS

- » 1/4 tbsp. butter
- » Two garlic cloves
- » 1/4 c. hot sauce
- » 1 tbsp. extra-virgin olive oil
- » 1 lb. shrimp tails removed
- » Kosher salt
- » Ground black pepper
- » One head romaine leaf
- » 1/4 red onion
- » One rib celery
- » 1/2 c. blue cheese

DIRECTIONS

1. Make buffalo sauce:
2. Dissolve the butter over medium heat in a small saucepan. Put the garlic and cook for 1 minute. Put hot sauce, and stir. Adjust to low.
3. Make shrimp:
4. Warm-up oil in a large skillet over medium heat. Put shrimp, salt, and pepper to season. Cook, around 2 minutes per side. Remove then put buffalo sauce, toss.
5. Assemble wraps:
6. Put a small scoop of shrimp to a roman leaf center, then top with red onion, celery, and blue cheese. Serve.

NUTRITION:

Calories: 242 Carbs: 7g Fat: 12g Protein: 25g

56. BROCCOLI BACON SALAD

COOKING: 15'   **PREPARATION: 15'**   **SERVINGS: 6**

INGREDIENTS

- » For the salad:
- » Kosher salt
- » heads broccoli
- » Two carrots
- » 1/2 red onion
- » 1/2 c. cranberries
- » 1/2 c. almonds
- » Six slices bacon
- » For the dressing:
- » 1/2 c. mayonnaise
- » 3 tbsp. apple cider vinegar
- » Kosher salt
- » Ground black pepper

DIRECTIONS

1. Boil 4 cups of salted water. Prepare a large bowl of ice water.
2. Put broccoli florets to the heated water, and cook within 1 to 2 minutes. Put the ice water in the prepared cup. Drain.
3. Combine broccoli, red onion, carrots, cranberries, nuts, and bacon in a large bowl.
4. Mix vinegar and mayonnaise in a bowl and put salt plus pepper.
5. Pour the broccoli mixture over the dressing. Mix and serve.

NUTRITION:

Calories: 280 Carbs: 9g Fat: 25g Protein: 6g

57. KETO EGG SALAD

COOKING: 15'   **PREPARATION: 15'**   **SERVINGS: 4**

INGREDIENTS

- » 3 tbsp. mayonnaise
- » 2 tsp. lemon juice
- » 1 tbsp. chives
- » Ground black pepper
- » Kosher salt
- » Six hard-boiled eggs
- » One avocado
- » Lettuce
- » Cooked bacon

DIRECTIONS

1. Mix the mayonnaise, lemon juice, and chives, put pepper and salt.
2. Add eggs and avocado to mix. Serve with bacon and lettuce.

NUTRITION:

Calories: 408 Carbs: 5g Fat: 39g Protein: 13g

58. LOADED CAULIFLOWER SALAD

COOKING: 30' **PREPARATION: 15'** **SERVINGS: 4**

INGREDIENTS

- » One large head cauliflower
- » Six slices bacon
- » ½ c. sour cream
- » ¼ c. mayonnaise
- » 1 tbsp. lemon juice
- » ½ tsp. garlic powder
- » Kosher salt
- » Ground black pepper
- » 1 ½ c. cheddar
- » ¼ c. chives

DIRECTIONS

1. Boil ¼ water, put cauliflower, cover pan, and steam within 4 minutes. Drain and cool.
2. Cook the pork around 3 minutes per side. Drain then cut.
3. Mix the sour cream, mayonnaise, lemon juice, and garlic powder in a big bowl. Toss the cauliflower florets. Put salt pepper, bacon, cheddar, and chives. Serve.

NUTRITION:

Calories: 440 Protein: 19g Carbohydrates: 13g Fiber: 4g Fat: 35g

59. CAPRESE ZOODLES

COOKING: 0' **PREPARATION: 15'** **SERVINGS: 4**

INGREDIENTS

- » Four zucchinis
- » 2 tbsp. extra-virgin olive oil
- » Kosher salt
- » Ground black pepper
- » 2 c. cherry tomatoes halved
- » 1 c. mozzarella balls
- » ¼ c. basil leaves
- » 2 tbsp. balsamic vinegar

DIRECTIONS

1. Creating zoodles out of zucchini using a spiralizer.
2. Mix the zoodles, olive oil, salt, and pepper. Marinate for 15 minutes.
3. Put the tomatoes, mozzarella, and basil and toss.
4. Drizzle, and drink with balsamic.

NUTRITION:

Calories: 417 Carbs: 11g Fat: 24g Protein: 36g

60. ZUCCHINI SUSHI

COOKING: 0'   **PREPARATION: 20'**   **SERVINGS: 6**

INGREDIENTS

- » Two zucchinis
- » 4 oz. cream cheese
- » 1 tsp. Sriracha hot sauce
- » 1 tsp. lime juice
- » 1 c. lump crab meat
- » ½ carrot
- » ½ avocado
- » ½ cucumber
- » 1 tsp. Toasted sesame seeds

DIRECTIONS

1. Slice each zucchini into thin flat strips. Put aside.
2. Combine cream cheese, sriracha, and lime juice in a medium-sized cup.
3. Place two slices of zucchini horizontally flat on a cutting board. Place a lean layer of cream cheese over it, then top the left with a slice of lobster, carrot, avocado, and cucumber.
4. Roll up zucchini. Serve with sesame seeds.

NUTRITION:

Calories: 980.3 Protein: 57.2g Carbs: 0.4g Fat: 81.3g Fiber: 0.1g

61. ASIAN CHICKEN LETTUCE WRAPS

COOKING: 15'   **PREPARATION: 15'**   **SERVINGS: 4**

INGREDIENTS

- » 3 tbsp. hoisin sauce
- » 2 tbsp. low-sodium soy sauce
- » 2 tbsp. rice wine vinegar
- » 1 tbsp. Sriracha
- » 1 tsp. sesame oil
- » 1 tbsp. extra-virgin olive oil
- » One onion
- » Two cloves garlic
- » 1 tbsp. grated ginger
- » 1 lb. ground chicken
- » ½ c. water chestnuts
- » Two green onions
- » Kosher salt
- » Ground black pepper
- » Large leafy lettuce
- » Cooked white rice

DIRECTIONS

1. Make the sauce:
2. Mix the hoisin sauce, soy sauce, rice wine vinegar, sriracha, and sesame oil in a small bowl.
3. Mix the olive oil in a large pan, put onions and cook within 5 minutes, then stir in garlic and ginger and cook 1-minute. Put ground chicken and cook.
4. Put in the sauce and cook within 1 to 2 minutes. Turn off heat and put in the green onions and chestnuts. Season with pepper and salt.
5. Add spoon rice of chicken mixture in the center of a lettuce leaf. Serve.

NUTRITION:

Calories: 315 Carbs: 5g Fat: 12g Protein: 34g

62. CALIFORNIA BURGER BOWLS

COOKING: 20'   **PREPARATION: 15'**   **SERVINGS: 4**

INGREDIENTS

- **For the dressing:**
- ½ c. extra-virgin olive oil
- 1/3 c. balsamic vinegar
- 3 tbsp. Dijon mustard
- 2 tsp. honey
- One clove garlic
- Kosher salt
- Ground black pepper
- **For the burger:**
- 1 lb. grass-fed organic ground beef
- 1 tsp. Worcestershire sauce
- ½ tsp. chili powder
- ½ tsp. onion powder
- Kosher salt
- Ground black pepper
- One package butterhead lettuce
- One medium red onion
- One avocado
- 2 tomatoes

DIRECTIONS

1. Make the dressing:
2. Mix the dressing items in a medium bowl.
3. **Make burgers:**
4. Combine beef and Worcestershire sauce, chili powder, and onion powder in another large bowl. Put pepper and salt, mix. Form into four patties.
5. Grill the onions within 3 minutes each. Remove and detach burgers from the grill pan. Cook within 4 minutes per side.
6. **Assemble:**
7. Put lettuce in a large bowl with ½ the dressing. Finish with a patty burger, grilled onions, ¼ slices of avocado, and tomatoes. Serve.

NUTRITION:

Calories: 407 Carbs: 33g Fat: 19g Protein: 26g

63. PARMESAN BRUSSELS SPROUTS SALAD

COOKING: 25'   **PREPARATION: 15'**   **SERVINGS: 6**

INGREDIENTS

- 5 tbsp. extra-virgin olive oil
- 5 tbsp. lemon juice
- ¼ c. parsley
- Kosher salt
- Ground black pepper
- 2 lb. Brussels sprouts
- ½ c. toasted almonds
- ½ c. pomegranate seeds
- Shaved Parmesan

DIRECTIONS

1. Mix olive oil, lemon juice, parsley, two teaspoons of salt, and one teaspoon of pepper.
2. Add the sprouts in Brussels and toss.
3. Let sit before serving within 20 minutes and up to 4 hours.
4. Fold in almonds and pomegranate seeds and garnish with a rasped parmesan. Serve.

NUTRITION:

Calories: 130 Carbs: 8g Fat: 9g Protein: 4g

64. CHICKEN TACO AVOCADOS

COOKING: 20' **PREPARATION: 15'** **SERVINGS: 6**

INGREDIENTS

- » **For the filling:**
- » 1 c. black beans
- » 1 c. canned corn
- » 4-oz. green chilies
- » 1 c. rotisserie chicken
- » 1 c. Cheddar
- » One package taco seasoning
- » 2 tbsp.
- » cilantro
- » Three ripe avocados

- » **For the dressing:**
- » 1 c. ranch dressing
- » ¼ c. lime juice
- » 1 tbsp. cilantro
- » 1 tsp. Kosher salt
- » 1 tsp. Ground black pepper

DIRECTIONS

1. Warm-up the broiler to cook.
2. **For the filling:**
3. Mix black beans, corn, ½ can of green chilies, shredded chicken, cheddar, taco seasoning, and fresh cilantro in a bowl. Halve three avocados and split, eliminating pit. Mash the flesh in a small bowl inside, and set aside. Fill the avocado boats with 1/3 cup of filling. Put cheddar and fresher cilantro, then broil within 2 minutes.
4. **Dressing:**
5. Mix ranch dressing, lime juice, remaining green chilies, cilantro, salt, and pepper. Fold in mashed avocados. Remove avocado. Serve with dressing and cilantro.

NUTRITION:

Calories: 324 Carbs: 16g Fat: 24g Protein: 15g

65. KETO QUESADILLAS

COOKING: 25' **PREPARATION: 15'** **SERVINGS: 4**

INGREDIENTS

- » 1 tbsp. extra-virgin olive oil
- » One bell pepper
- » ½ yellow onion
- » ½ tsp. chili powder
- » Kosher salt
- » Ground black pepper
- » 3 c. Monterey Jack
- » 3 c. cheddar
- » 4 c. chicken
- » One avocado
- » One green onion
- » Sour cream

DIRECTIONS

1. Warm-up oven to 400 F, and line two medium parchment paper baking sheets.
2. Warm-up oil in a medium skillet. Put the onion and pepper, chili powder, salt, and pepper. Cook for 5 minutes.
3. Stir cheeses in a medium-sized dish. Put 1 ½ cups of mixed cheese to prepared baking sheets. Form a circle, the size of a tortilla flour.
4. Bake the cheeses within 8 to 10 minutes. Put a batter of onion-pepper, shredded chicken, and slices of avocado to one half each. Cool and fold one side of the "tortilla" cheese over the side with the fillings. Bake within 3 to 4 more minutes.
5. Serve with green onion and sour cream.

NUTRITION:

Calories: 473 Carbs: 5g Fat: 41g Protein: 21g

66. NO-BREAD ITALIAN SUBS

COOKING: 15'   **PREPARATION: 15'**   **SERVINGS: 6**

INGREDIENTS

- ½ c. mayonnaise
- 2 tbsp. red wine vinegar
- 1 tbsp. extra-virgin olive oil
- One small garlic clove, grated
- 1 tsp. Italian seasoning
- Six slices ham
- 12 salami slices
- 12 pepperoni slices
- Six provolone slices
- 1 c. romaine
- ½ c. roasted red peppers

DIRECTIONS

1. Make creamy Italian dressing:
2. Mix the mayo, vinegar, butter, garlic, and Italian seasoning.
3. Assemble sandwiches:
4. Stack a ham slice, two salami pieces, two pepperoni slices, and a provolone slice.
5. Put a handful of romaine and a couple of roasted red peppers. Put creamy Italian sauce, then roll in and eat.

NUTRITION:

Calories: 390 Protein: 16g Carbohydrates: 3g — Fat: 34g

67. BASIL AVOCADO FRAIL SALAD WRAPS & SWEET POTATO CHIPS

COOKING: 30'   **PREPARATION: 15'**   **SERVINGS: 4**

INGREDIENTS

- **For the sweet potato chips:**
- Kosher salt
- Ground black pepper
- cooking spray
- 2 -3 medium potatoes
- **For the shrimp salad:**
- ¼ small red onion
- 20 large frails
- 1 ½ c. halved grape tomatoes
- cooking spray
- Two avocados
- Four fresh basil leaves
- Two large heads butterhead lettuce
- **For the marinade:**
- 2 lemon juice
- Two cloves garlic
- Three basil leaves
- 2 tbsp. white wine vinegar
- 3 tbsp. extra-virgin olive oil
- ½ tsp. paprika
- Kosher salt
- Ground black pepper

DIRECTIONS

1. For sweet potato chips:
2. Warm-up the oven to 375, then grease a large baking sheet. Put the sweet potatoes wedge with salt and pepper.
3. Roast within 15 minutes, then flip and roast for 15 minutes. Cool and put aside.
4. For shrimp salad:
5. Grease a large skillet, cook the shrimp, occasionally stirring, within 2 minutes per side. Set aside.
6. For marinade:
7. Mix the lemon juice, garlic, basil, vinegar, butter, and paprika, put salt and pepper.
8. Stir the tomatoes, onion, avocados, and basil. Fold in the shrimps. Mix.
9. Serve with lettuce cups.

NUTRITION:

Calories: 80 Carbs: 19g Fat: 0g Protein: 1g

68. CAULIFLOWER LEEK SOUP

COOKING: 45'
PREPARATION: 15'
SERVINGS: 2

INGREDIENTS

- » ½ tablespoons olive oil
- » ½ tablespoon garlic
- » ½ tablespoons butter
- » 2 cups Vegetable Broth
- » 1 leek
- » Salt
- » 1 cup cauliflower
- » black pepper
- » ¼ cup heavy cream

DIRECTIONS

1. Put the oil and butter in the pan to heat. Add garlic, cauliflower, and leek pieces and cook within 5 minutes on low.
2. Add vegetable broth and boil. Cover the pan and cook on low within 45 minutes.
3. Remove then blend the soup in a mixer. Put heavy cream, salt, pepper, and blend more.
4. Serve with salt and pepper.

NUTRITION:

Calories: 155 kcal Fats: 13.1 g Carbohydrates: 8.3 g Proteins: 2.4 g

69. SUGAR-FREE BLUEBERRY COTTAGE CHEESE PARFAITS

COOKING: 5'
PREPARATION: 5'
SERVINGS: 2

INGREDIENTS

- » 225 g cheese, low fat
- » 1/8 tablespoon cinnamon
- » ¼ vanilla extract
- » 6 drops stevia, liquid
- » 150 g berries

DIRECTIONS

1. Blend cheese, vanilla extract, cinnamon, and stevia into the blender.
2. Remove and pour these into bowls.
3. Put the berries on top of the cheese parfaits. Serve.

NUTRITION:

Calories: 125 kcal Fats: 2.2 g Carbohydrates: 12.5 g Proteins: 14.8g Fiber: 1.5 g

70. LOW-CALORIE CHEESY BROCCOLI QUICHE

COOKING: 30'　　　**PREPARATION: 25'**　　　**SERVINGS: 2**

INGREDIENTS

- » 1/3 tablespoon butter
- » Black pepper
- » 4 oz. broccoli
- » ¼ teaspoon garlic powder
- » 2 tablespoon full-fat cream
- » 1/8 cup scallions
- » Kosher salt
- » ¼ cup cheddar cheese
- » 2 eggs

DIRECTIONS

1. Warm-up the oven to 360 degrees F, then grease the baking dish with butter.
2. Put broccoli and 4 to 8 tablespoons water and place the bowl in the microwave within 3 minutes. Mix and again bake within 3 minutes.
3. Beat the eggs in a bowl. Pour all leftover items with broccoli.
4. Put all mixture in the baking dish. Bake within 30 minutes. Slice and serve.

NUTRITION:

Calories: 196 kcal Fats: 14g Carbohydrates: 5 g Proteins: 12g Fiber: 2 g

71. LOW-CARB BROCCOLI LEEK SOUP

COOKING: 15'　　　**PREPARATION: 15'**　　　**SERVINGS: 2**

INGREDIENTS

- » ½ leek
- » 100 g cream cheese
- » 150 g broccoli
- » ½ cup heavy cream
- » 1 cup of water
- » ¼ tablespoon black pepper
- » ½ vegetable bouillon cube
- » ¼ cup basil
- » 1 teaspoon garlic
- » Salt
- »

DIRECTIONS

1. Put water into a pan and put broccoli chopped, leek chopped, and salt. Boil on high.
2. Simmer on low. Put the remaining items, simmer for 1 minute. Remove.
3. Blend the soup mixture into a blender. Serve.

NUTRITION:

Calories: 545 kcal Fats: 50 g Carbohydrates: 10 g Proteins: 15g

72. LOW-CARB CHICKEN TACO SOUP

COOKING: 12'   **PREPARATION: 10'**   **SERVINGS: 2**

INGREDIENTS

- » 1 cup chicken broth
- » ½ cup tomatoes
- » ½ cup boneless chicken
- » 4 green chilies
- » ½ package cream cheese
- » 1 tablespoon seasoning

DIRECTIONS

1. Put chicken broth, boneless ch·icken, cheese, tomatoes, and green chilies in a pressure cooker.
2. Cook within 10 minutes. Remove. Shred the chicken.
3. Put shredded chicken in the soup and stir. Put Italian seasoning. Serve.

NUTRITION:

Calories: 239 Fats: 12 g Carbohydrates: 3 g Proteins: 26 g

73. KETO CHICKEN & VEGGIES SOUP

COOKING: 30'   **PREPARATION: 5'**   **SERVINGS: 2**

INGREDIENTS

- » ¼ tablespoon olive oil
- » 1 cup chicken broth
- » ½ onion
- » ¼ tablespoon seasoning, Italian
- » 2 bell peppers
- » 1 spoon Bay leaves
- » ½ tablespoon garlic
- » Sea salt
- » ¼ cup green beans
- » Black pepper
- » ½ cup tomatoes
- » 2 chicken breast pieces

DIRECTIONS

1. Massage the chicken with salt and pepper and grill within 10 minutes.
2. Put onions and bell pepper into heated oil and simmer within 5-6 minutes on low.
3. Add all leftover items and simmer within 15 minutes on low. Remove. Serve.

NUTRITION:

Calories: 79 Fats: 2g Carbohydrates: 11 g Proteins: 2g — Fiber: 3 g

74. LOW-CARB SEAFOOD SOUP WITH MAYO

COOKING: 40' **PREPARATION: 15'** **SERVINGS: 2**

INGREDIENTS

- » ¼ tablespoon olive oil
- » ½ chopped onion
- » ¼ tablespoon garlic
- » 2 cup fish broth
- » 1 tomato
- » thyme
- » Salt
- » Garlic Mayo
- » 3 oz. Whitefish
- » 1/3 cup olive oil
- » 1/8 cup shrimps
- » 1/3 garlic clove
- » 1/8 cup mussels
- » 1 egg,
- » 1/8 cup scallops
- » ½ tablespoon lemon juice
- » 1/3 bay leaf
- » Salt
- » ½ lime

DIRECTIONS

1. Cook onions and garlic in heated olive oil. Put broth, bay leaf, tomatoes, and salt. After boiling, cover within 20 minutes on low flame.
2. Add all fixing and cook within 4 minutes.
3. Blend garlic mayo in the blender and put olive oil.
4. Put the mayo on the top middle and serve with thyme and lime.

NUTRITION:

Calories: 592 kcal Fats: 47g Net Carbohydrates: 8 g Proteins: 27 g

75. KETO TORTILLA CHIPS

COOKING: 40' **PREPARATION: 10'** **SERVINGS: 2**

INGREDIENTS

- » ¼ cube of mozzarella cheese
- » ¼ teaspoon cumin powder
- » 20 g almond flour
- » 1 teaspoon coriander
- » 1 tablespoon cream cheese
- » Chili powder
- » 1 egg
- » Salt

DIRECTIONS

1. Microwave the mozzarella cheese, cream cheese, and flour within 30 seconds. Stir and set for 30 seconds more.
2. Put spices and egg into the cheese mixture to make the dough.
3. Put the dough in two pieces of parchment paper in a large rectangular form.
4. Remove the parchment paper. Bake within 15 minutes to 400-degree F.
5. Bake the other side of the dough in the same way.
6. Remove and cut into rectangular chips. Bake again within 2 minutes and serve.

NUTRITION:

Calories: 198 Fats: 16 g Carbohydrates: 4 g Proteins: 11 g

76. CHICKEN ZUCCHINI ALFREDO

COOKING: 30' **PREPARATION: 15'** **SERVINGS: 2**

INGREDIENTS

- » 100 g chicken breast
- » Basil
- » 100 g zucchini
- » 90 g cauliflower
- » 40 g cream cheese
- » Mayo
- » Black pepper
- » 1 teaspoon olive oil
- » 1 teaspoon garlic

DIRECTIONS

1. Marinate chicken with basil, salt, and pepper. Grill the chicken and set aside.
2. Add oil, garlic, and zucchini and cook within 8 to 10 minutes.
3. Put cream cheese in the zucchini with salt and pepper.
4. Let the cauliflower steam in the water. Mash the steamed cauliflower and put salt, pepper, and herbs.
5. Serve with mashed cauliflowers and enjoy an excellent lunch.

NUTRITION:

Calories: 262.4 Fats: 9.8 g Carbohydrates: 13.7 g Proteins: 30.2g Fiber: 3.8 g

77. LOW CARBS CHICKEN CHEESE

COOKING: 20' **PREPARATION: 10'** **SERVINGS: 2**

INGREDIENTS

- » 150 g chicken breast
- » Salt
- » ½ tablespoon Italian seasoning
- » Pepper
- » ½ teaspoon paprika
- » ½ onion
- » ¼ teaspoon onion powder
- » 1 teaspoon garlic
- » ½ tablespoon olive oil
- » ½ fire-roasted pepper
- » 425 g tomato
- » Red pepper flakes
- » ½ tablespoon parsley
- » ¼ cup mozzarella cheese

DIRECTIONS

1. Marinate the chicken with salt, pepper, onion powder, and seasoning. Cook the chicken on low within 15 minutes.
2. Put the onion and all fixing except cheese and simmer within 7 minutes.
3. Put this sauce into a dish and place the cheese on the top of the chicken pieces. Warm-up within 1 to 2 minutes. Garnish with parsley and serve.

NUTRITION:

Calories: 309 Fats: 9 g Carbohydrates: 9 g Proteins: 37g Fiber: 3 g

78. LEMON CHICKEN SPAGHETTI SQUASH BOATS

COOKING: 1H 10'   PREPARATION: 10'   SERVINGS: 2

INGREDIENTS

- » ½ spaghetti squash
- » ½ onion
- » 1 tablespoon olive oil
- » 1 tablespoon garlic
- » 1 chicken breast
- » 300 g cherry tomatoes
- » Sea Salt
- » ½ cup chicken broth
- » Black pepper
- » ½ tablespoon lime
- » 1 cup spinach

DIRECTIONS

1. Combine the olive oil, salt, and pepper into the half squash. Bake within 40 minutes.
2. Stir fry the chicken pieces in olive oil.
3. Remove the chicken and pour 1 tablespoon more olive oil with onions. Put garlic and stir. Put salt, pepper, and tomatoes, and simmer.
4. Put the lemon juice and chicken broth, cook within 15 minutes.
5. Put chicken and spinach and cook within 3 to 4 minutes.
6. Shred the baked squash. Pour the sauce on the top of the shredded squash and serve.

NUTRITION:

Calories: 234 kcal Fats: 10 g Carbohydrates: 10 g Proteins: 26 g Fiber: 3 g

79. STUFFED PORTOBELLO MUSHROOMS

COOKING: 10'   PREPARATION: 5'   SERVINGS: 2

INGREDIENTS

- » ¼ tablespoon butter
- » Balsamic glaze
- » 1 clove garlic
- » 100 g mozzarella cheese
- » 1 teaspoon parsley
- » ¼ cup tomatoes
- » 2 large Portobello mushrooms

DIRECTIONS

1. Set the oven to 400-degree F. Warm-up the butter and stir garlic.
2. Grease the bottoms of the mushrooms with butter and place the butter side down the baking dish.
3. Fill in the mushrooms with the cheese slices and tomato slices. Broil in the microwave.
4. Top the mushrooms with the salt, basil, and balsamic glaze. Serve.

NUTRITION:

Calories: 101 kcal Fats: 5 g Carbohydrates: 12 g Proteins: 2 g

80. LOW CARBS MEXICAN STUFFED BELL PEPPERS

COOKING: 20' **PREPARATION: 10'** **SERVINGS: 2**

INGREDIENTS

- » 1 large bell pepper
- » ¼ teaspoon chipotle chili
- » 1 teaspoon coconut oil
- » Cinnamon
- » 250 g grounded beef
- » 1/8 cup Tomato puree
- » 1 large onion
- » 1-ounce cheddar cheese
- » 1 teaspoon grounded cumin
- » Cilantro leaves
- » ½ tablespoon chili powder

DIRECTIONS

1. Bake the bell peppers in a baking dish for 5 minutes. Cook grounded beef and cook within 10 minutes.
2. Put onions and mushrooms and cook.
3. Put cumin, chili powder, cinnamon, chipotle, and salt, then cook. Remove and put tomato puree, then stir.
4. Fill the peppers with beef mixture and with cheese plus cilantro.
5. Microwave within 1 minute then serve.

NUTRITION:

Calories: 247 kcal Fats: 15 g Carbohydrates: 9 g Proteins: 22 g Fiber: 4 g

81. LOW-CARB BROCCOLI MASH

COOKING: 5' **PREPARATION: 10'** **SERVINGS: 2**

INGREDIENTS

- » 325 g broccoli
- » ½ clove garlic
- » 2 tablespoons parsley
- » Salt
- » 40 g butter
- » Pepper

DIRECTIONS

1. Put salt into the water and boil. Put broccoli florets and cook within a few minutes. Remove the water and separate the soft broccoli.
2. Place all fixing in a blender and pulse. Serve.

NUTRITION:

Calories: 210 kcal Fats: 18 g Carbohydrates: 7 g Proteins: 5 g Fiber: 18 g

82. ROASTED TRI-COLOR VEGETABLES

COOKING: 30'   **PREPARATION: 10'**   **SERVINGS: 2**

INGREDIENTS

- » 150 g Brussels sprouts
- » Black pepper grounded
- » 75 g cherry tomatoes
- » ½ teaspoon dried thyme
- » 75 g mushrooms, diced
- » 3 tablespoons Olive oil
- » Salt

DIRECTIONS

1. Warm-up the microwave oven to 360-degree F. Put all vegetables in a baking dish.
2. Mix in salt, pepper, and oil. Bake within 20 minutes. Serve.

NUTRITION:

Calories: 208 kcal Fats: 18 g Carbohydrates: 6 g Proteins: 4 g Fiber: 4g

CHAPTER 6. SNACKS

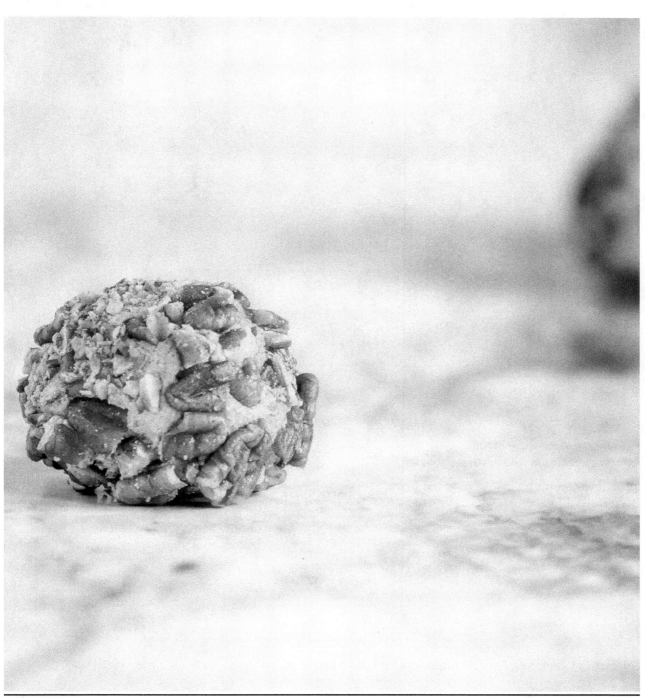

83. PARMESAN CHEESE STRIPS

COOKING: 30' **PREPARATION: 15'** **SERVINGS: 12**

INGREDIENTS

- » 1 cup parmesan cheese
- » 1 tsp. dried basil

DIRECTIONS

1. Heat-up the oven to 350 Fahrenheit.
2. Form small piles of the parmesan cheese on the baking sheet. Flatten and sprinkle dried basil on top of the cheese. Bake within 5 to 7 minutes. Serve.

NUTRITION:

Calories: 31 Fat: 2g Protein: 2g Carbohydrates: 6.21g

84. PEANUT BUTTER POWER GRANOLA

COOKING: 40' **PREPARATION: 15'** **SERVINGS: 2**

INGREDIENTS

- » 1 cup shredded coconut
- » 1 ½ cups almonds
- » 1 ½ cups pecans
- » 1/3 cup swerve sweetener
- » 1/3 cup vanilla whey protein powder
- » 1/3 cup peanut butter
- » ¼ cup sunflower seeds
- » ¼ cup butter
- » ¼ cup water

DIRECTIONS

1. Heat-up the oven to 300 Fahrenheit.
2. Process the almonds and pecans using a food processor. Transfer and add the sunflower seeds, shredded coconut, vanilla, sweetener, and protein powder.
3. Dissolve the peanut butter and butter in the microwave.
4. Mix the melted butter in the nut mixture. Put in the water to create a lumpy mixture.
5. Scoop out the batter and place it on the baking sheet. Bake within 30 minutes. Serve!

NUTRITION:

Calories: 338 Fat: 30g Carbohydrates: 5g Protein: 9.6g Fiber: 5g

85. HOMEMADE GRAHAM CRACKERS

COOKING: 1H 10' **PREPARATION: 15'** **SERVINGS: 10**

INGREDIENTS

- » 1 egg
- » 2 cups almond flour
- » 1/3 cup swerve brown
- » 2 tsp. cinnamon
- » 1 tsp. baking powder
- » 2 tbsp. melted butter
- » 1 tsp. vanilla extract
- » Salt

DIRECTIONS

1. Heat-up the oven to 300 Fahrenheit.
2. Mix the almond flour, cinnamon, sweetener, baking powder, and salt.
3. Put in the egg, molasses, melted butter, and vanilla extract. Mix to form a dough.
4. Roll out the dough evenly. Cut the dough into the shapes.
5. Bake within 20 to 30 minutes. Cool within 30 minutes and then put back in for another 30 minutes, 200 Fahrenheit. Serve.

NUTRITION:

Calories: 156 Fat: 13.35g Carbohydrates: 6.21g Protein: 5.21g Fiber: 2.68g

86. KETO NO-BAKE COOKIES

COOKING: 2' **PREPARATION: 15'** **SERVINGS: 18**

INGREDIENTS

- » 2/3 cup natural peanut butter
- » 1 cup coconut, unsweetened
- » 2 tbsp. real butter
- » 4 drops of vanilla lakanto

DIRECTIONS

1. Dissolve the butter in the microwave. Remove and put in the peanut butter. Stir.
2. Add the sweetener and coconut. Mix. Spoon it onto a pan lined with parchment paper
3. Freeze for 10 minutes. Cut and serve.

NUTRITION:

Calories: 80 Fat: 0g Carbohydrates: 0g Protein: 0g

87. SWISS CHEESE CRUNCHY NACHOS

COOKING: 20' **PREPARATION: 15'** **SERVINGS: 2**

INGREDIENTS

- » ½ cup Swiss cheese
- » ½ cup cheddar cheese
- » 1/8 cup cooked bacon

DIRECTIONS

1. Heat-up the oven to 300 Fahrenheit.
2. Spread the Swiss cheese on the parchment. Sprinkle it with bacon and top it with the cheese.
3. Bake within 10 minutes. Cool and cut into triangle strips.
4. Broil within 2 to 3 minutes. Serve.

NUTRITION:

Calories: 280 Fat: 21.8g Protein: 18.6g Net Carbohydrates: 2.44g

88. HOMEMADE THIN MINTS

COOKING: 60' **PREPARATION: 15'** **SERVINGS: 20**

INGREDIENTS

- » 1 egg
- » 1 3/4 cups almond flour
- » 1/3 cup cocoa powder
- » 1/3 cup swerve sweetener
- » 2 tbsp. butter melted
- » 1 tsp. Baking powder
- » ½ tsp. Vanilla extract
- » ¼ tsp. Salt
- » 1 tbsp. coconut oil
- » 7 oz sugar-free dark chocolate
- » 1 tsp. peppermint extract

DIRECTIONS

1. Heat-up the oven to 300 Fahrenheit.
2. Mix the cacao powder, sweetener, almond flour, salt, and baking powder. Then put the beaten egg, vanilla extract, and butter.
3. Knead the dough and roll it on the parchment paper. Cut into a cookie. Bake the cookies within 20 to 30 minutes.
4. For the coating, dissolve the oil and chocolate. Stir in the peppermint extract.
5. Dip the cookie in the coating, chill, and serve.

NUTRITION:

Calories: 116g Fat: 10.41g Carbohydrates: 6.99g Protein: 8g Cholesterol: 5mg

89. MOZZARELLA CHEESE POCKETS

COOKING: 25' **PREPARATION: 15'** **SERVINGS: 8**

INGREDIENTS

- » 1 egg
- » 8 mozzarella cheese sticks
- » 1 ¾ cup mozzarella cheese
- » ¾ cup almond flour
- » 1 oz. cream cheese
- » ½ cup crushed pork rinds

DIRECTIONS

1. Grate the mozzarella cheese.
2. Mix the almond flour, mozzarella, and the cream cheese. Microwave within 30 seconds.
3. Put in the egg and mix to form a dough.
4. Put the dough in between two wax papers and roll it into a semi-rectangular shape.
5. Cut them into smaller rectangle pieces and wrap them around the cheese sticks.
6. Roll the stick onto crushed pork rinds.
7. Bake within 20 to 25 minutes at 400 degrees Fahrenheit. Serve.

NUTRITION:

Calories: 272 Fat: 22g Net Carbohydrates: 2.4g Protein: 17g

90. NO-BAKE COCONUT COOKIES

COOKING: 10' **PREPARATION: 15'** **SERVINGS: 8**

INGREDIENTS

- » 3 cups unsweetened shredded coconut
- » ½ cup sweetener
- » 3/8 cup coconut oil
- » 3/8 tsp. salt
- » 2 tsp. vanilla
- » Topping: coconut shreds

DIRECTIONS

1. Process all the fixing in a food processor. Form into shape. Put the topping.
2. Chill and serve.

NUTRITION:

Calories: 329 Carbohydrates: 4.1g Protein: 2.1g Fat: 30g

91. CHEESY CAULIFLOWER BREADSTICKS

COOKING: 45'   **PREPARATION: 15'**   **SERVINGS: 8**

INGREDIENTS

- » 4 eggs
- » 4 cups cauliflower riced
- » 2 cups mozzarella cheese
- » 4 cloves minced garlic
- » 3 tsp. oregano
- » Salt
- » Pepper

DIRECTIONS

1. Warm-up oven to 425 Fahrenheit.
2. Process cauliflower in a food processor. Microwave within 10 minutes. Cool and drain; put the eggs, oregano, garlic, salt, pepper, and mozzarella. Mix.
3. Separate the mixture into individual sticks. Bake within 25 minutes. Remove and sprinkle mozzarella on top. Bake again within 5 minutes. Serve.

NUTRITION:

Calories: 121 Carbohydrates: 4g Protein: 13g Fat: 11g

92. EASY PEANUT BUTTER CUPS

COOKING: 1H 35'   **PREPARATION: 15'**   **SERVINGS: 12**

INGREDIENTS

- » ½ cup peanut butter
- » ¼ cup butter
- » 3 oz. cacao butter
- » 1/3 cup powdered swerve sweetener
- » ½ tsp. vanilla extract
- » 4 oz. sugar-free dark chocolate

DIRECTIONS

1. Dissolve the peanut butter, butter, and cacao butter in low heat.
2. Add the vanilla and sweetener. Put the mixture in the muffin cups. Chill. Put the chocolate in a bowl and steam.
3. Take out the muffin and drizzle in the chocolate on top. Chill again within 15 minutes. Serve.

NUTRITION:

Calories: 200 Fat: 19g Carbohydrates: 6g Protein: 2.9g Fiber: 3.6g

93. FRIED GREEN BEANS ROSEMARY

COOKING: 5' **PREPARATION: 10'** **SERVINGS: 2**

INGREDIENTS

» green beans
» 3 tsp. minced garlic
» 2 tbsps. Rosemary
» ½ tsp. Salt
» 1 tbsp. butter

DIRECTIONS

1. Warm-up an Air Fryer to 390°F.
2. Put the chopped green beans then brush with butter. Sprinkle salt, minced garlic, and rosemary over then cook within 5 minutes. Serve.

NUTRITION:

Calories: 72 Fat: 6.3g Protein: 0.7g Carbs: 4.5g

94. CRISPY BROCCOLI POPCORN

COOKING: 10' **PREPARATION: 15'** **SERVINGS: 4**

INGREDIENTS

» 2 c. broccoli florets
» 2 c. coconut flour
» 4 egg yolks
» ½ tsp. Salt
» ½ tsp. Pepper
» ¼ c. butter

DIRECTIONS

1. Dissolve butter, then let it cool. Break the eggs in it.
2. Put coconut flour to the liquid, then put salt and pepper. Mix.
3. Warm-up an Air Fryer to 400°F.
4. Dip a broccoli floret in the coconut flour mixture, then place it in the Air Fryer.
5. Cook the broccoli florets 6 minutes. Serve.

NUTRITION:

Calories: 202 Fat: 17.5g Protein: 5.1g Carbs: 7.8g

95. CHEESY CAULIFLOWER CROQUETTES

COOKING: 16'   **PREPARATION: 10'**   **SERVINGS: 4**

INGREDIENTS

- » 2 c. cauliflower florets
- » 2 tsp. Garlic
- » ½ c. onion
- » ¾ tsp. Mustard
- » ½ tsp. Salt
- » ½ tsp. pepper
- » 2 tbsps. Butter
- » ¾ c. cheddar cheese

DIRECTIONS

1. Microwave the butter. Let it cool.
2. Process the cauliflower florets using a processor. Transfer to a bowl then put chopped onion and cheese.
3. Put minced garlic, mustard, salt, and pepper, then pour melted butter over. Shape the cauliflower batter into medium balls.
4. Warm-up an Air Fryer to 400°F and cook within 14 minutes. Serve.

NUTRITION:

Calories: 160 Fat: 13g Protein: 6.8g Carbs: 5.1g

96. SPINACH IN CHEESE ENVELOPES

COOKING: 30'   **PREPARATION: 15'**   **SERVINGS: 8**

INGREDIENTS

- » 3 c. cream cheese
- » 1½ c. coconut flour
- » 3 egg yolks
- » 2 eggs
- » ½ c. cheddar cheese
- » 2 c. steamed spinach
- » ¼ tsp. Salt
- » ½ tsp. Pepper
- » ¼ c. onion

DIRECTIONS

1. Whisk cream cheese, put egg yolks. Stir in coconut flour until becoming a soft dough.
2. Put the dough on a flat surface then roll until thin. Cut the thin dough into 8 squares.
3. Beat the eggs, then place it in a bowl. Put salt, pepper, and grated cheese.
4. Put chopped spinach and onion to the egg batter.
5. Put spinach filling on a square dough then fold until becoming an envelope. Glue with water.
6. Warm-up an Air Fryer to 425°F (218°C). Cook within 12 minutes.
7. Remove and serve!

NUTRITION:

Calories: 365 Fat: 34.6g Protein: 10.4g Carbs: 4.4g

97. CHEESY MUSHROOM SLICES

COOKING: 15'　　**PREPARATION: 8-10'**　　**SERVINGS: 8**

INGREDIENTS

- » 2 c. mushrooms
- » 2 eggs
- » ¾ c. almond flour
- » ½ c. cheddar cheese
- » 2 tbsps. Butter
- » ½ tsp. Pepper
- » ¼ tsp. Salt

DIRECTIONS

1. Process chopped mushrooms in a food processor then add eggs, almond flour, and cheddar cheese.
2. Put salt and pepper then pour melted butter into the food processor. Transfer.
3. Warm-up an Air Fryer to 375°F (191°C).
4. Put the loaf pan on the Air Fryer's rack then cook within 15 minutes. Slice and serve.

NUTRITION:

Calories: 365 Fat: 34.6g Protein: 10.4g Carbs: 4.4g

98. ASPARAGUS FRIES

COOKING: 10'　　**PREPARATION: 10'**　　**SERVINGS: 4**

INGREDIENTS

- » 10 organic asparagus spears
- » 1 tablespoon Organic roasted red pepper
- » ¼ Almond flour
- » ½ teaspoon Garlic powder
- » ½ teaspoon Smoked paprika
- » 2 tablespoons parsley
- » ½ cup Parmesan cheese, full-fat
- » 2 organic eggs
- » 3 tablespoons mayonnaise, full-fat

DIRECTIONS

1. Warm-up oven to 425 degrees F.
2. Process cheese in a food processor, add garlic and parsley, and pulse for 1 minute.
3. Add almond flour, pulse for 30 seconds, transfer, and put paprika.
4. Whisk eggs into a shallow dish.
5. Dip asparagus spears into the egg batter, then coat with parmesan mixture and place it on a baking sheet. Bake in the oven within 10 minutes.
6. Put the mayonnaise in a bowl, add red pepper and whisk, then chill. Serve with prepared dip.

NUTRITION:

Calories: 453 Fat: 33.4 g Protein: 19.1 g Net Carbs: 5.5 g

99. KALE CHIPS

COOKING: 12' **PREPARATION: 5'** **SERVINGS: 4**

INGREDIENTS

- » 1 organic kale
- » 1 tablespoon seasoned salt
- » 2 tablespoons olive oil

DIRECTIONS

1. Warm-up oven to 350 degrees F.
2. Put kale leaves into a large plastic bag and add oil. Shake and then spread on a large baking sheet.
3. Bake within 12 minutes. Serve with salt.

NUTRITION:

Calories: 163 Fat: 10 g Protein: 2 g Net Carbs: 14 g

100. GUACAMOLE

COOKING: 0' **PREPARATION: 10'** **SERVINGS: 4**

INGREDIENTS

- » 2 organic avocados pitted
- » 1/3 organic red onion
- » 1 organic jalapeño
- » ½ teaspoon salt
- » ½ teaspoon ground pepper
- » 2 tablespoons tomato salsa
- » 1 tablespoon lime juice
- » ½ organic cilantro

DIRECTIONS

1. Slice the avocado flesh horizontally and vertically.
2. Mix in onion, jalapeno, and lime juice in a bowl.
3. Put salt and black pepper, add salsa, and mix. Fold in cilantro and serve.

NUTRITION:

Calories: 16.5 Fat: 1.4 g Protein: 0.23 g Net Carbs: 0.5 g

101. ZUCCHINI NOODLES

COOKING: 5' **PREPARATION: 6'** **SERVINGS: 2**

INGREDIENTS

- » 2 zucchinis, spiralized into noodles
- » 2 tablespoons butter, unsalted
- » 1 ½ tablespoon garlic
- » ¾ cup Parmesan cheese
- » ½ sea salt
- » ¼ teaspoon ground black pepper
- » ¼ teaspoon red chili flakes

DIRECTIONS

1. Sauté butter and garlic within 1 minute.
2. Put zucchini noodles, cook within 5 minutes, then put salt and black pepper.
3. Transfer then top with cheese and sprinkle with red chili flakes. Serve.

NUTRITION:

Calories: 298 Fat: 26.1 g Protein: 5 g Net Carbs: 2.3 g Fiber: 0.1 g

102. CAULIFLOWER SOUFFLE

COOKING: 12' **PREPARATION: 10'** **SERVINGS: 6**

INGREDIENTS

- » 1 cauliflower, florets
- » 2 eggs
- » 2 tablespoons heavy cream
- » 2 ounces cream Cheese
- » ½ cup sour cream
- » ½ cup Asiago cheese
- » 1 cup cheddar cheese
- » ¼ cup Chives
- » 2 tablespoons butter, unsalted
- » 6 bacon slices, sugar-free
- » 1 cup of water

DIRECTIONS

1. Pulse eggs, heavy cream, sour cream, cream cheese, and cheeses in a food processor.
2. Put cauliflower florets, pulse for 2 seconds, then add butter and chives and pulse for another 2 seconds.
3. Put in water in a pot, and insert a trivet stand.
4. Put the cauliflower batter in a greased round casserole dish then put the dish on the trivet stand.
5. Cook within 12 minutes at high. Remove, top with bacon, and serve.

NUTRITION:

Calories: 342 Fat: 28 g Protein: 17 g — Net Carbs: 5 g

103. NO-CHURN ICE CREAM

COOKING: 0'　　　**PREPARATION: 10'**　　　**SERVINGS: 3**

INGREDIENTS　　　　　　　**DIRECTIONS**

- » Pinch salt
- » 1 cup heavy whipping cream
- » ¼ tsp. xanthan gum
- » 2 tbsp. zero-calorie sweetener powder
- » 1 tsp. vanilla extract
- » 1 tbsp. vodka

1. Put the xanthan gum, heavy cream, vanilla extract, sweetener, vodka, and salt to a jar and mix.
2. Blend the batter to the immersion blender within 2 minutes. Put the batter back in the jar, cover it, and chill within 4 hours. Stir the cream batter in 40 minutes intervals. Serve.

NUTRITION:

Calories: 291 Carbs: 3.2g Protein: 1.6g Fat: 29.4g Cholesterol: 109mg

104. CHEESECAKE CUPCAKES

COOKING: 15'　　　**PREPARATION: 10'**　　　**SERVINGS: 12**

INGREDIENTS　　　　　　　**DIRECTIONS**

- » 1 tsp. vanilla extract
- » ½ cup almond meal
- » ¾ cup granulated no-calorie sucralose sweetener
- » ¼ cup melted butter
- » 2 eggs
- » 2 8 oz pack softened cream cheese

1. Warm-up oven to 350 degrees F.
2. Mix butter and almond meal put into the bottom of the muffin cup.
3. Mix vanilla extract, cream cheese, sucralose sweetener, and egg in an electric mixer. Put this batter to the top of the muffin cups.
4. Bake within 17 minutes. Cool and serve.

NUTRITION:

Calories: 209 Carbs: 3.5g Protein: 4.9g Fat: 20g Cholesterol: 82mg

105. CHOCOLATE PEANUT BUTTER CUPS

COOKING: 3'   **PREPARATION: 15'**   **SERVINGS: 12**

INGREDIENTS

- » 1 oz roasted peanut, salted
- » 1 cup of coconut oil
- » ¼ tsp. Kosher salt
- » ½ cup natural peanut butter
- » ¼ tsp. vanilla extract
- » 2 tbsp. heavy cream
- » 1 tsp. liquid stevia
- » 1 tbsp. cocoa powder

DIRECTIONS

1. Dissolve coconut oil within 5 minutes, then put peanut butter, salt, heavy cream, cocoa powder, vanilla extract, and liquid stevia to the pan. Stir.
2. Put the batter into muffin molds. Put the salted peanuts on top. Chill within an hour. Serve.

NUTRITION:

Calories: 246 Carbs: 3.3g Protein: 3.4g Fat: 26g

106. PEANUT BUTTER COOKIES

COOKING: 15'   **PREPARATION: 15'**   **SERVINGS: 12**

INGREDIENTS

- » 1 tsp. vanilla extract, sugar-free
- » 1 cup peanut butter
- » 1 egg
- » ½ cup natural sweetener, low-calorie

DIRECTIONS

1. Heat-up the oven to 350 degrees F.
2. Mix peanut butter, vanilla extract, sweetener, and egg to form a dough.
3. Mold the dough into balls. Bake within 15 minutes. Cool and serve.

NUTRITION:

Calories: 133 Carbs: 12.4g Protein: 5.9g Fat: 11.2g

107. LOW-CARB ALMOND COCONUT SANDIES

COOKING: 12'   **PREPARATION: 15'**   **SERVINGS: 18**

INGREDIENTS

- » ⅓ tsp. stevia powder
- » 1 cup coconut, unsweetened
- » 1 tsp. Himalayan sea salt
- » 1 cup almond meal
- » 1 tbsp. vanilla extract
- » ⅓ cup melted coconut oil
- » 2 tbsp. water
- » 1 egg white

DIRECTIONS

1. Warm-up oven to 325 F.
2. Mix Himalayan sea salt, unsweetened coconut, stevia powder, almond meal, vanilla extract, coconut oil, water, and egg white. Put aside within 10 minutes.
3. Mold into little balls. Press down on the balls. Bake within 15 minutes. Cool and serve.

NUTRITION:

Calories: 107 Carbs: 2.7g Protein: 1.9g Fat: 10.5g

108. CREME BRULE

COOKING: 34'   **PREPARATION: 15**   **SERVINGS: 4**

INGREDIENTS

- » 5 tbsp. natural sweetener, low calorie
- » 4 egg yolks
- » 2 cups heavy whipping cream
- » 1 tsp. vanilla extract

DIRECTIONS

1. Heat-up the oven to 325 degrees F. Mix the vanilla extract and egg yolks in it.
2. Simmer 1 tbsp. of natural sweetener and heavy cream to the pan and mix. Put the ramekins with batter in a glass baking dish and add hot water.
3. Bake within 30 minutes. Put 1 tbsp. natural sweetener on top. Serve.

NUTRITION:

Calorie: 466 Carbs: 16.9g Protein: 5.1g Fat: 48.4g

109. CHOCOLATE FAT BOMB

COOKING: 0'   **PREPARATION: 15'**   **SERVINGS: 10**

INGREDIENTS

- » 1.4 oz pack chocolate pudding mix, sugar-free
- » 8 oz package cream cheese
- » Coconut oil

DIRECTIONS

1. Mix the chocolate pudding mix, cream cheese, and coconut oi using an electric mixer.
2. Put this batter into a mold to form into mounds. Cover and chill within 30 minutes. Serve.

NUTRITION:

Calories: 231Carbs: 3.5g Protein: 1.9g Fat: 24.3g

110. COCOA MUG CAKE

COOKING: 5'   **PREPARATION: 15'**   **SERVINGS: 2**

INGREDIENTS

- » 2 tbsp. melted coconut oil
- » 6 tbsp. almond flour
- » 2 eggs
- » 2 tbsp. cocoa powder, unsweetened
- » Salt
- » 2 tsp. natural sweetener, low-calorie
- » ½ tsp. baking powder

DIRECTIONS

1. Mix salt, almond flour, baking powder, cocoa powder, natural sweetener.
2. Beat the eggs using an electric mixer. Put the coconut oil and stir. Put this egg batter into the bowl containing baking powder. Whisk.
3. Put the batter into mugs. Microwave to high within 1 minute. Serve.

NUTRITION:

Calories: 338 Carbs: 8.6g Protein: 12.3g Fat: 30.9g

111. DARK CHOCOLATE ESPRESSO PALEO AND KETO MUG CAKE

COOKING: 15'   PREPARATION: 5'   SERVINGS: 2

INGREDIENTS

» 1 tbsp. brewed espresso
» 4 oz dark chocolate chips
» 1 egg
» 1 tbsp. coconut oil
» baking soda
» 2 tbsp. water
» 1 tbsp. coconut flour
» 1 tbsp. almond flour

DIRECTIONS

1. Put both the coconut oil and chocolate chips in a mug. Put baking soda, water, coconut flour, and almond flour. Microwave and cook within 1 minute and 30 seconds. Cool and serve.

NUTRITION:

Calories: 793 Carbs: 83.7g Protein: 14 Fat: 52.2g

112. KETO MATCHA MINT BARS

COOKING: 0'   PREPARATION: 15'   SERVINGS: 12

DIRECTIONS

» 6 drops stevia
» 1 cup almond flour,
» ¼ tsp. peppermint extract
» 3 tbsp. melted butter
» 3 tbsp. cocoa powder
» 1 tbsp. cocoa powder, unsweetened
» 3 tbsp. warmed coconut oil
» 1 tbsp. stevia powder
» 1 tsp. vanilla extract
» 1 cup coconut butter
» 1 tsp. peppermint extract
» 2 ripe avocados
» 1 tbsp. matcha
» 3 tbsp. stevia powder

1. Mix almond flour, stevia powder, cocoa powder, and butter. Press down on it till a crust is formed. Chill within 15 minutes.
2. For the filling:
3. Mix 3 tbsp. of stevia powder, coconut butter, vanilla extract, matcha, avocados, and 1 tsp. peppermint extract using an electric mixer. Put this on the crust. Chill.
4. Mix liquid stevia, coconut oil, 1 tbsp. cocoa powder, and 1 tsp. peppermint extract into the crust. Chill within 30 minutes.

NUTRITION:

Calories: 276 Carbs: 12.6g Protein: 4.3g Fat: 26.1g

113. KETO NO-CHURN BLUEBERRY MAPLE ICE CREAM

COOKING: 0'   **PREPARATION: 15'**   **SERVINGS: 2**

INGREDIENTS

- » Salt
- » 1 cup heavy whipping cream
- » ¼ tsp. xanthan gum
- » ⅓ 10 oz pack blueberries frozen
- » ½ tsp. maple extract
- » 2 tbsp. natural sweetener, low calorie
- » 1 tbsp. vodka

DIRECTIONS

1. Put heavy cream, salt, blueberries, xanthan gum, natural sweetener, maple extract, and vodka in a jar. Process this mixture within 75 seconds with an immersion blender.
2. Chill in 35 minutes, stirring occasionally. Serve.

NUTRITION:

Calories: 304 Carbs: 13.4g Protein: 1.8g Fat: 29.6g

CHAPTER 7. DINNER RECIPES

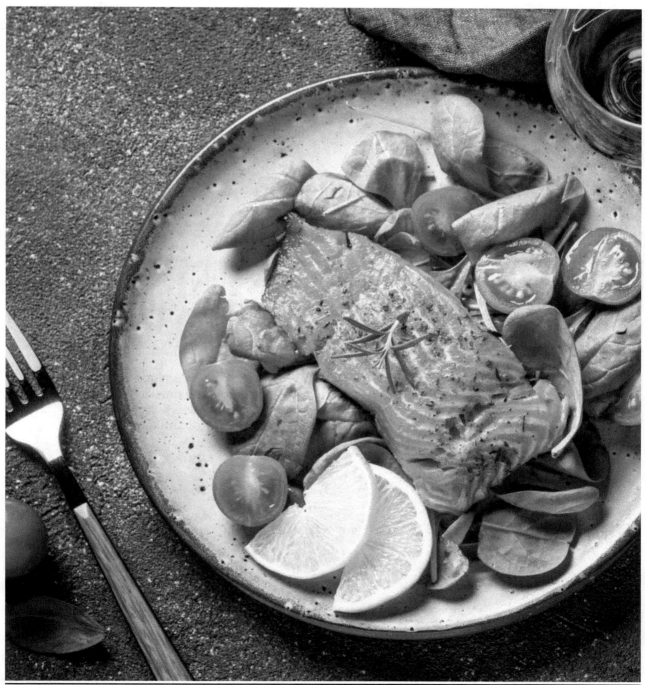

114. BAKED ZUCCHINI NOODLES WITH FETA

COOKING: 15'　　**PREPARATION: 15'**　　**SERVINGS: 4**

INGREDIENTS

- » 1 quartered plum tomato
- » 2 spiralized zucchini
- » 8 cubes Feta cheese
- » 1 tsp. Pepper
- » 1 tbsp. Olive oil

DIRECTIONS

1. Set the oven temperature to reach 375° Fahrenheit.
2. Slice the noodles with a spiralizer and put the olive oil, tomatoes, pepper, and salt.
3. Bake within 10 to 15 minutes. Transfer then put cheese cubes, toss. Serve.

NUTRITION:

Carbohydrates: 5 grams Protein: 4 grams Total Fats: 8 grams Calories: 105

115. BRUSSELS SPROUTS WITH BACON

COOKING: 40'　　**PREPARATION: 15'**　　**SERVINGS: 6**

INGREDIENTS

- » 16 oz. Bacon
- » 16 oz. Brussels sprouts
- » Black pepper

DIRECTIONS

1. Warm the oven to reach 400° Fahrenheit.
2. Slice the bacon into small lengthwise pieces. Put the sprouts and bacon with pepper.
3. Bake within 35 to 40 minutes. Serve.

NUTRITION:

Carbohydrates: 3.9 grams Protein: 7.9 grams Total Fats: 6.9 grams Calories: 113

116. BUNLESS BURGER - KETO STYLE

COOKING: 25' **PREPARATION: 15'** **SERVINGS: 6**

INGREDIENTS

- » 1lb. Ground beef
- » 1 tbsp. Worcestershire sauce
- » 1 tbsp. Steak Seasoning
- » 2 tbsp. Olive oil
- » 4 oz. Onions

DIRECTIONS

1. Mix the beef, olive oil, Worcestershire sauce, and seasonings.
2. Grill the burger. Prepare the onions by adding one tablespoon of oil in a skillet to med-low heat. Sauté. Serve.

NUTRITION:

Carbohydrates: 2 grams Protein: 26 grams Total Fats: 40 grams Calories: 479

117. COFFEE BBQ PORK BELLY

COOKING: 60' **PREPARATION: 15'** **SERVINGS: 4**

INGREDIENTS

- » 1.5 cups Beef stock
- » 2lb. Pork belly
- » 4 tbsp. Olive oil
- » Low-carb barbecue dry rub
- » 2 tbsp. Instant Espresso Powder

DIRECTIONS

1. Set the oven at 350° Fahrenheit.
2. Heat-up the beef stock in a small saucepan.
3. Mix in the dry barbecue rub and espresso powder.
4. Put the pork belly, skin side up in a shallow dish and drizzle half of the oil over the top.
5. Put the hot stock around the pork belly. Bake within 45 minutes.
6. Sear each slice within three minutes per side. Serve.

NUTRITION:

Net Carbohydrates: 2.6 grams Protein: 24 grams Total Fats: 68 grams Calories: 644

118. GARLIC & THYME LAMB CHOPS

COOKING: 10'   **PREPARATION: 15'**   **SERVINGS: 6**

INGREDIENTS

- » 6-4 oz. Lamb chops
- » 4 whole garlic cloves
- » 2 thyme sprigs
- » 1 tsp. Ground thyme
- » 3 tbsp. Olive oil

DIRECTIONS

1. Warm-up a skillet. Put the olive oil. Rub the chops with the spices.
2. Put the chops in the skillet with the garlic and sprigs of thyme.
3. Sauté within 3 to 4 minutes and serve.

NUTRITION:

Calories: 31 Fat: 2g Protein: 2g Carbohydrates: 6.21g

119. JAMAICAN JERK PORK ROAST

COOKING: 4H   **PREPARATION: 15'**   **SERVINGS: 12**

INGREDIENTS

- » 1 tbsp. Olive oil
- » 4 lb. Pork shoulder
- » .5 cup Beef Broth
- » .25 cup Jamaican Jerk spice blend

DIRECTIONS

1. Rub the roast well the oil and the jerk spice blend. Sear the roast on all sides. Put the beef broth.
2. Simmer within four hours on low. Shred and serve.

NUTRITION:

Net Carbohydrates: 0 grams Protein: 23 grams Total Fats: 20 grams Calories: 282

120. KETO MEATBALLS

COOKING: 20'   **PREPARATION: 15'**   **SERVINGS: 10**

INGREDIENTS

- » 1 egg
- » .5 cup Grated parmesan
- » .5 cup Shredded mozzarella
- » 1 lb. Ground beef
- » 1 tbsp. garlic

DIRECTIONS

1. Warm-up the oven to reach 400. Combine all of the fixings.
2. Shape into meatballs. Bake within 18-20 minutes. Cool and serve.

NUTRITION:

Net Carbohydrates: 0.7 grams Protein: 12.2 grams Total Fats: 10.9 grams Calories: 153

121. MIXED VEGETABLE PATTIES - INSTANT POT

COOKING: 10'   **PREPARATION: 15'**   **SERVINGS: 4**

INGREDIENTS

- » 1 cup cauliflower florets
- » 1 bag vegetables
- » 1.5 cups Water
- » 1 cup Flax meal
- » 2 tbsp. Olive oil

DIRECTIONS

1. Steam the veggies to the steamer basket within 4 to 5 minutes. Mash in the flax meal. Shape into 4 patties. Cook the patties within 3 minutes per side. Serve.

NUTRITION:

Net Carbohydrates: 3 grams Protein: 4 grams Total Fats: 10 grams Calories: 220

122. ROASTED LEG OF LAMB

COOKING: 1H 30'   **PREPARATION: 15'**   **SERVINGS: 6**

INGREDIENTS

- » .5 cup Reduced-sodium beef broth
- » 2 lb. lamb leg
- » 6 garlic cloves
- » 1 tbsp. rosemary leaves
- » 1 tsp. Black pepper

DIRECTIONS

1. Warm-up oven temperature to 400 Fahrenheit.
2. Put the lamb in the pan and put the broth and seasonings.
3. Roast 30 minutes and lower the heat to 350° Fahrenheit. Cook within one hour.
4. Cool and serve.

NUTRITION:

Net Carbohydrates: 1 gram Protein: 22 grams Total Fats: 14 grams Calories: 223

123. SALMON PASTA

COOKING: 1H 30'   **PREPARATION: 15'**   **SERVINGS: 2**

INGREDIENTS

- » 2 tbsp. Coconut oil
- » 2 Zucchinis
- » 8 oz. Smoked salmon
- » .25 cup Keto-friendly mayo

DIRECTIONS

1. Make noodle-like strands from the zucchini.
2. Warm-up the oil, put the salmon and sauté within 2 to 3 minutes.
3. Stir in the noodles and sauté for 1 to 2 more minutes.
4. Stir in the mayo and serve.

NUTRITION:

Net Carbohydrates: 3 grams Protein: 21 grams Total Fats: 42 grams Calories: 470

124. SKILLET FRIED COD

COOKING: 30'   **PREPARATION: 15'**   **SERVINGS: 4**

INGREDIENTS

- » 6 garlic cloves
- » 3 tbsp. Ghee
- » 4 cod fillets
- » Optional: Garlic powder

DIRECTIONS

1. Toss half of the garlic into a skillet with the ghee.
2. Put the fillets in the pan, put garlic, pepper, and salt.
3. Turn it over, and add the remainder of the minced garlic. Cook.
4. Serve with garlic.

NUTRITION:

Net Carbohydrates: 1 gram Protein: 21 grams Total Fats: 7 grams Calories: 160

125. SLOW-COOKED KALUA PORK & CABBAGE

COOKING: 11H   **PREPARATION: 15'**   **SERVINGS: 12**

INGREDIENTS

- » 3 lb. pork shoulder butt
- » 1 medium cabbage
- » 7 strips bacon
- » 1 tbsp. Coarse sea salt

DIRECTIONS

1. Trim the fat from the roast.
2. Layer most of the bacon in the cooker. Put salt over the roast and add to the slow cooker on top of the bacon. Cook on low within eight to ten hours. Put in the cabbage, and cook within an hour.
3. Shred the roast. Serve with cabbage and slow cooker juice.

NUTRITION:

Net Carbohydrates: 4 grams Protein: 22 grams Total Fats: 13 grams Calories: 227

126. STEAK PINWHEELS

COOKING: 25' **PREPARATION: 15'** **SERVINGS: 6**

INGREDIENTS

- » 2 lb. Flank steak
- » 8 oz. pkg. Mozzarella cheese
- » 1 bunch Spinach

DIRECTIONS

1. Warm-up the oven to reach 350° Fahrenheit.
2. Slice the steak into six portions. Beat until thin with a mallet.
3. Shred the cheese using a food processor and sprinkle the steak. Roll it up and tie with cooking twine.
4. Line the pan with the pinwheels and place it on a layer of spinach. Bake within 25 minutes.

NUTRITION:

Net Carbohydrates: 2 grams Protein: 55 grams Total Fats: 20 grams Calories: 414

127. TANGY SHRIMP

COOKING: 15' **PREPARATION: 15'** **SERVINGS: 2**

INGREDIENTS

- » 3 garlic cloves
- » .25 cup olive oil
- » .5lb. Jumbo shrimp
- » 1 lemon
- » Cayenne pepper

DIRECTIONS

1. Sauté the garlic and cayenne with the olive oil. Peel and devein the shrimp. Cook within 2 to 3 minutes per side. Put pepper, salt, and lemon wedges. Use the rest of the garlic oil for a dipping sauce. Serve.

NUTRITION:

Net Carbohydrates: 3 grams Protein: 23 grams Total Fats: 27 grams Calories: 335

128. CHICKEN SALAD WITH CHAMPAGNE VINEGAR

COOKING: 10' **PREPARATION: 15'** **SERVINGS: 3**

INGREDIENTS

» ½ cup of sliced red onion
» ½ cup of champagne vinegar
» 1 package of Chipotle Adobo flavor
» 4 cups of mixed greens
» 4 cups of sweet butter lettuce
» ½ cup of cooked; then crumbled bacon
» 1 cup of halved cherry tomatoes
» ½ cup of almond flour
» ½ sliced Avocado
» 1 cup of avocado Lime Green Goddess Dressing
» 2 sliced hard-boiled eggs

DIRECTIONS

1. Put the red onion and the vinegar in a bowl. Open the bag of the chipotle adobo flavor, then toss the almond flour in the bag; then add in the chicken and shake it very well. Toss the chicken in your Air Fryer basket and lock the lid. Set the timer to about 8 to 10 minutes at a temperature of about 390° F. When the timer beeps; turn off your Air Fryer. Transfer the chicken to a bowl and add in the lettuce, the bacon, the greens, the tomatoes, and the avocado. Toss your ingredients very well with the dressing.
2. Top your salad with the pickled onion, the hard-boiled eggs, and the baked chicken shakers!

NUTRITION:

Calories: 189 Carbs: 11g Protein: 8.9g Fats: 4.6g

129. MEXICAN BEEF SALAD

COOKING: 12' **PREPARATION: 15'** **SERVINGS: 6**

INGREDIENTS

» 1-pound grass-fed ground beef
» 1 tbsp. taco seasoning
» 1 1/3 cups grape tomatoes, halved
» ½ cup scallion, chopped
» 1/3 cup salsa
» 1 tsp. olive oil, divided
» 8 ounces lettuce, chopped
» 1 large cucumber, chopped
» ¾ cup cheddar cheese, shredded
» 1/3 cup sour cream

DIRECTIONS

1. Warm-up oil over high heat and stir fry the beef for about 8-10 minutes, breaking up the pieces with a spatula. Stir in the taco seasoning and remove from the heat. Set aside to cool slightly. Meanwhile, in a large bowl, add remaining ingredients and mix well. Add the ground beef and toss to coat well. Serve immediately.

NUTRITION:

Calories: 263 Carbs: 7g Protein: 28.1g Fat: 13.1g

130. CHERRY TOMATOES TILAPIA SALAD

COOKING: 18' **PREPARATION: 15'** **SERVINGS: 3**

INGREDIENTS

» A cup of mixed greens
» 1 cup of cherry tomatoes
» ⅓ Cup of diced red onion
» 1 medium avocado
» 2 to 3 Tortilla Crusted Tilapia fillet

DIRECTIONS

1. Spray the tilapia fillet with a little bit of cooking spray. Put the fillets in your Air Fryer basket. Lock the lid of your Air Fryer and set the timer to about 18 minutes and the temperature to about 390° F. When the timer beeps; turn off your Air Fryer and transfer the fillet to a bowl. Add about half of the fillets in a large bowl, then toss it with the tomatoes, the greens, and the red onion. Add the lime dressing and mix again. When the timer beeps, turn off your Air Fryer and transfer the fish to the veggie salad. Serve and enjoy your salad!

NUTRITION:

Calories: 271 Carbs: 10.1g Protein: 18.5g Fats: 8g

131. CRUNCHY CHICKEN MILANESE

COOKING: 10' **PREPARATION: 15'** **SERVINGS: 2**

INGREDIENTS

» Chicken breasts (2, skinless, boneless)
» ½ cup coconut flour
» 1 egg, lightly beaten
» ½ cup crushed pork rinds
» 2 tablespoons olive oil

DIRECTIONS

1. Pound the chicken breasts using a heavy mallet. Prepare two separate prep plates and one small, shallow bowl. On plate 1, put the coconut flour, cayenne pepper, pink salt, and pepper. Mix together. On plate 2, put the crushed pork rinds. Warm-up the olive oil, then dredge chicken breasts in flour mixture, then egg and finish with pork rinds. Set a skillet with oil over medium heat and add your coated chicken. Cook the chicken for 10 minutes and serve.

NUTRITION:

Calories: 604 Carbs: 17g Protein: 65g Fats: 29g

132. PARMESAN BAKED CHICKEN

COOKING: 20'   **PREPARATION: 15'**   **SERVINGS: 2**

INGREDIENTS

- » 2 tablespoons ghee
- » 2 boneless skinless chicken breasts
- » ½ cup mayonnaise
- » ¼ cup grated Parmesan cheese
- » ¼ cup crushed pork rinds

DIRECTIONS

1. Preheat the oven to 425°F. Put both chicken breasts in a large baking dish and coat it with the ghee. Pat dry the chicken breasts with a paper towel, season with pink salt and pepper, and place in the prepared baking dish. In a small bowl, mix to combine the mayonnaise, Parmesan cheese, and Italian seasoning. Slather the mayonnaise mixture evenly over the chicken breasts and sprinkle the crushed pork rinds on top of the mayonnaise mixture. Bake until the topping is browned, about 20 minutes, and serve.

NUTRITION:

Calories: 850 Carbs: 2g Protein: 60g Fats: 67g

133. CHEESY BACON AND BROCCOLI CHICKEN

COOKING: 1 H   **PREPARATION: 15'**   **SERVINGS: 6**

INGREDIENTS

- » 2 boneless skinless chicken breasts
- » 4 bacon slices
- » 6 ounces cream cheese, room temp.
- » 2 cups frozen broccoli florets thawed
- » ½ cup shredded Cheddar cheese

DIRECTIONS

1. Warm-up the oven to 375 degrees F, then choose a baking dish that is large enough to hold both chicken breasts and coat it with the ghee. Pat dry the chicken breasts with a paper towel and season with pink salt and pepper. Place the chicken breasts and the bacon slices in the baking dish and bake for 25 minutes. Shred the chicken. Season it again with pink salt and pepper. Place the bacon on a paper towel–lined plate to crisp up and then crumble it. In a medium bowl, mix to combine the cream cheese, shredded chicken, broccoli, and half of the bacon crumbles. Transfer the chicken mixture, and top with the cheddar and the remaining half of the bacon crumbles. Bake about 35 minutes and serve.

NUTRITION:

Calories: 935 Carbs: 10g Protein: 75g Fats: 66g

134. BUTTERY GARLIC CHICKEN

COOKING: 40' **PREPARATION: 15'** **SERVINGS: 2**

INGREDIENTS

- » 2 tablespoons ghee melted
- » 2 boneless skinless chicken breasts
- » 4 tablespoons butter
- » 2 garlic cloves minced
- » ¼ cup grated Parmesan cheese

DIRECTIONS

1. Warm-up the oven to 375 degrees F, then choose a baking dish that is large enough to hold both chicken breasts and coat it with the ghee. Pat dry the chicken breasts and season with pink salt, pepper, and Italian seasoning. Place the chicken in the baking dish. Dissolve the butter in a skillet. Put the minced garlic and cook within 5 minutes, then remove the butter-garlic mixture from the heat and pour it over the chicken breasts. Roast the chicken in the oven for 30 to 35 minutes, until cooked through. Sprinkle some of the Parmesan cheese on top of each chicken breast. Let it rest in the baking dish within 5 minutes, then spoon the butter sauce over the chicken, and serve.

NUTRITION:

Calories: 642 Carbs: 2g Protein: 57g Fats: 45g

135. CREAMY SLOW COOKER CHICKEN

COOKING: 4H 15' **PREPARATION: 15'** **SERVINGS: 2**

INGREDIENTS

- » 2 boneless skinless chicken breasts
- » 1 cup Alfredo Sauce
- » ¼ cup chopped sun-dried tomatoes
- » ¼ cup Parmesan cheese, grated
- » 2 cups fresh spinach

DIRECTIONS

1. Dissolve the ghee in a skillet, then put the chicken and cook, about 4 minutes on each side. With the crock insert in place, transfer the chicken to your slow cooker. Set your slow cooker to low. In a small bowl, mix the Alfredo sauce, sun-dried tomatoes, Parmesan cheese, salt, and pepper. Pour the sauce over the chicken. Cover and cook on low within 4 hours. Add the fresh spinach. Cover and cook for 5 minutes more, until the spinach is slightly wilted, and serve.

NUTRITION:

Calories: 900 Carbs: 9g Protein: 70g Fats: 66g

136. BRAISED CHICKEN THIGHS WITH KALAMATA OLIVES

COOKING: 40'   **PREPARATION: 15'**   **SERVINGS: 2**

INGREDIENTS

- » 4 chicken thighs, skin on
- » ½ cup chicken broth
- » 1 lemon, ½ sliced and ½ juiced
- » ½ cup pitted Kalamata olives
- » 2 tablespoons butter

DIRECTIONS

1. Warm-up the oven to 375 degrees F, then dry chicken, and season to taste. In a medium oven-safe skillet or high-sided baking dish over medium-high heat, melt butter. When the butter has melted and is hot, add the chicken thighs, skin-side down, and leave them for about 8 minutes, or until the skin is brown and crispy. Turn over the chicken and cook for 2 minutes on the second side. Around the chicken thighs, pour in the chicken broth, and add the lemon slices, lemon juice, and olives. Bake in the oven for about 30 minutes, until the chicken is cooked through. Add the butter to the broth mixture. Divide the chicken and olives between two plates and serve.

NUTRITION:

Calories: 567 Carbs: 4g Protein: 33g Fats: 47g

137. BAKED GARLIC AND PAPRIKA CHICKEN LEGS

COOKING: 55'   **PREPARATION: 15'**   **SERVINGS: 2**

INGREDIENTS

- » 1 lb. chicken drumsticks, skin on
- » 2 tablespoons paprika
- » 2 garlic cloves minced
- » ½ pound fresh green beans
- » 1 tablespoon olive oil

DIRECTIONS

1. Set oven to 350°F. Combine all the ingredients in a large bowl, toss to combine, and transfer to a baking dish. Bake for 60 minutes until crisp and thoroughly cooked.

NUTRITION:

Calories: 700 Carbs: 10g Protein: 63g Fats: 45g

138. CHICKEN CURRY WITH MASALA

COOKING: 30' **PREPARATION: 15'** **SERVINGS: 4**

INGREDIENTS

- » 2 tbsp. of oil
- » 2 tbsp. of minced jalapeño
- » 1 ½ pound of diced boneless skinless chicken thighs
- » 1 tsp. of garam masala
- » ¼ cup of chopped cilantro
- » 2 tbsp. of diced ginger
- » 1 cup of chopped tomatoes
- » 2 tsp. of turmeric
- » 1 tsp. of cayenne
- » 2 tbsp. of lemon juice
- » 1 tsp. of garam masala

DIRECTIONS

1. Heat your Air Fryer to a temperature of about 400° F. Grease the Air Fryer pan with the cooking spray. Add the jalapenos and the ginger. Add in the chicken and the tomatoes and stir. Add the spices and 1 tbsp. of oil and 1 tbsp. of water. Place the pan in Air Fryer and set the temperature to 365° F. now, set the timer to 30 minutes. When the timer beeps, turn off your Air Fryer. Serve and enjoy your lunch!

NUTRITION:

Calories: 254 Carbs: 9g Protein: 27.8g Fats: 14g

139. CHICKEN QUESADILLA

COOKING: 5' **PREPARATION: 15'** **SERVINGS: 2**

INGREDIENTS

- » 1 tablespoon olive oil
- » 2 low-carbohydrate tortillas
- » ½ cup shredded Mexican blend cheese
- » 2 ounces shredded chicken
- » 2 tablespoons sour cream

DIRECTIONS

1. Warm-up the olive oil in a large skillet, then put a tortilla, then top with ¼ cup of cheese, the chicken, the Tajin seasoning, and the remaining ¼ cup of cheese. Top with the second tortilla. Once the bottom tortilla gets golden, and the cheese begins to melt, after about 2 minutes, flip the quesadilla over. The second side will cook faster, about 1 minute. Once the second tortilla is crispy and golden, transfer the quesadilla to a cutting board and let sit for 2 minutes. Cut the quesadilla into 4 wedges using a pizza cutter or chef's knife. Transfer half the quesadilla to each of two plates. Put 1 tablespoon of sour cream and serve hot.

NUTRITION:

Calories: 414 Carbs: 24g Protein: 26g Fats: 28g

140. SLOW COOKER BARBECUE RIBS

COOKING: 4H   **PREPARATION: 15'**   **SERVINGS: 2**

INGREDIENTS

- 1lb. pork ribs
- Pink salt
- Freshly Ground black pepper
- 1.25 oz. package dry rib-seasoning rub
- ½ cup sugar-free barbecue sauce

DIRECTIONS

1. With the crock insert in place, preheat your slow cooker to high. Generously season the pork ribs with pink salt, pepper, and dry rib-seasoning rub. Stand the ribs up along the walls of the slow-cooker insert, with the bonier side facing inward. Pour the barbecue sauce on both sides of the ribs, using just enough to coat. Cover, cook for 4 hours, and serve.

NUTRITION:

Calories: 956 Carbs: 5g Protein: 68g Fats: 72g

141. BARBACOA BEEF ROAST

COOKING: 40'   **PREPARATION: 15'**   **SERVINGS: 6**

INGREDIENTS

- 1 lb. beef chuck roast
- 4 chipotle peppers in adobo sauce
- 6oz. can green jalapeño chilis
- 2 tablespoons apple cider vinegar
- ½ cup beef broth

DIRECTIONS

1. With the crock insert in place, preheat your slow cooker to low. Massage the beef chuck roast on both sides with pink salt and pepper. Put the roast in the slow cooker. Pulse the chipotle peppers and their adobo sauce, jalapeños, and apple cider vinegar in a blender. Add the beef broth and pulse a few more times. Pour the chili mixture over the top of the roast. Cover and cook on low within 8 hours, then shred the meat. Serve hot.

NUTRITION:

Calories: 723 Carbs: 7g Protein: 66g Fats: 46g

142. BEEF & BROCCOLI ROAST

COOKING: 4 H 30'　　**PREPARATION: 15'**　　**SERVINGS: 2**

INGREDIENTS

- » 1 lb. beef chuck roast
- » ½ cup beef broth
- » ¼ cup soy sauce
- » 1 teaspoon toasted sesame oil
- » 1 (16-ounce) bag frozen broccoli

DIRECTIONS

1. With the crock insert in place, preheat your slow cooker to low. On a cutting board, season the chuck roast with pink salt and pepper, and slice the roast thin. Put the sliced beef in your slow cooker. Combine sesame oil and beef broth in a small bowl then pour over the beef. Cover and cook on low for 4 hours. Add the frozen broccoli and cook for 30 minutes more. If you need more liquid, add additional beef broth. Serve hot.

NUTRITION:

Calories: 803 Carbs: 18g Protein: 74g Fats: 49g

143. CAULIFLOWER AND PUMPKIN CASSEROLE

COOKING: 1H 30'　　**PREPARATION: 15'**　　**SERVINGS: 4**

INGREDIENTS

- » 2 tbsp. olive oil
- » ¼ medium yellow onion, minced
- » 6 cups chopped forage kale into small pieces (about 140 g)
- » 1 little clove garlic, minced
- » Salt and freshly ground black pepper
- » ½ cup low sodium chicken broth
- » 2 cups of 1.5 cm diced pumpkin (about 230 g)
- » 2 cups of 1.5 cm diced zucchini (about 230 g)
- » 2 tbsp. mayonnaise
- » 3 cups frozen, thawed brown rice
- » 1 cup grated Swiss cheese
- » 1/3 cup grated Parmesan
- » 1 cup panko flour
- » 1 large beaten egg
- » Cooking spray

DIRECTIONS

1. Preheat oven to 200 ° C. Heats the oil in a large non-stick skillet over medium heat. Add onions and cook, occasionally stirring, until browned and tender (about 5 minutes). Add the cabbage, garlic, ½ teaspoon salt, and ½ teaspoon pepper and cook until the cabbage is light (about 2 minutes).
2. Put the stock and cook within 5 minutes, then put the squash, zucchini, and ½ teaspoon Salt and mix well. Continuously cooking within 8 minutes. Remove from heat and add mayonnaise.
3. In a bowl, combine cooked vegetables, brown rice, cheese, ½ cup flour, and large egg and mix well. Spray a 2-liter casserole with cooking spray. Put the mixture to the pan and cover with the remaining flour, ¼ teaspoon salt, and a few pinches of pepper. Bake until the squash and zucchini are tender and the top golden and crispy (about 35 minutes). Serve hot.
4. Advanced Preparation Tip: Freeze the casserole for up to 2 weeks. Cover with aluminum foil and heat at 180 ° C until warm (35 to 45 minutes).

NUTRITION:

Calories: 83 Carbs: 11g Fat: 3g Protein: 5g

144. THAI BEEF SALAD TEARS OF THE TIGER

COOKING: 30'   **PREPARATION: 15'**   **SERVINGS: 4**

INGREDIENTS

- » 800 g of beef tenderloin
- » For the marinade:
- » 2 tablespoons of soy sauce
- » 1 tablespoon soup of honey
- » 1 pinch of the pepper mill
- » For the sauce:
- » 1 small bunch of fresh coriander
- » 1 small bouquet of mint
- » 3 tablespoons soup of fish sauce
- » lemon green
- » 1 clove of garlic
- » tablespoons soup of sugar palm
- » 1 bird pepper or ten drops of Tabasco
- » 1 small glass of raw Thai rice to make grilled rice powder
- » 200 g of arugula or young shoots of salad

DIRECTIONS

1. Cut the beef tenderloin into strips and put it in a container. Sprinkle with 2 tablespoons soy sauce, 1 tablespoon honey, and pepper. Soak thoroughly and let marinate 1 hour at room temperature.
2. Meanwhile, prepare the roasted rice powder. Pour a glass of Thai rice into an anti-adhesive pan. Dry color the rice, constantly stirring to avoid burning. When it has a lovely color, get rid of it on a plate and let it cool.
3. When it has cooled, reduce it to powder.
4. Wash and finely chop mint and coriander. Put in a container and add lime juice, chopped garlic clove, 3 tablespoons Nuoc mam, 3 tablespoons brown sugar, 3 tablespoons water, 1 tablespoon sauce soy, and a dozen drop of Tabasco. Mix well and let stand the time that the sugar melts and the flavors mix.
5. Place a bed of salad on a dish. Cook the beef strips put them on the salad. Sprinkle with the spoonful of sauce and roasted rice powder. To be served as is or with a Thai cooked white rice scented.

NUTRITION:

Calories: 137 Carbs: 33g Fat: 0g Protein: 0g

145. STUFFED APPLES WITH SHRIMP

COOKING: 30'   **PREPARATION: 15'**   **SERVINGS: 4**

INGREDIENTS

- » 6 medium apples
- » 1 lemon juice
- » 2 tablespoons butter
- » Filling:
- » 300 gr of shrimp
- » 1 onion minced
- » ½ cup chopped parsley
- » 2 tbsp. flour
- » 1 can of cream/cream
- » 100 gr of curd
- » 1 tablespoon butter
- » 1 tbsp. pepper sauce
- » Salt to taste

DIRECTIONS

1. Cut a cap from each apple, remove the seeds a little from the pulp on the sides, and put the pulp in the bottom, leaving a cavity.
2. Pass a little lemon and some butter on the apples, bake them in the oven. Remove from oven, let cool and bring to freeze.
3. Prepare the shrimp sauce in a pan by mixing the butter with the flour, onion, parsley, and pepper sauce.
4. Then add the prawn shrimp to the sauce. When boiling, mix the cream cheese and sour cream.
5. Stuff each apple. Serve hot or cold, as you prefer.

NUTRITION:

Calories: 75 Carbs: 0g Fat: 1g Protein: 6g

146. GRILLED CHICKEN SALAD WITH ORANGES

COOKING: 15'   **PREPARATION: 15'**   **SERVINGS: 4**

INGREDIENTS

- » 75 ml (1/3 cup) orange juice
- » 30 ml (2 tablespoons) lemon juice
- » 45 ml (3 tablespoons) of extra virgin olive oil
- » 15 ml (1 tablespoon) Dijon mustard
- » 2 cloves of garlic, chopped
- » 1 ml (¼ teaspoon) Salt
- » Freshly ground pepper
- » 1 lb. (450 g) skinless chicken breast, trimmed
- » 25 g (¼ cup) pistachio or flaked almonds, toasted
- » 600 g (8c/5 oz) of mesclun, rinsed and dried
- » 75 g (½ cup) minced red onion
- » 2 medium oranges, peeled, quartered and sliced

DIRECTIONS

1. Place the orange juice, lemon juice, oil, mustard, garlic, salt, and pepper in a small bowl or jar with an airtight lid; whip or shake to mix. Reserve 75 milliliters of this salad vinaigrette and 45 milliliters for basting.
2. Place the rest of the vinaigrette in a shallow glass dish or resealable plastic bag. Add the chicken and turn it over to coat. Cover or close and marinate in the refrigerator for at least 20 minutes or up to two hours.
3. Preheat the barbecue over medium heat. Lightly oil the grill by rubbing it with a crumpled paper towel soaked in oil. Grill the chicken 10 to 15 centimeters (four to six inches) from the heat source, basting the cooked sides with the basting vinaigrette until it is no longer pink in the center, and Instant-read thermometer inserted in the thickest part records 75 ° C (170 ° F), four to six minutes on each side. Transfer then let it rest for five minutes.
4. Meanwhile, grill almonds in a small, dry pan on medium-low heat, stirring constantly, until lightly browned, about two to three minutes. Transfer them to a bowl and let them cool.
5. Place the salad and onion mixture in a large bowl then mix with the vinaigrette reserved for the salad. Slice chicken and spread on salads. Sprinkle orange slices on top and sprinkle with pistachios.

NUTRITION:

Calories: 290 Carbs: 21g Fat: 14g Protein: 25g

147. RED CURRY WITH VEGETABLES

COOKING: 30'   **PREPARATION: 15'**   **SERVINGS: 4**

INGREDIENTS

- » 600 g sweet potatoes
- » 200 g canned chickpeas
- » 2 leek whites
- » 2 tomatoes
- » 100 g of spinach shoots
- » 40 cl of coconut milk
- »
- » 1 jar of Greek yogurt
- » 1 lime
- » 3 cm fresh ginger
- » 1 small bunch of coriander
- » ½ red onion
- » 2 cloves garlic
- » 4 tbsp. red curry paste
- » Salt

DIRECTIONS

1. Cut the sweet potatoes into pieces. Clean the leek whites and cut them into slices. Peel and seed the tomatoes.
2. Mix the Greek yogurt with a drizzle of lime juice, chopped onion, salt, and half of the coriander leaves.
3. In a frying pan, heat 15 cl of coconut milk until it reduces and forms many small bubbles. Brown curry paste with chopped ginger and garlic.
4. Add vegetables, drained chickpeas, remaining coconut milk, and salt. Cook for 20 min covered, then 5 min without lid for the sauce to thicken.
5. When serving, add spinach sprouts and remaining coriander. Serve with the yogurt sauce.

NUTRITION:

Calories: 105 Carbs: 13g Fat: 4g Protein: 3g

148. BAKED TURKEY BREAST WITH CRANBERRY SAUCE

COOKING: 1H 30'   PREPARATION: 15'   SERVINGS: 3

INGREDIENTS

- » 2 kilos of whole turkey breast
- » 1 tablespoon olive oil
- » ¼ cup onion
- » 2 cloves of garlic
- » thyme
- » poultry seasonings
- » coarse-grained salt
- » 2 butter spoons
- » ¼ cup minced shallot
- » ¼ cup chopped onion
- » 1 clove garlic
- » 2 tablespoons flour
- » 1 ½ cups of blueberries
- » 2 cups apple cider
- » 2 tablespoons maple honey
- » peppers

DIRECTIONS

1. Grind in the blender ¼ cup onion, 2 garlic with herbs. Grease the breast with oil.
2. Put in the baking tray, add a cup of citron and bake at 350 Fahrenheit (180 ° C) to have a thermometer record 165 Fahrenheit (75 ° C) inside, about an hour, add ½ cup of water if necessary.
3. Bring the citron to a boil, add the blueberries, and leave a few minutes. In the butter (2 tablespoons), fry the onion (¼ cup), shallot, and garlic (1 clove).
4. Add the flour to the onion and shallot and leave a few minutes. Add the citron, cranberries, and honey and leave on low heat. Season with salt and pepper, let the blueberries get soft. If you want to strain, use the processor.
5. Let it thicken slightly.
6. Slice the thin turkey breast and serve with the blueberry sauce.

NUTRITION:

Calories: 220 Carbs: 6g Fat: 7g Protein: 23g

149. ITALIAN KETO CASSEROLE

COOKING: 1H   PREPARATION: 15'   SERVINGS: 4

INGREDIENTS

- » 200 g Shirataki noodles
- » 2 tbsp. olive oil
- » 1 small onion, diced
- » 2 garlic cloves, finely chopped
- » 1 tsp. dried marjoram
- » 450 g ground beef
- » 1 tsp. Salt
- » ½ tsp. ground pepper
- » 2 chopped tomatoes
- » 1 cup of fat cream
- » 340 g ricotta cheese
- » ⅓ cup grated parmesan
- » 1 egg
- » ¼ cup parsley, roughly chopped

DIRECTIONS

1. Preheat the oven to 190 degrees.
2. Prepare the shirataki noodles as indicated on the packaging, strain well, and set aside.
3. Cook oil, onion, garlic, marjoram, and fry for 2-3 minutes, until the onion is soft.
4. Add ground beef, salt and pepper, and simmer, stirring, while the mixture is browned.
5. Add tomatoes and fat cream, and cook for 5 minutes.
6. Remove from heat and mix with noodles. Transfer the mixture to a baking dish.
7. Mix ricotta, parmesan, egg, and parsley. Spoon over the casserole.
8. Bake about 35-45 minutes until golden brown.

NUTRITION:

Calories: 275 Carbs: 0g Fat: 0g Protein: 0g

150. SALMON KETO CUTLETS

COOKING: 10'　　　**PREPARATION: 15'**　　　**SERVINGS: 4**

INGREDIENTS

- » 450 g canned salmon
- » ½ cup almond flour
- » ¼ cup shallots, finely chopped
- » 2 tbsp. parsley, finely chopped
- » 1 tbsp. dried chopped onions
- » 2 large eggs
- » Zest of 1 lemon
- » 1 clove garlic, finely chopped
- » ½ tsp. Salt
- » ½ tsp. ground white pepper
- » 3 tbsp. olive oil

DIRECTIONS

1. Put all the fixing except the oil in a large bowl and mix well.
2. Form 8, identical cutlets.
3. Fry salmon cutlets in portions, adding more oil as needed, for 2-3 minutes on each side.
4. Serve the cutlets warm or cold with lemon wedges and low carbohydrate mayonnaise.

NUTRITION:

Calories: 300 Carbs: 0g Fat: 19g Protein: 35g

151. BAKED CAULIFLOWER

COOKING: 60'　　　**PREPARATION: 15'**　　　**SERVINGS: 2**

INGREDIENTS

- » 1 medium cauliflower
- » 113 g of salted butter
- » ⅓ cup finely grated parmesan
- » 3 tbsp. Dijon mustard
- » 2 minced garlic cloves
- » Zest of 1 lemon
- » ½ tsp. Salt
- » ½ tsp. ground pepper
- » 28 g fresh Parmesan
- » 1 tbsp. finely chopped parsley

DIRECTIONS

1. Preheat the oven to 190 degrees.
2. Put the cauliflower in a small baking dish.
3. Put the remaining ingredients in a small saucepan, except for fresh parmesan and parsley, and put on low heat until they melt. Whip together.
4. Lubricate cauliflower ⅓ of the oil mixture.
5. Bake for 20 minutes, then remove from the oven and pour another quarter of the oil mixture.
6. Bake for another 20 minutes and pour over the remaining oil mixture.
7. Cook for another 20-30 minutes until the core is soft.
8. Put on a plate, sprinkle a drop of oil from the mold, grate fresh parmesan and sprinkle with parsley.

NUTRITION:

Calories: 1 Carbs: 4g Fat: 11g Protein: 1g

152. RISOTTO WITH MUSHROOMS

COOKING: 25'   **PREPARATION: 15'**   **SERVINGS: 2**

INGREDIENTS

- » 2 tbsp. olive oil
- » 2 minced garlic cloves
- » 1 small onion, finely diced
- » 1 tsp. Salt
- » ½ tsp. ground white pepper
- » 200 g chopped mushrooms
- » ¼ cup chopped oregano leaves
- » 255 g cauliflower "rice"
- » ¼ cup vegetable broth
- » 2 tbsp. butter
- » ⅓ cup grated parmesan

DIRECTIONS

1. Sauté oil, garlic, onions, salt, and pepper, and sauté for 5-7 minutes until the onions become transparent.
2. Add mushrooms and oregano, and cook for 5 minutes.
3. Add cauliflower rice and vegetable broth, then reduce heat to medium. Cook the risotto, frequently stirring, for 10-15 minutes, until the cauliflower is soft.
4. Remove from heat, and mix with butter and parmesan.
5. Try and add more seasoning if you want.

NUTRITION:

Calories: 206 Carbs: 31g Fat: 7g Protein: 4g

153. LOW CARB GREEN BEAN CASSEROLE

COOKING: 60'   **PREPARATION: 15'**   **SERVINGS: 4**

INGREDIENTS

- » 2 tbsp. butter
- » 1 small chopped onion
- » 2 minced garlic cloves
- » 226.8 g chopped mushrooms
- » ½ tsp. Salt
- » ½ tsp. ground pepper
- » ½ cup chicken stock
- » ½ cup of fat cream
- » ½ tsp. xanthan gum
- » 453.59 g green beans (with cut ends)
- » 56.7 g crushed cracklings

DIRECTIONS

1. Preheat the oven to 190 degrees.
2. Add oil, onion, and garlic to a non-stick pan over high heat. Fry until onion is transparent.
3. Add mushrooms, salt, and pepper. Cook for 7 minutes until the mushrooms are tender.
4. Add chicken stock and cream, and bring to a boil. Sprinkle with xanthan gum, mix and cook for 5 minutes.
5. Add the string beans to the creamy mixture and pour it into the baking dish.
6. Cover with foil and bake for 20 minutes.
7. Remove the foil, sprinkle with greaves and bake for another 10-15 minutes.

NUTRITION:

Calories: 244 Carbs: 6g Fat: 18g Protein: 8g

154. AVOCADO LOW CARB BURGER

COOKING: 25'   **PREPARATION: 15'**   **SERVINGS: 4**

INGREDIENTS

- » 1 avocado
- » 1 leaf lettuce
- » 2 slices of prosciutto or any ham
- » 1 slice of tomato
- » 1 egg
- » ½ tbsp. olive oil for frying
- » For the sauce:
- » 1 tbsp. low carb mayonnaise
- » ¼ tsp. low carb hot sauce
- » ¼ tsp. mustard
- » ¼ tsp. Italian seasoning
- » ½ tsp. sesame seeds (optional

DIRECTIONS

1. In a small bowl, combine keto-friendly mayonnaise, mustard, hot sauce, and Italian seasoning.
2. Heat ½ tablespoon of olive oil in a pan and cook an egg. The yolk must be fluid.
3. Cut the avocado in half, remove the peel and bone. Cut the narrowest part of the avocado so that the fruit can stand on a plate.
4. Fill the hole in one half of the avocado with the prepared sauce.
5. Top with lettuce, prosciutto strips, a slice of tomato, and a fried egg.
6. Cover with the other half of the avocado and sprinkle with sesame seeds (optional).

NUTRITION:

Calories: 416 Carbs: 15g Fat: 24g Protein: 35g

155. PROTEIN GNOCCHI WITH BASIL PESTO

COOKING: 30'   **PREPARATION: 15'**   **SERVINGS: 4**

INGREDIENTS

- » 400g Potatoes, boiling
- » 60 g Nutri-Plus protein powder, neutral
- » 50 g wheat flour
- » ½ tsp. Salt
- » Nutmeg
- » 2 tbsp. Flour for the work surface
- » One bunch basil
- » 30 g pine nuts
- » clove of garlic
- » 100 ml olive oil
- » Salt and pepper

DIRECTIONS

1. The recipe is a bit tricky. So, take your time.
2. Slice the potatoes into small pieces, and cook 20-25 minutes. Let the potatoes cool off.
3. Put the pieces of potato, the protein powder, the flour, and the spices together in a blender and mix everything properly.
4. Put flour on the work surface and divide the dough into four parts.
5. Form long, round snakes out of the dough.
6. Slice the snakes every 1.5-2 cm, press briefly with a fork to keep the pesto better, and you're done with the raw gnocchi.
7. Now put the gnocchi together in lightly boiling water for 3-4 minutes and wait until they float up. Serve.

NUTRITION:

Calories: 250 Carbs: 33g Fat: 11g Protein: 7g

156. SUMMERY BOWLS WITH FRESH VEGETABLES AND PROTEIN QUARK

COOKING: 10' **PREPARATION: 15'** **SERVINGS: 4**

INGREDIENTS

- » 100g green salad
- » 100 g radish
- » 200g kohlrabi
- » 70g carrots
- » 70g Red lenses
- » 50g tomatoes
- » Two spring onions
- » 20g Nuts/seeds
- » 150 g soy yogurt
- » 2 tbsp. mixed herbs
- » One teaspoon lemon juice
- » 20 g Nutri-Plus Shape & Shake, neutral
- » One pinch of salt and pepper

DIRECTIONS

1. Wash the salad and the vegetables and peel the kohlrabi.
2. Simmer the red lentils for about 7 minutes.
3. In time, grate the vegetables.
4. Mix the soy yogurt with the lemon juice, the protein powder, salt, and the herbs.
5. Arrange all ingredients together in a deep plate or bowl and top with the spring onions and nuts.

NUTRITION:

Calories: 357 Carbs: 10g Fat: 1g Protein: 80g

157. BEEF AND KALE PAN

COOKING: 20' **PREPARATION: 10'** **SERVINGS: 4**

INGREDIENTS

- » 1-pound beef stew meat, cubed
- » 1 red onion, chopped
- » 1 tablespoon olive oil
- » 2 garlic cloves, minced
- » 1 cup kale, torn
- » 1 cup beef stock
- » 1 teaspoon chili powder
- » ½ teaspoon sweet paprika
- » 1 teaspoon rosemary, dried
- » 1 tablespoon cilantro, chopped

DIRECTIONS

1. Ensure that you heat the pan; add the onion and the garlic, stir and sauté for 2 minutes.
2. Add the meat and brown it for 5 minutes.
3. Put the rest of the fixing, simmer, then cook over medium heat for 13 minutes more.
4. Divide the mix between plates and serve for lunch.

NUTRITION:

Calories: 160g Fat: 10g Fiber: 3g Carbs: 1g Protein: 12g

158. SALMON AND LEMON RELISH

COOKING: 1 H **PREPARATION: 10'** **SERVINGS: 2**

INGREDIENTS

- » 2 medium salmon fillets
- » Black pepper and salt to taste
- » A drizzle of olive oil
- » 1 shallot, chopped
- » 1 tablespoon lemon juice
- » 1 big lemon
- » ¼ cup olive oil
- » 2 tablespoons parsley, finely chopped

DIRECTIONS

1. Grease salmon fillets with olive oil, put salt and pepper, place on a lined baking sheet, standing in the oven at 400 degrees F, and bake for 1 hour.
2. Stir 1 tablespoon lemon juice, salt, and pepper in a bowl, and leave aside for 10 minutes.
3. Cut the whole lemon in wedges and then very thinly.
4. Put this to shallots, parsley, and ¼ cup olive oil and stir.
5. Break the salmon into medium pieces and serve with the lemon relish on the side.

NUTRITION:

Calories: 200g Fat: 10g Fiber: 1g Carbs: 5g Protein: 20g

159. MUSTARD GLAZED SALMON

COOKING: 20' **PREPARATION: 10'** **SERVINGS: 1**

INGREDIENTS

- » 1 big salmon fillet
- » Black pepper and salt to taste
- » 2 tablespoons mustard
- » 1 tablespoon coconut oil
- » 1 tablespoon maple extract

DIRECTIONS

1. Mix maple extract with mustard in a bowl.
2. Massage salmon with salt and pepper and half of the mustard mix
3. Heat-up a pan to high heat, place salmon flesh side down and cook for 5 minutes.
4. Rub salmon with the rest of the mixture, transfer to a baking dish, place in the oven at 425 degrees F and bake for 15 minutes.
5. Serve with a tasty side salad.
6. Enjoy!

NUTRITION:

Calories: 240g Fat: 7g Fiber: 1g Carbs: 5g Protein: 23g

160. TURKEY AND TOMATOES

COOKING: 30' **PREPARATION: 10'** **SERVINGS: 4**

INGREDIENTS

- » 2 shallots, chopped
- » 1 tablespoon ghee, melted
- » 1 cup chicken stock
- » 1-pound turkey breast, skinless, boneless and cubed
- » 1 cup cherry tomatoes, halved
- » 1 tablespoon rosemary, chopped

DIRECTIONS

1. Ensure that the pan containing ghee is heated, add the shallots, and the meat and brown for 5 minutes.
2. Put the rest of the fixing, simmer, and cook over medium heat for 25 minutes, stirring often.
3. Divide into bowls and serve.

NUTRITION:

Calories: 150g Fat: 4g Fiber: 1g Carbs: 3g Protein: 10g

161. GRILLED SQUID AND TASTY GUACAMOLE

COOKING: 10' **PREPARATION: 10'** **SERVINGS: 2**

INGREDIENTS

- » 2 medium squid, tentacles separated and tubes scored lengthwise
- » A drizzle of olive oil
- » Juice from 1 lime
- » Black pepper and salt to taste
- » For the guacamole:
- » 2 avocados, pitted, peeled and chopped
- » Some coriander springs, chopped
- » 2 red chilies, chopped
- » 1 tomato, chopped
- » 1 red onion, chopped
- » Juice from 2 limes

DIRECTIONS

1. Season squid and squid tentacles with salt, pepper, drizzle some olive oil and massage generously. Grill for 2 minutes in medium-high. Cook for 2 minutes more.
2. Add juice from 1 lime, toss to coat, and keep warm. Put the avocado in a bowl and mash using a fork.
3. Add coriander, chilies, tomato, onion, and juice from 2 limes and stir well everything.
4. Divide squid on plates, top with guacamole, and serve.

NUTRITION:

Calories: 500g Fat: 43g Fiber: 6g Carbs: 7g Protein: 20g

162. SALMON BOWLS

COOKING: 15'   **PREPARATION: 10'**   **SERVINGS: 4**

INGREDIENTS

- » 1-pound salmon fillets, boneless, skinless, and roughly cubed
- » 1 cup chicken stock
- » 2 spring onions, chopped
- » 1 tablespoon olive oil
- » 1 cup kalamata olives, pitted and halved
- » 1 avocado, pitted, peeled, and roughly cubed
- » 1 cup baby spinach
- » ¼ cup cilantro, chopped
- » 1 tablespoon basil, chopped
- » 1 teaspoon lime juice

DIRECTIONS

1. Ensure that you heat the pan, add the spring onions and the salmon, toss gently, then cook for 5 minutes.
2. Add the olives and the other ingredients, and then cook over medium heat for 10 minutes more.
3. Divide the mix into bowls and serve for lunch.
4.

NUTRITION:

Calories: 254 Fat: 17 Fiber: 1.9 Carbs: 6.1 Protein: 20

163. SHRIMP AND CAULIFLOWER DELIGHT

COOKING: 15'   **PREPARATION: 10'**   **SERVINGS: 2**

INGREDIENTS

- » 1 tablespoon ghee
- » 1 tablespoon parsley
- » 1 cauliflower head, florets separated
- » 1-pound shrimp, peeled and deveined
- » ¼ cup of coconut milk
- » 8 ounces mushrooms, roughly chopped
- » A pinch of red pepper flakes
- » Black pepper and salt to taste
- » 2 garlic cloves, minced
- » 4 bacon slices
- » ½ cup beef stock
- » 1 tablespoon chives, chopped

DIRECTIONS

1. Heat-up a pan, add bacon, cook until it's crispy, transfer to paper towels, and leave aside.
2. Heat-up 1 tablespoon bacon fat on another pan over medium-high heat, add shrimp, and cook for 2 minutes on each side and transfer to a bowl.
3. Cook mushrooms, stir, and cook for 3-4 minutes. Put garlic, pepper flakes, cook for 1 minute.
4. Put beef stock, salt, pepper, and return shrimp to pan. Stir. Mince cauliflower in the food processor. Cook for 5 minutes.
5. Add ghee and butter, stir and blend using an immersion blender. Put salt and pepper, stir.
6. Top with shrimp mixture and serve with parsley and chives sprinkled all over. Enjoy!

NUTRITION:

Calories: 245g Fat: 7g Fiber: 4g Carbs: 6g Protein: 20g

164. SCALLOPS AND FENNEL SAUCE

COOKING: 10'   **PREPARATION: 10'**   **SERVINGS: 6**

INGREDIENTS

- » 6 scallops
- » 1 fennel, trimmed, leaves chopped and bulbs cut in wedges
- » Juice from ½ lime
- » 1 lime, cut in wedges
- » Zest from 1 lime
- » 1 egg yolk
- » 3 tablespoons ghee, melted and heated up
- » ½ tablespoons olive oil
- » Black pepper and salt to the taste

DIRECTIONS

1. Season scallops with salt and pepper, put in a bowl and mix with half of the lime juice and half of the zest and toss to coat.
2. In a bowl, mix the egg yolk with some salt and pepper, the rest of the lime juice, and the rest of the lime zest and whisk well.
3. Add melted ghee and stir very well. Also, add fennel leaves and stir.
4. Brush fennel wedges with oil, place on heated grill over medium-high heat, cook for 2 minutes, flip and cook for 2 minutes more.
5. Add scallops on the grill, cook for 2 minutes, flip and cook for 2 minutes more.
6. Divide fennel and scallops on plates, drizzle fennel, and ghee mix and serve with lime wedges on the side. Enjoy!

NUTRITION:

Calories: 400g Fat: 24g Fiber: 4g Carbs: 12g Protein: 25g

165. SALMON STUFFED WITH SHRIMP

COOKING: 25'   **PREPARATION: 10'**   **SERVINGS: 2**

INGREDIENTS

- » 2 salmon fillets
- » A drizzle of olive oil
- » 5 ounces tiger shrimp, peeled, deveined, and chopped
- » 6 mushrooms, chopped
- » 3 green onions, chopped
- » 2 cups spinach
- » ¼ cup macadamia nuts, toasted and chopped
- » Black pepper and salt to taste
- » A pinch of nutmeg
- » ¼ cup mayonnaise

DIRECTIONS

1. Heat-up a pan and add mushrooms, onions, salt, and pepper, stir and cook for 4 minutes.
2. Add macadamia nuts, stir and cook for 2 minutes.
3. Add spinach, stir and cook for 1 minute.
4. Add shrimp, stir and cook for 1 minute.
5. Take off heat, leave aside for a few minutes, add mayo and nutmeg and stir well.
6. Make an incision lengthwise in each salmon fillet, sprinkle salt and pepper, divide spinach and shrimp mix into incisions, and place on a working surface.
7. Grease the pan with oil over medium-high heat, add stuffed salmon, skin side down, cook for 1 minute, reduce temperature, cover pan and cook for 8 minutes.
8. Broil for 3 minutes, divide among plates, and serve.
9. Enjoy!

NUTRITION:

Calories: 430g Fat: 30g Fiber: 3g Carbs: 7g Protein: 50g

166. CHEESY PORK CASSEROLE

COOKING: 40'   **PREPARATION: 10'**   **SERVINGS: 4**

INGREDIENTS

- » 1 cup cheddar cheese, grated
- » 2 eggs, whisked
- » 1-pound pork loin, cubed
- » 2 tablespoons avocado oil
- » 2 shallots, chopped
- » 3 garlic cloves, minced
- » 1 cup red bell peppers
- » ¼ cup heavy cream
- » 1 tablespoon chives, chopped
- » ½ teaspoon cumin, ground

DIRECTIONS

1. Ensure that you heat the pan; add the shallots and the garlic and sauté for 2 minutes.
2. Add the bell peppers and the meat, toss, then cook for 5 minutes more.
3. Add the cumin, salt, pepper, toss, and take off the heat.
4. In a bowl, mix the eggs with the cream and the cheese, whisk and pour over the pork mix.
5. Cook with chives on top at 380 degrees F for 30 minutes.
6. Divide the mix between plates and serve for lunch.

NUTRITION:

Calories: 455g Fat: 34g Fiber: 3g Carbs: 3g — Protein: 33g

167. INCREDIBLE SALMON DISH

COOKING: 15'   **PREPARATION: 10'**   **SERVINGS: 4**

INGREDIENTS

- » 3 cups of ice water
- » 2 teaspoons sriracha sauce
- » 4 teaspoons stevia
- » 3 scallions, chopped
- » Black pepper and salt to taste
- » 2 teaspoons flaxseed oil
- » 4 teaspoons apple cider vinegar
- » 3 teaspoons avocado oil
- » 4 medium salmon fillets
- » 4 cups baby arugula
- » 2 cups cabbage, finely chopped
- » 1 and ½ teaspoon Jamaican jerk seasoning
- » ¼ cup pepitas, toasted
- » 2 cups watermelon radish, julienned

DIRECTIONS

1. Put ice water in a bowl, add scallions, and leave aside.
2. In another bowl, mix sriracha sauce with stevia and stir well.
3. Transfer 2 teaspoons of this mix to a bowl and mix with half of the avocado oil, flaxseed oil, vinegar, salt and pepper, and whisk.
4. Sprinkle jerk seasoning over salmon, rub with sriracha and stevia mix, and season with salt and pepper.
5. Heat-up a pan with the rest of the avocado oil over medium-high heat, add salmon, flesh side down, cook for 4 minutes, flip and cook for 4 minutes more and divide among plates.
6. In a bowl, mix radishes with cabbage and arugula.
7. Add salt, pepper, sriracha, and vinegar mix and toss well.
8. Add this to salmon fillets, drizzle the remaining sriracha, and stevia sauce all over and top with pepitas and drained scallions.
9. Enjoy!

NUTRITION:

Calories: 160g Fat: 6g Fiber: 1g Carbs: 1g Protein: 12g

CHAPTER 8. DESSERTS

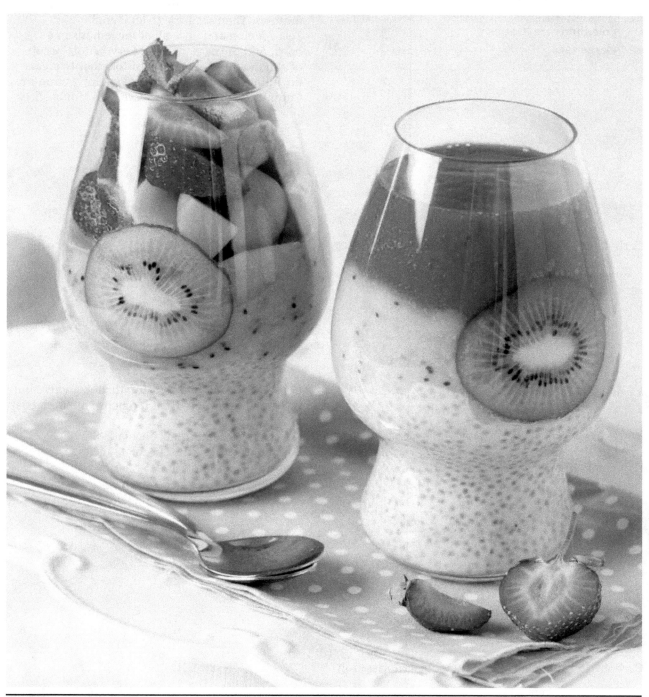

168. SUGAR-FREE LEMON BARS

COOKING: 45'   **PREPARATION: 15'**   **SERVINGS: 8**

INGREDIENTS

» ½ cup butter, melted
» 1¾ cup almond flour, divided
» 1 cup powdered erythritol, divided
» 3 medium-size lemons
» 3 large eggs

DIRECTIONS

1. Prepare the parchment paper and baking tray. Combine butter, 1 cup of almond flour, ¼ cup of erythritol, and salt. Stir well. Bake for about 20 minutes. Then set aside to let it cool.
2. Zest 1 lemon and juice all of the lemons in a bowl. Add the eggs, ¾ cup of erythritol, ¾ cup of almond flour, and salt. Stir together to create the filling. Put it on top, then cook for 25 minutes. Cut into small pieces and serve with lemon slices.

NUTRITION:

Carbohydrates: 4 g Fat: 26 g Protein: 8 g Calories: 272

169. CREAMY HOT CHOCOLATE

COOKING: 5'   **PREPARATION: 5'**   **SERVINGS: 4**

INGREDIENTS

» 6 oz. dark chocolate, chopped
» ½ cup unsweetened almond milk
» ½ cup heavy cream
» 1 tbsp. erythritol
» ½ tsp. vanilla extract

DIRECTIONS

1. Combine the almond milk, erythritol, and cream in a small saucepan. Heat it (choose medium heat and cook for 1-2 minutes).
2. Add vanilla extract and chocolate. Stir continuously until the chocolate melts.
3. Pour into cups and serve.

NUTRITION:

Carbohydrates: 4g Fat: 18g Protein: 2g Calories: 193

170. DELICIOUS COFFEE ICE CREAM

COOKING: 5' **PREPARATION: 10'** **SERVINGS: 1**

INGREDIENTS

- » 6 ounces coconut cream, frozen into ice cubes
- » 1 ripe avocado, diced and frozen
- » ½ cup coffee expresso
- » 2 tbsp. sweetener
- » 1 tsp. vanilla extract
- » 1 tbsp. water
- » Coffee beans

DIRECTIONS

1. Take out the frozen coconut cubes and avocado from the fridge. Slightly melt them for 5-10 minutes.
2. Add the sweetener, coffee expresso, and vanilla extract to the coconut-avocado mix and whisk with an immersion blender until it becomes creamy (for about 1 minute). Pour in the water and blend for 30 seconds.
3. Top with coffee beans and enjoy!

NUTRITION:

Carbohydrates: 20.5 g Fat: 61 g Protein: 6.3 g Calories: 596

171. FATTY BOMBS WITH CINNAMON AND CARDAMOM

COOKING: 35' **PREPARATION: 10'** **SERVINGS: 10**

INGREDIENTS

- » ½ cup unsweetened coconut, shredded
- » 3 oz unsalted butter
- » ¼ tsp. ground green cinnamon
- » ¼ ground cardamom
- » ½ tsp. vanilla extract

DIRECTIONS

1. Roast the unsweetened coconut (choose medium-high heat) until it begins to turn lightly brown.
2. Combine the room-temperature butter, half of the shredded coconut, cinnamon, cardamom, and vanilla extract in a separate dish. Cool the mix in the fridge for about 5-10 minutes.
3. Form small balls and cover them with the remaining shredded coconut.
4. Cool the balls in the fridge for about 10-15 minutes.

NUTRITION:

Carbohydrates: 0.4 g Fat: 10 g Protein: 0.4 g Calories: 90

172. RASPBERRY MOUSSE

COOKING: 4 H   **PREPARATION: 10'**   **SERVINGS: 8**

INGREDIENTS

- » 3 oz fresh raspberry
- » 2 cups heavy whipping cream
- » 2 oz pecans, chopped
- » ¼ tsp. vanilla extract
- » ½ lemon, the zest

DIRECTIONS

1. Pour the whipping cream into the dish and blend until it becomes soft.
2. Put the lemon zest and vanilla into the dish and mix thoroughly.
3. Put the raspberries and nuts into the cream mix and stir well.
4. Cover the dish with plastic wrap and put it in the fridge for 3 hours.
5. Top with raspberries and serve.

NUTRITION:

Carbohydrates: 3 g Fat: 26 g Protein: 2 g Calories: 255

173. CHOCOLATE SPREAD WITH HAZELNUTS

COOKING: 5'   **PREPARATION: 5'**   **SERVINGS: 6**

INGREDIENTS

- » 2 tbsp. cacao powder
- » 5 oz hazelnuts, roasted and without shells
- » 1 oz unsalted butter
- » ¼ cup of coconut oil

DIRECTIONS

1. Whisk all the spread ingredients with a blender. Serve.

NUTRITION:

Carbohydrates: 2 g Fat: 28 g Protein: 4 g Calories: 271

174. QUICK AND SIMPLE BROWNIE

COOKING: 5' **PREPARATION: 20'** **SERVINGS: 2**

INGREDIENTS

- » 3 tbsp. Keto chocolate chips
- » 1 tbsp. unsweetened cacao powder
- » 2 tbsp. salted butter
- » 2¼ tbsp. powdered sugar

DIRECTIONS

1. Combine 2 tbsp. of chocolate chips and butter, melt them in a microwave for 10-15 minutes. Add the remaining chocolate chips, stir and make a sauce.
2. Add the cacao powder and powdered sugar to the sauce and whisk well until you have a dough.
3. Place the dough on a baking sheet, form the Brownie.
4. Put your Brownie into the oven (preheated to 350°F).
5. Bake for 5 minutes.

NUTRITION:

Carbohydrates: 9 g Fat: 30 g Protein: 13 g Calories: 100

175. CUTE PEANUT BALLS

COOKING: 20' **PREPARATION: 20'** **SERVINGS: 18**

INGREDIENTS

- » 1 cup salted peanuts, chopped
- » 1 cup peanut butter
- » 1 cup powdered sweetener
- » 8 oz keto chocolate chips

DIRECTIONS

1. Combine the chopped peanuts, peanut butter, and sweetener in a separate dish. Stir well and make a dough. Divide it into 18 pieces and form small balls. Put them in the fridge for 10-15 minutes.
2. Use a microwave to melt your chocolate chips.
3. Plunge each ball into the melted chocolate.
4. Return your balls in the fridge. Cool for about 20 minutes.

NUTRITION:

Carbohydrates: 7 g Fat: 17 g Protein: 7 g Calorie: 194

176. CHOCOLATE MUG MUFFINS

COOKING: 2'   **PREPARATION: 5'**   **SERVINGS: 4**

INGREDIENTS

- » 4 tbsp. almond flour
- » 1 tsp. baking powder
- » 4 tbsp. granulated erythritol
- » 2 tbsp. cocoa powder
- » ½ tsp. vanilla extract
- » 2 pinches of salt
- » 2 eggs beaten
- » 3 tbsp. butter, melted
- » 1 tsp. coconut oil, for greasing the mug
- » ½ oz sugar-free dark chocolate, chopped

DIRECTIONS

1. Mix the dry ingredients in a separate bowl. Add the melted butter, beaten eggs, and chocolate to the bowl. Stir thoroughly.
2. Divide your dough into 4 pieces. Put these pieces in the greased mugs and put them in the microwave. Cook for 1-1.5 minutes (700 watts).
3. Let them cool for 1 minute and serve.

NUTRITION:

Carbohydrates: 2 g Fat: 19 g Protein: 5 g Calories: 208

177. KETO PEANUT BUTTER CUP STYLE FUDGE

COOKING: 30'   **PREPARATION: 10'**   **SERVINGS: 36**

INGREDIENTS

- » 1 ½ cup natural peanut butter
- » ¼ cup butter
- » 3/4 cup powdered swerve sweetener
- » 1 tsp. vanilla extract
- » 1/8 tsp. Salt (omit if butter is salted)
- » 3 tbsp. peanuts chopped
- » Flaked sea salt for topping

DIRECTIONS

1. Line a baking sheet with parchment pepper for easy removal.
2. Add peanut butter, vanilla, and butter in a pan and heat over medium heat until melted and smooth.
3. Turn off the heat and stir in sweetener and salt, combine to mix well.
4. Spread the mixture in the prepared baking sheet in even layered.
5. Chill for 20-30 minutes, cut into 36 slices.
6. Sprinkle with sea salt or other toppings of your choice, keep in an airtight container.

NUTRITION:

Calories: 79 Fats: 7g Carbohydrates: 2g Protein: 2g

178. KETO AND DAIRY-FREE VANILLA CUSTARD

COOKING: 5'   **PREPARATION: 11'**   **SERVINGS: 4**

INGREDIENTS

- » 6 egg yolks
- » ½ cup unsweetened almond milk
- » 1 tsp. vanilla extract
- » ¼ cup melted coconut oil

DIRECTIONS

1. Mix egg yolks, almond milk, vanilla in a metal bowl.
2. Gradually stir in the melted coconut oil.
3. Boil water in a saucepan, place the mixing bowl over the saucepan.
4. Whisk the mixture constantly and vigorously until thickened for about 5 minutes.
5. Remover from the saucepan, serve hot or chill in the fridge.

NUTRITION:

Calories: 215.38 Fats: 21g Carbohydrates: 1g Protein: 4g

179. KETO TRIPLE CHOCOLATE MUG CAKE

COOKING: 60'   **PREPARATION: 15'**   **SERVINGS: 2**

INGREDIENTS

- » 1 ½ tbsp. coconut flour
- » ½ tsp. baking powder
- » 2 tbsp. cacao powder
- » 2 tbsp. powdered sweetener
- » 1 medium egg
- » 5 tbsp. double/heavy cream
- » 2 tbsp. sugar-free chocolate chips
- » ¼ tsp. vanilla extract optional

DIRECTIONS

1. Mix all dry fixing- coconut flour, baking powder, cacao powder, and a bowl.
2. Whisk together the egg, cream, and vanilla extract, pour the mixture in the dry ingredients.
3. Add the chocolate chips in the mixture and let the batter rest for a minute.
4. Grease the ramekins with the melted butter, pour the batter in the ramekins.
5. Place in the microwave and microwave for 1 ½ minute until cooked through.

NUTRITION:

Calories: 250 Carbohydrates: 9.7g Protein: 6g Fat: 22g

180. KETO CHEESECAKE STUFFED BROWNIES

COOKING: 30'   **PREPARATION: 11'**   **SERVINGS: 16**

INGREDIENTS

» **For the Filling:**
» 8 oz (225g) cream cheese
» ¼ cup sweetener
» 1 large egg
» **For the Brownie:**
» 3 oz (85g) low carb milk chocolate
» 5 tbsp. butter
» 3 large eggs
» ½ cup sweetener
» ¼ cup cocoa powder
» ½ cup almond flour

DIRECTIONS

1. Heat-up oven to 350 °F, line a brownie pan with parchment.
2. In a mixing bowl, whisk together cream cheese, egg, and sweetener until smooth, set aside.
3. Place chocolate and butter in a microwave-safe bowl and microwave at 30 seconds interval.
4. Whisk frequently until smooth, allow to cool for a few minutes.
5. Whisk together the remaining eggs and sweetener until fluffy.
6. Mix in the almond flour plus cocoa powder until soft peaks form.
7. Mix in the chocolate and butter mixture and beat with a hand mixer for a few seconds.
8. Fill the prepared pan with ¾ of the batter, then top with the cream cheese and the brownie batter. Bake the cheesecake brownie until mostly set for about 25-30 minutes.
9. The jiggling parts of the cake will firm when you remove it from the oven.

NUTRITION:

Calories: 143.94 Fat: 13.48g
Carbohydrates: 1.9g Protein: 3.87g

181. KETO RASPBERRY ICE CREAM

COOKING: 0'   **PREPARATION: 45'**   **SERVINGS: 8**

INGREDIENTS

» 2 cups heavy whipping cream
» 1 cup raspberries
» ½ cup powdered erythritol
» 1 pasteurized egg yolk

DIRECTIONS

1. Process all the ice cream ingredients in a food processor.
2. Add blended mixture into the ice cream maker.
3. Turn on the ice cream machine and churn according to the manufacturer's directions.

NUTRITION:

Calories: 120 Fats: 23g Carbohydrates: 4g Protein: 0g

182. CHOCOLATE MACADAMIA NUT FAT BOMBS

COOKING: 30'   **PREPARATION: 11'**   **SERVINGS: 4**

INGREDIENTS

- » 1⅓ oz (38g) sugar-free dark chocolate
- » 1 tbsp. coconut oil
- » coarse salt or sea salt
- » 1½ oz (42g) raw macadamia nuts halves

DIRECTIONS

1. Put three macadamia nut halves in each of 8 wells of the mini muffin pan.
2. Microwave the chocolate chips for about a few seconds.
3. Whisk until smooth, add coconut oil and salt, mix until well combined.
4. Fill the mini muffin pan with the chocolate mixture to cover the nuts completely.
5. Refrigerate the muffin pan until chilled and firm for about 30 minutes.

NUTRITION:

Calories: 153 Fat: 1g Carbohydrates: 2g Protein: 4g

183. KETO PEANUT BUTTER CHOCOLATE BARS

COOKING: 10'   **PREPARATION: 11**   **SERVINGS: 8**

INGREDIENTS

- » **For the Bars:**
- » 3/4 cup (84 g) Superfine Almond Flour
- » 2 oz (56.7 g) Butter
- » ¼ cup (45.5 g) Swerve, Icing sugar style
- » ½ cup Peanut Butter
- » 1 tsp. Vanilla extract
- » **For the Topping:**
- » ½ cup (90 g) Sugar-Free Chocolate Chips

DIRECTIONS

1. Combine all the ingredients for the bars and spread into a small 6-inch pan.
2. Microwave the chocolate in the microwave oven for 30 seconds and whisk until smooth.
3. Pour the melted chocolate in over the bars ingredients.
4. Refrigerate for at least an hour or two until the bars firmed. Keep in an airtight container.

NUTRITION:

Calories: 246 Fats: 23g Carbohydrates: 7g Protein: 7g

184. SALTED TOFFEE NUT CUPS

INGREDIENTS

» 5 oz (141g) low-carb milk chocolate
» 3 tbsp. + 2 tbsp. sweetener
» 3 tbsp. cold butter
» ½ oz (14g) raw walnuts, chopped
» Sea salt to taste

DIRECTIONS

1. Microwave the chocolate in 45 seconds intervals and continue whisk until chocolate melted.
2. Line the cupcake pan with 5 paper liners and add chocolate to the bottom of the cupcake.
3. Spread the chocolate to coat the bottom of the cupcake evenly, freeze to harden.
4. In a heat-proof bowl, heat the cold butter and sweetener on power 8 for three minutes.
5. Stir the butter every 20 seconds to prevent the burning.
6. Mix in the 2 tbsp. of sweetener and whisk to thicken. Fold in the walnuts.
7. Fill the chocolate cups with the toffee mixture quickly.
8. Top the cupcakes with the remaining chocolate and refrigerate to firm for 20-30 minutes.
9. Remove from the cups and sprinkle with sea salt!

NUTRITION:

Calories: 194 Fat: 18g Carbohydrates: 2g
Protein: 2.5g

185. CRISP MERINGUE COOKIES

INGREDIENTS

» 4 large egg whites
» ¼ tsp. cream of tartar
» ½ tsp. almond extract
» 6 tbsp. Swerve Confectioners
» Pinch of salt

DIRECTIONS

1. Preheat oven to 210 °F (100 °C).
2. Whip egg whites, cream of tartar in a mixing bowl on medium speed until foamy.
3. While whipping, gradually add the swerve confectioners ¼ tsp. at a time.
4. When all the swerve added ultimately, then turn the mixer up to high speed and whip.
5. Add in the almond extract and whip until very stiff.
6. Pour the batter in a piping bag with a French star tip and pipe the batter onto the lined baking
7. Sheet. Bake the meringue for 40 minutes.
8. Serve immediately, enjoy!

NUTRITION:

Calories: 4 Fats: 0.01g Carbohydrates: 0.09g Protein: 0.08g

186. INSTANT POT MATCHA CHEESECAKE

COOKING: 55'   **PREPARATION: 11'**   **SERVINGS: 6**

INGREDIENTS

- » Cheesecake:
- » 16 oz (450g) cream cheese, room temperature
- » ½ cup sweetener
- » 2 tsp. coconut flour
- » ½ tsp. vanilla extract
- » 2 tbsp. heavy whipping cream
- » 1 tbsp. matcha powder
- » 2 large eggs, room temperature

DIRECTIONS

1. In a mixing bowl, combine cream cheese, Swerve, coconut flour, vanilla extract, whipping cream, and matcha powder until well combined. Stir in the eggs one at a time.
2. Add the cheesecake batter into the prepared springform pan.
3. Pour 1 ½ cups of water into the bottom of the Instant Pot. Put the trivet in the instant pot.
4. Place the springform on the top of the trivet, sealing, and securing the instant pot's lid.
5. Set the instant pot on high pressure, set the timing for 35 minutes.
6. Once the cooking time is up, release the pressure naturally.
7. Transfer the cheesecake on a cooling rack and allow it to cool the cake for 30 minutes.
8. Top with your favorite toppings, enjoy!

NUTRITION:

Calories: 350 Fats: 33.2g Carbohydrates: 5.8g
— Protein: 8.4g

187. MATCHA SKILLET SOUFFLE

COOKING: 5'   **PREPARATION: 5'**   **SERVINGS: 1**

INGREDIENTS

- » 3 large eggs
- » 2 tbsp. sweetener
- » 1 tsp. vanilla extract
- » 1 tbsp. matcha powder
- » 1 tbsp. butter
- » 7 whole raspberries
- » 1 tbsp. coconut oil
- » 1 tbsp. unsweetened cocoa powder
- » ¼ cup whipped cream

DIRECTIONS

1. Broil, then heat-up a heavy-bottom pan over medium heat.
2. Whip the egg whites with one tablespoon of Swerve confectioners. Once the peaks form to add in the matcha powder, whisk again.
3. With a fork, break up the yolks. Mix in the vanilla, then add a little amount of the whipped whites. Carefully fold the remaining of the whites into the yolk mixture.
4. Dissolve the butter in a pan, put the souffle mixture to the pan. Reduce the heat to low and top with raspberries. Cook until the eggs double in size and set.
5. Transfer the pan to the oven and keep an eye on it. Cook until golden browned.
6. Melt the coconut oil and combine with cocoa powder and the remaining Swerve.
7. Drizzle the chocolate mixture across the top.

NUTRITION:

Calories 578 Fats: 50.91g Carbohydrates: 5.06g Protein: 20.95g

188. FLOURLESS KETO BROWNIES

COOKING: 25'   **PREPARATION: 10'**   **SERVINGS: 4**

INGREDIENTS

- » 5 oz (141g) low-carb milk chocolate
- » 4 tbsp. butter
- » 3 large eggs
- » ½ cup Swerve
- » ¼ cup mascarpone cheese
- » ¼ cup unsweetened cocoa powder, divided
- » ½ tsp. Salt

DIRECTIONS

1. Heat oven to 375 °F (190 °C) and line a baking sheet with parchment. In a glass bowl over medium heat, melt the 5 oz. chocolate for 30 seconds, stirring until smooth.
2. Stir in the butter and microwave the bowl for another ten seconds. Repeat the process until smooth. Put aside.
3. Beat the eggs and sweetener in a large mixing bowl until eggs became pale and the mixture fluffy.
4. Stir in the mascarpone cheese and whisk until smooth.
5. Gently sift in the half cocoa powder and salt, combine.
6. Sift the remaining cocoa powder and whisk until combined and form the mixture into a batter.
7. Heat the chocolate again if it firmed and whisk in the mixture until creamy.
8. Add the mixture to the prepared baking pan and bake until no longer jiggle for about 25 minutes.
9. Allow to cool before serving, enjoy!

NUTRITION:

Calories: 86.94 Fat: 8g Carbohydrates: 2.9g — Protein: 2.18g

189. TROPICAL CHOCOLATE MOUSSE BITES

COOKING: 2'   **PREPARATION: 5'**   **SERVINGS: 1**

INGREDIENTS

- » 10.5 oz (300 g) sugar-free dark chocolate
- » 1 oz (30 g) coconut oil
- » ½ cup heavy whipping cream
- » 1 tbsp. shredded coconut
- » 1 tbsp. lemon zest

DIRECTIONS

1. Chill the molds in the freezer.
2. Microwave the chocolate and coconut oil in 10-second intervals, stirring continuously until smooth.
3. In a separate mixing bowl, whip the cream until medium-stiff peaks form.
4. Stir in the lemon zest and shredded coconut and fold into the cream.
5. Gradually stir in the 1/3 of the melted chocolate into the cream until well combined, reserving 2/3 for the molds. Place the mousse in the fridge to cool.
6. Pour the remaining melted chocolate into the chilled molds to form a thick layer on the sides.
7. Refrigerate the molds for 10-15 minutes.
8. Fill the cooled ice molds with the mousse batter, leaving some space for the chocolate topping.
9. Pour the remaining melted chocolate over the mousse and refrigerate and molds for 10-15 minutes.
10. Keep in the airtight container in the fridge.

NUTRITION:

Calories: 174.67 Fats: 13.75g
Carbohydrates: 1.02g — Protein: 1.98g

190. COCONUT RASPBERRY SLICE

COOKING: 20'   **PREPARATION: 11'**   **SERVINGS: 12**

INGREDIENTS

- » 3.8 oz (110g) butter melted
- » 2 oz (50g) coconut flour
- » 4 tbsp. granulated sweetener
- » 2 tsp. vanilla or more
- » 1 tsp. baking powder
- » 8 eggs - medium
- » 4 oz (120 g) frozen raspberries

DIRECTIONS

1. Mix the melted butter, coconut flour, sweetener, vanilla, and baking powder in a bowl until smooth.
2. Put the eggs, whisk in between each one.
3. Add the mixture to a rectangle baking dish, lined with baking parchment.
4. Top with each frozen raspberry evenly onto the cake.
5. Bake the raspberry fingers at 180C/350F for 20-25 minutes until cooked through in the center.
6. Allow cooling, for raspberry fingers, cut down in the center, then cut across.

NUTRITION:

Calories: 146 Fats: 11.5g Carbohydrates: 6g Protein: 4.7g

191. WHITE CHOCOLATE BARK

COOKING: 10'   **PREPARATION: 11'**   **SERVINGS: 12**

INGREDIENTS

- » 2 oz (56g) cacao butter
- » 1/3 cup sweetener
- » 1 tsp. vanilla powder
- » ½ tsp. hemp seed powder
- » Pinch of Salt
- » 1 tsp. toasted pumpkin seeds

DIRECTIONS

1. Finely chop, measure cacao butter and melt in a double boiler over a pan of boiling water.
2. Mix the remaining items in a bowl. Grease a plate or bowl
3. With coconut oil, mix the melted butter into the remaining ingredients, combine well.
4. Pour the mixture into the greased plate or bowl, freeze until firm for 15 minutes.
5. Remove the dish from the freezer and break the frozen mix into 12 even pieces.
6. Chill and serve.

NUTRITION:

Calories: 23.92 Fats: 2.36g Carbohydrates: 0.11g
Protein: 0.13g

192. KETO HOT CHOCOLATE

COOKING: 10'   **PREPARATION: 5'**   **SERVINGS: 1**

INGREDIENTS

» ½ c. heavy cream, divided
» ½ tsp. vanilla extract, divided
» 1 ¼ c. water
» 2 tbsp. cocoa powder, unsweetened
» 4 tsp. erythritol or comparable measure of preferred sweetener, divided

DIRECTIONS

1. Mix half of the heavy cream, half of the erythritol, and half of the vanilla extract in a bowl. Using a hand mixer, beat the mixture until it becomes light and fluffy. Set to chill in the refrigerator while you prepare the cocoa.
2. Warm a medium saucepan over medium-low heat and combine two tablespoons of water, the cocoa powder, and the remainder of the erythritol. Stir.
3. Kick the heat back up to medium.
4. Once smooth, add the remaining heavy cream and water. Stir continuously to combine.
5. Stir the vanilla into the mixture and allow it to get nice and hot, to your preference.
6. Pour the mixture into your favorite mug and serve topped with about two tablespoons of your whipped cream in the refrigerator.

NUTRITION:

Calories: 320 Carbohydrates: 9 grams Fat: 31 grams
Protein: 1 gram

193. CARROT CAKE CHIA PUDDING

COOKING: 0'   **PREPARATION: 15'**   **SERVINGS: 4**

INGREDIENTS

» ¼ c. chia seeds
» ½ tsp. erythritol or comparable measure of preferred sweetener
» 1 ½ tsp. Cinnamon, ground
» ¼ tsp. Nutmeg, ground
» ¼ tsp. ginger, ground
» 1 c. carrot, grated
» 1 tsp. vanilla extract
» 1 c. Greek yogurt, plain
» ½ c. pecans, toasted
» 1 1/3 c. almond milk, unsweetened

DIRECTIONS

1. Mix chia seeds with seasonings, carrot, and almond milk in a bowl. Stir to combine thoroughly.
2. Let chill for 30 minutes so the chia seeds can swell. The mixture will become very thick like a pudding.
3. Remove mixture from the refrigerator and stir the yogurt into it.
4. Top with toasted pecans.
5. Serve chilled!

NUTRITION:

Calories: 123 Carbohydrates: 6 grams Fat: 15 grams
Protein: 9 grams

194. CARROT CAKE ENERGY BALLS

COOKING: 0' **PREPARATION: 15'** **SERVINGS: 8**

INGREDIENTS

» ¼ c. coconut, shredded & unsweetened
» ¼ c. sugar-free maple syrup
» ½ c. carrot, grated
» ½ tsp. cinnamon, ground
» 1 c. almond flour
» 1/3 c. coconut flour
» 1/8 tsp. ginger, ground
» 1/8 tsp. nutmeg, ground
» 3 tbsp. erythritol or comparable measure of preferred sweetener

DIRECTIONS

1. Combine all fixing except for the shredded coconut and pulse until a thick dough is formed.
2. If the dough is too wet, add a little extra flour and pulse. If the dough is too dry, add a bit more of water and pulse.
3. Once the dough has reached the desired consistency, take about a tablespoon of dough at a time and roll it into a smooth ball.
4. Roll each ball through the shredded coconut to coat thoroughly and set on the baking sheet in an even layer.
5. Once you've rolled out all your balls, set them in the refrigerator for 30 minutes to become firm.
6. Keep stored in the refrigerator, in an airtight container for a snack, or serve chilled to guests!

NUTRITION:

Calories: 105 Carbohydrates: 3 grams Fat: 9 grams Protein: 1 gram

195. CARAMEL PECAN MUFFINS

COOKING: 20' **PREPARATION: 10'** **SERVINGS: 8**

INGREDIENTS

» **For the Muffins:**
» ¼ c. coconut flour
» ¼ c. coconut milk, canned & unsweetened
» ½ c. almond flour
» 1 ½ scoops vanilla protein powder of choice
» 1 ½ tbsp. coconut oil, melted
» 1 lb. egg, beaten
» 1 tsp. baking powder
» 1/8 tsp. sea salt
» 3 tbsp. erythritol
» or comparable measure of preferred sweetener
» **For the Filling:**
» ¼ c. water
» ¼ c. erythritol
» 1 egg, yolk only
» 2 tbsp. Coconut oil
» ½ tsp. Vanilla extract
» ¼ tsp. Yacon syrup
» ¼ tsp. Sea salt
» ¼ tsp. Cinnamon, ground
» ½ c. pecans, chopped

DIRECTIONS

1. Heat-up the oven to 350° Fahrenheit.
2. In a large sauté pan, combine all the filling ingredients (except the pecans). Warm them over medium heat, continually stirring until it begins to bubble.
3. Allow the filling to bubble for about 30 seconds, kill the heat, and set the pan on a cold burner or trivet. The mixture should have a slight thickness but will be a little thinner than the traditional caramel.
4. Stir the pecans into the filling until thoroughly incorporated and set aside.
5. In a large mixing bowl, combine all dry ingredients for the muffins, whisking to combine.
6. In a smaller bowl, combine the wet ingredients for the muffins and whisk to combine.
7. Mix the wet and the dry fixing. Beat.
8. Once the mixture is smooth, scoop a little batter into each cup to cover the bottoms.
9. Spoon a teaspoon of the filling into each muffin liner then top each with the bowl's remaining batter.
10. Add small dollops of caramel to each muffin's tops, using a toothpick, give each a quick swirl to give the muffin a swirled and delicious top.
11. Bake within 18 to 22 minutes, then cool for about minutes before removing from the tin.
12. Serve warm!

NUTRITION:

Calories: 95 Carbohydrates: 12 grams Fat: 13 grams
Protein: 4 grams

196. CINNAMON ROLL COOKIES

COOKING: 6'   **PREPARATION: 25'**   **SERVINGS: 16**

INGREDIENTS

- For the Cookies:
- ¼ c. coconut flour
- ¼ c. erythritol or comparable measure of preferred sweetener
- ¼ tsp. xanthan gum
- ½ tsp. vanilla extract
- ¾ c. almond flour
- 1 tbsp. egg whites
- 1/8 tsp. baking soda
- 1/8 tsp. sea salt
- 3 tbsp. butter, cubed
- For the Filling:
- ½ tbsp. butter, melted
- ½ tsp. cinnamon, ground
- 2 tsp. erythritol or comparable measure of preferred sweetener
- For the Frosting:
- 1 tbsp. coconut oil
- 1 tsp. erythritol or comparable measure of preferred sweetener
- 1/8 tsp. vanilla extract
- 3 tbsp. cream cheese

NUTRITION:

Calories: 55

Carbohydrates: 4 grams

Fat: 5 grams Protein: 1 gram

DIRECTIONS

1. Mix all the dry ingredients for the cookie dough in a bowl.
2. Drop the cubes of butter into the dough and use your hands to crumble it into the mixture of dry ingredients.
3. Stir the wet ingredients into the dough mix and combine until a smooth dough begins to form. You may need to let it stand for about five minutes once it's soft to allow it to firm up.
4. On a baking sheet, place a piece of parchment paper.
5. Turn your cookie dough out onto the parchment paper and shape it into a long rectangular sheet. You may need to place parchment paper on top of the dough to make it easier to roll out. Try to ensure that it is of even thickness (about half an inch) all the way through.
6. Chill the baking sheet, then allow the dough to chill and firm up for about 20 minutes.
7. Grease the dough with melted butter, then put the filling ingredients over the dough, spreading them evenly.
8. Take hold of one of the short sides of the dough and roll it up tightly.
9. Cut the dough into disks about a quarter of an inch thick and place onto a baking sheet lined with parchment paper.
10. Chill the baking sheet for another 20 minutes and set the oven to preheat to 350° Fahrenheit.
11. Bake the cookies for 7 minutes or until an inserted toothpick comes out clean.
12. Mix all the fixing for the frosting and dip, drizzle into the cookies.
13. Serve and enjoy!

197. ZUCCHINI COOKIES

COOKING: 12'   **PREPARATION: 10'**   **SERVINGS: 10**

INGREDIENTS

- 1 egg, beaten
- tsp. vanilla extract
- zucchini, grated ned
- nd flour
- llium husk
- nthan
- ground
- ½ c. sugar-free chocolate chips
- ¼ tsp. Sea salt
- ¼ tsp. nutmeg, ground
- 1/3 c. butter softened
- 2/3 c. erythritol or comparable measure of preferred sweetener

ams Fat: 10 grams

DIRECTIONS

1. Heat-up the oven to 350° Fahrenheit and line a baking sheet with parchment paper.
2. In a medium mixing bowl, combine sweetener, eggs, vanilla, and butter. Mix until thoroughly combined.
3. Add zucchini to the bowl and mix once more.
4. Stir the psyllium husk powder (or xanthan gum), cinnamon, nutmeg, salt, and baking powder into the bowl and form a smooth batter.
5. Using your spoon or spatula, fold the sugar-free chocolate chips into the batter.
6. Make 10 evenly-sized blobs of dough on your cookie sheet, taking care to space them evenly. Flatten each chunk just a little bit, so the dough is more cookie-shaped.
7. Bake for 11 to 12 minutes or until the edges begin to crisp up.
8. Let stand for about 10 minutes, then move to a cooling rack.
9. Serve and enjoy!

128

194. CARROT CAKE ENERGY BALLS

COOKING: 0'   **PREPARATION: 15'**   **SERVINGS: 8**

INGREDIENTS

» ¼ c. coconut, shredded & unsweetened
» ¼ c. sugar-free maple syrup
» ½ c. carrot, grated
» ½ tsp. cinnamon, ground
» 1 c. almond flour
» 1/3 c. coconut flour
» 1/8 tsp. ginger, ground
» 1/8 tsp. nutmeg, ground
» 3 tbsp. erythritol or comparable measure of preferred sweetener

DIRECTIONS

1. Combine all fixing except for the shredded coconut and pulse until a thick dough is formed.
2. If the dough is too wet, add a little extra flour and pulse. If the dough is too dry, add a bit more of water and pulse.
3. Once the dough has reached the desired consistency, take about a tablespoon of dough at a time and roll it into a smooth ball.
4. Roll each ball through the shredded coconut to coat thoroughly and set on the baking sheet in an even layer.
5. Once you've rolled out all your balls, set them in the refrigerator for 30 minutes to become firm.
6. Keep stored in the refrigerator, in an airtight container for a snack, or serve chilled to guests!

NUTRITION:

Calories: 105 Carbohydrates: 3 grams Fat: 9 grams Protein: 1 gram

195. CARAMEL PECAN MUFFINS

COOKING: 20'   **PREPARATION: 10'**   **SERVINGS: 8**

INGREDIENTS

» **For the Muffins:**
» ¼ c. coconut flour
» ¼ c. coconut milk, canned & unsweetened
» ½ c. almond flour
» 1 ½ scoops vanilla protein powder of choice
» 1 ½ tbsp. coconut oil, melted
» 1 lb. egg, beaten
» 1 tsp. baking powder
» 1/8 tsp. sea salt
» 3 tbsp. erythritol
» or comparable measure of preferred sweetener
» **For the Filling:**
» ¼ c. water
» ¼ c. erythritol
» 1 egg, yolk only
» 2 tbsp. Coconut oil
» ½ tsp. Vanilla extract
» ¼ tsp. Yacon syrup
» ¼ tsp. Sea salt
» ¼ tsp. Cinnamon, ground
» ½ c. pecans, chopped

DIRECTIONS

1. Heat-up the oven to 350° Fahrenheit.
2. In a large sauté pan, combine all the filling ingredients (except the pecans). Warm them over medium heat, continually stirring until it begins to bubble.
3. Allow the filling to bubble for about 30 seconds, kill the heat, and set the pan on a cold burner or trivet. The mixture should have a slight thickness but will be a little thinner than the traditional caramel.
4. Stir the pecans into the filling until thoroughly incorporated and set aside.
5. In a large mixing bowl, combine all dry ingredients for the muffins, whisking to combine.
6. In a smaller bowl, combine the wet ingredients for the muffins and whisk to combine.
7. Mix the wet and the dry fixing. Beat.
8. Once the mixture is smooth, scoop a little batter into each cup to cover the bottoms.
9. Spoon a teaspoon of the filling into each muffin liner, then top each with the bowl's remaining batter.
10. Add small dollops of caramel to each muffin's tops and, using a toothpick, give each a quick swirl to give the muffin a swirled and delicious top.
11. Bake within 18 to 22 minutes, then cool for about 10 minutes before removing from the tin.
12. Serve warm!

NUTRITION:

Calories: 95 Carbohydrates: 12 grams Fat: 13 grams
Protein: 4 grams

196. CINNAMON ROLL COOKIES

COOKING: 6'   **PREPARATION: 25'**   **SERVINGS: 16**

INGREDIENTS

- » For the Cookies:
- » ¼ c. coconut flour
- » ¼ c. erythritol or comparable measure of preferred sweetener
- » ¼ tsp. xanthan gum
- » ½ tsp. vanilla extract
- » ¾ c. almond flour
- » 1 tbsp. egg whites
- » 1/8 tsp. baking soda
- » 1/8 tsp. sea salt
- » 3 tbsp. butter, cubed
- » For the Filling:
- » ½ tbsp. butter, melted
- » ½ tsp. cinnamon, ground
- » 2 tsp. erythritol or comparable measure of preferred sweetener
- » For the Frosting:
- » 1 tbsp. coconut oil
- » 1 tsp. erythritol or comparable measure of preferred sweetener
- » 1/8 tsp. vanilla extract
- » 3 tbsp. cream cheese

DIRECTIONS

1. Mix all the dry ingredients for the cookie dough in a bowl.
2. Drop the cubes of butter into the dough and use your hands to crumble it into the mixture of dry ingredients.
3. Stir the wet ingredients into the dough mix and combine until a smooth dough begins to form. You may need to let it stand for about five minutes once it's soft to allow it to firm up.
4. On a baking sheet, place a piece of parchment paper.
5. Turn your cookie dough out onto the parchment paper and shape it into a long rectangular sheet. You may need to place parchment paper on top of the dough to make it easier to roll out. Try to ensure that it is of even thickness (about half an inch) all the way through.
6. Chill the baking sheet, then allow the dough to chill and firm up for about 20 minutes.
7. Grease the dough with melted butter, then put the filling ingredients over the dough, spreading them evenly.
8. Take hold of one of the short sides of the dough and roll it up tightly.
9. Cut the dough into disks about a quarter of an inch thick and place onto a baking sheet lined with parchment paper.
10. Chill the baking sheet for another 20 minutes and set the oven to preheat to 350° Fahrenheit.
11. Bake the cookies for 7 minutes or until an inserted toothpick comes out clean.
12. Mix all the fixing for the frosting and dip, drizzle into the cookies.
13. Serve and enjoy!

NUTRITION:

Calories: 55

Carbohydrates: 4 grams

Fat: 5 grams Protein: 1 gram

197. ZUCCHINI COOKIES

COOKING: 12'   **PREPARATION: 10'**   **SERVINGS: 10**

INGREDIENTS

- » 1 egg, beaten
- » 2 tsp. vanilla extract
- » ½ c. zucchini, grated & drained
- » 1 c. almond flour
- » ¼ tsp. Psyllium husk powder or xanthan gum
- » ½ tsp. baking powder
- » 1 tsp. Cinnamon, ground
- » ½ c. sugar-free chocolate chips
- » ¼ tsp. Sea salt
- » ¼ tsp. nutmeg, ground
- » 1/3 c. butter softened
- » 2/3 c. erythritol or comparable measure of preferred sweetener

DIRECTIONS

1. Heat-up the oven to 350° Fahrenheit and line a baking sheet with parchment paper.
2. In a medium mixing bowl, combine sweetener, eggs, vanilla, and butter. Mix until thoroughly combined.
3. Add zucchini to the bowl and mix once more.
4. Stir the psyllium husk powder (or xanthan gum), cinnamon, nutmeg, salt, and baking powder into the bowl and form a smooth batter.
5. Using your spoon or spatula, fold the sugar-free chocolate chips into the batter.
6. Make 10 evenly-sized blobs of dough on your cookie sheet, taking care to space them evenly. Flatten each chunk just a little bit, so the dough is more cookie-shaped.
7. Bake for 11 to 12 minutes or until the edges begin to crisp up.
8. Let stand for about 10 minutes, then move to a cooling rack.
9. Serve and enjoy!

NUTRITION:

Calories: 105 Carbohydrates: 2 grams Fat: 10 grams

Protein: 2 grams

198. MINT CHOCOLATE PIE

COOKING: 0' **PREPARATION: 15'** **SERVINGS: 10**

INGREDIENTS

- ¼ c. almond flour
- ½ c. erythritol or comparable measure of preferred sweetener, powdered
- ½ c. mint, fresh & chopped
- 2 drops green food coloring
- 2 ½ c. heavy cream, divided
- 2 tsp. gelatin powder, unflavored
- 3 tbsp. water
- 4 eggs, yolks only
- 4 tbsp. butter, melted
- 5 tbsp. erythritol or comparable measure of preferred sweetener, granulated
- 6 tbsp. cocoa powder, unsweetened

DIRECTIONS

1. Mix almond flour, granulated erythritol, and cocoa powder in a bowl. Whisk to combine thoroughly.
2. Stir butter into the mixture until nice and crumbly.
3. Press the mixture into a pie plate, making sure to push it up the dish's sides.
4. Set the crust to chill in the refrigerator until you're ready for it.
5. Warm 1 ½ cups of the cream cheese and the mint in medium heat, stirring thoroughly to keep smooth.
6. When the mixture is hot, kill the heat, cover the pan, and let it stand on a cold burner or trivet for 30 minutes.
7. Pour the cream cheese mixture through a strainer into a mixing bowl. Use a plastic or silicone spatula to push the cream through the strainer without the leaves. Set the cream aside.
8. Whisk the water and gelatin until it's fully dissolved in medium-heat. Slowly stir the cream mixture into the water and continue to whisk until the mixture is entirely smooth and hot all the way through.
9. In another bowl, beat the egg yolks and powdered erythritol. Beat until smooth.
10. Take one cup of the cream mixture and slowly stir it into the egg yolks, constantly whisking so they don't seize.
11. Once the cream's cup is thoroughly mixed in, mix the egg mixture into the remainder of the cream over heat and whisk until it thickens to a puddling-like consistency.
12. Stir the food coloring (optional) into the mix and beat until peaks form in the cream.
13. Fill the pie crust with the creamy mixture and use your spoon or spatula to smooth the top.
14. Chill for about three hours, then slice and serve chilled!

NUTRITION:

Calories: 161 Carbohydrates: 2 grams Fat: 14 grams Protein: 5 grams

199. CHOCOLATE TRUFFLE BALLS

COOKING: 0' **PREPARATION: 15'** **SERVINGS: 12**

INGREDIENTS

- ½ c. butter, melted
- ½ c. erythritol or comparable measure of preferred sweetener
- 1 ¼ c. almond flour
- 1 ½ tsp. vanilla extract
- 1 pinch salt
- 1 tbsp. coconut oil
- 3 oz. sugar-free chocolate, chopped
- 6 tbsp. cocoa powder

DIRECTIONS

1. In a medium mixing bowl, combine the erythritol, almond flour, salt, and cocoa powder. Whisk to combine
2. Stir the butter and vanilla into the mixture and allow the dough to form.
3. Mix until the desired consistency is reached.
4. Use a spoon, take enough dough out of the bowl to form one-inch balls, roll them in your palms, and lay them in one even layer on the parchment paper.
5. Chill the balls about an hour to allow them to be firm enough to stand up to chocolate dipping.
6. In a double boiler or a heat-resistant glass bowl over boiling water, warm the chocolate and the coconut oil, continually stirring to make a coating.
7. Once the mixture is smooth, remove it from the boiler and place it on a trivet.
8. Gently dip and roll each ball in the coating (using two forks is a great way to move the balls and pull them out without burning your fingers), then place back on the parchment.
9. Once all the balls are coated, place all the truffles into the refrigerator for about an hour to stiffen.
10. If you have chocolate coating leftover, set it to cool until the truffles are done chilling.
11. Put back the batter to the double boiler to melt once again, then drizzle the remaining chocolate on top of the truffle balls.
12. Chill and serve.

NUTRITION:

Calories: 87 Carbohydrates: 7 grams Fat: 8 grams Protein: 2 grams

200. PEANUT BUTTER CHOCOLATE CUPCAKES

COOKING: 20' **PREPARATION: 15'** **SERVINGS: 12**

INGREDIENTS

- » 1 c. peanut flour
- » ¾ c. cocoa powder, unsweetened
- » 2 tsp. baking powder
- » 1 pinch Salt
- » 4 egg whites
- » ¾ c. erythritol or comparable measure of preferred sweetener, powdered
- » ½ tsp. stevia powdered
- » ½ tbsp. vanilla extract
- » 12 tbsp. butter, melted
- » ¾ c. almond milk, unsweetened
- » 1 ½ c. sugar-free peanut butter

DIRECTIONS

1. Heat-up the oven to 350° Fahrenheit, then line a muffin tin with paper liners.
2. In a bowl, mix the flour, baking powder, cocoa powder, and salt. Whisk to combine.
3. In another bowl, mix eggs, sweeteners, and vanilla.
4. Whisk the melted butter and almond milk in with the other wet ingredients.
5. Mix all the dry ingredients into the wet and create a smooth batter with no lumps.
6. Spoon the batter into the cups (they won't rise too much).
7. Bake for 18 to 20 minutes or until an inserted toothpick comes out clean.
8. Let cool for about five minutes in the muffin tin, then set them out on wire racks to cool completely.
9. Using two tablespoons for each cupcake, frost with peanut butter.
10. Serve and enjoy!

NUTRITION:

Calories: 340 Carbohydrates: 6.5 grams Fat: 30.5 grams Protein: 12.5 grams

CHAPTER 9. 30 DAYS MEAL PLAN FOR WOMEN

Day	Breakfast	Lunch	Snack	Dinner	Dessert
1	Almond Coconut Egg Wraps	Turkey & Cream Cheese Sauce	Parmesan Cheese Strips	Baked Zucchini Noodles with Feta	Sugar-Free Lemon Bars
2	Bacon & Avocado Omelet	Baked Salmon & Pesto	Peanut Butter Power Granola	Brussels Sprouts with Bacon	Creamy Hot Chocolate
3	Bacon & Cheese Frittata	Keto Chicken with Butter & Lemon	Homemade Graham Crackers	Bunless Burger- Keto Style	Delicious Coffee Ice Cream
4	Bacon & Egg Breakfast Muffins	Garlic Chicken	Keto no Bake Cookies	Coffee BBQ Pork Belly	Fatty Bombs with Cinnamon and Cardamom
5	Bacon Hash	Salmon Skewers & Wrapped with Prosciutto	Swiss Cheese Crunchy Nachos	Garlic & Thyme Lamb Chops	Raspberry Mousse

6	Bagel with Cheese	Buffalo Drumsticks & Chili Aioli	Homemade Thin Mints	Jamaican Jerk Pork Roast	Quick & Simple Brownie
7	Baked Apples	Slow Cooked Roasted Pork & Creamy Gravy	Mozzarella Cheese Pockets	Keto Meatballs	Cute Peanut Balls
8	Baked Eggs in the Avocado	Bacon-Wrapped Meatloaf	No-Bake Coconut Cookies	Mixed Vegetables Patties-Instant Pot	Chocolate Mug Muffins
9	Banana Pancakes	Lamb Chops & Herb Butter	Cheesy Cauliflower Breadsticks	Roasted Leg of Lamb	Chocolate Spreads with Hazelnuts
10	Breakfast Skillet	Crispy Cuban Pork Roast	Easy Peanut Butter Cups	Salmon Pasta	Keto Peanut Butter Cup Style Fudge
11	Brunch BLT Wrap	Keto Barbecued Ribs	Fried Green Beans Rosemary	Skillet Fried Cod	Keto and Fairy-Free Vanilla Custard
12	Cheesy Bacon & Egg Cups	Turkey Burgers & Tomato Butter	Crispy Broccoli Popcorn	Slow-Cooked Kalua Pork & Cabbage	Keto Triple Chocolate Mug Cake
13	Coconut Keto Porridge	Keto Hamburger	Cheesy Cauliflower Croquettes	Steak Pinwheels	Keto Cheesecake Stuffed Brownies
14	Cream Cheese Eggs	Chicken Wings & Blue Cheese Dressing	Spinach in Cheese Envelopes	Tangy Shrimp	Keto Raspberry Ice Cream

15	Creamy Basil Baked Sausage	Salmon Burgers with Lemon Butter & Mash	Cheesy Mushroom Slices	Chicken Salad with Champagne Vinegar	Chocolate Macadamia Nut Fat Bombs
16	Banana Waffles	Egg Salad Recipe	Asparagus Fries	Mexican Beef Salad	Keto Peanut Butter Chocolate Bars
17	Keto Cinnamon Coffee	Taco Stuffed Avocados	Kale Chips	Cherry Tomatoes Tilapia Salad	Salted Toffee Nut Cups
18	Keto Waffles & Blueberries	Buffalo Shrimp Lettuce Wraps	Guacamole	Crunchy Chicken Milanese	Crisp Meringue Cookies
19	Baked Avocado Eggs	Broccoli Bacon Salad	Zucchini Noodles	Parmesan Baked Chicken	Instant Pot Matcha Cookies
20	Mushroom Omelet	Keto Egg Salad	Cauliflower Souffle	Cheesy Bacon and Broccoli Chicken	Matcha Skillet Souffle
21	Chocolate Sea Salt Smoothie	Loaded Cauliflower Salad	No-Churn Ice Cream	Buttery Garlic Chicken	Flourless Keto Brownies
22	Zucchini Lasagna	Caprese Zoodles	Cheesecake Cupcakes	Creamy Slow Cooker Chicken	Tropical Chocolate Mousse Bites
23	Vegan Keto Scramble	Zucchini Sushi	Chocolate Peanut Butter Cups	Braised Chicken Thighs with Kalamata Olives	Coconut Raspberry Slice

24	Bavarian Cream with Vanilla and Hazelnuts	Asian Chicken Lettuce Wraps	Low-Carb Almond Coconut Sandies	Baked Garlic and Paprika Chicken Legs	White Chocolate Bark
25	Vanilla Mousse	California Burger Bowls	Crème Brulee	Chicken Curry with Masala	Keto Hot Chocolate
26	Blueberry Mousse	Parmesan Brussels Sprouts Salad	Chocolate Fat Bomb	Chicken Quesadilla	Carrot Cake Chia Pudding
27	Strawberry Bavarian	Chicken Taco Avocados	Cocoa Mug Cake	Slow Cooker BBQ Ribs	Carrot Cake Energy Balls
28	Almond Mousse	Keto Quesadillas	Dark Chocolate Espresso Paleo & Keto Mug Cake	Barbacoa Beef Roast	Caramel Pecan Muffins
29	Nougat	No-Bread Italian Subs	Keto Matcha Mint Bars	Beef & Broccoli Roast	Cinnamon Roll Cookies
30	Chocolate Crepes	Basil Avocado frail Salad Wraps & Sweet Potato Chips	Keto No-Churn Blueberry Maple Ice cream	Cauliflower and Pumpkin Casserole	Zucchini Cookies

CHAPTER 10. 30 DAYS MEAL PLAN FOR MEN

Day	Breakfast	Lunch	Snack	Dinner	Dessert
1	Rusk with Walnut Cream	Cauliflower Leek Soup	Chocolate Fat Bomb	Thai Beef salad Tears of the Tiger	Mint Chocolate Pie
2	Bavarian Coffee with Hazelnuts	Sugar-free Blueberry Cottage Cheese Parfaits	Cocoa Mug Cake	Stuffed Apples with Shrimp	Chocolate Truffle Balls
3	Strawberry Butter Bavarian	Low-Calorie Cheesy Broccoli Leek Soup	Dark Chocolate Espresso Paleo & Keto Mug Cake	Grilled Chicken Salad with Oranges	Peanut Butter Chocolate Cupcakes
4	Cheese Platters	Low Carb Chicken Taco Soup	Keto Matcha Mint Bars	Red Curry with Vegetables	Caramel Pecan Muffins
5	Hazelnut Bavarian with Hot Coffee Drink	Keto Chicken & Veggies Soup	Keto No-Churn Blueberry Maple Ice Cream	Baked Turkey Breast with Cranberry Sauce	Cinnamon Roll Cookies
6	Muffins with Coffee Drink	Low Carb Seafood Soup with Mayo	Keto-Friendly Crackers	Italian Keto Casserole	Zucchini Cookies

7	French toast with Coffee Drink	Keto Tortilla Chips	Parmesan Cheese Strips	Salmon Keto cutlets	Sugar-Free Lemon Bars
8	Almond Coconut Egg Wraps	Chicken Zucchini Alfredo	Peanut Butter Power Granola	Baked Cauliflower	Creamy Hot Chocolate
9	Bacon & Avocado Omelet	Low Carbs Chicken Cheese	Homemade Graham Crackers	Risotto with Mushrooms	Delicious Coffee Ice Cream
10	Bacon & Cheese Frittata	Lemon Chicken Spaghetti Squash Boats	Keto no Bake Cookies	Low Carb Green Bean Casserole	Fatty Bombs with Cinnamon and Cardamom
11	Bacon & Egg Breakfast Muffins	Stuffed Portobello Mushrooms	Swiss Cheese Crunchy Nachos	Avocado Low Carb Burger	Raspberry Mousse
12	Bacon Hash	Low Carbs Mexican Stuffed Bell Peppers	Homemade Thin Mints	Protein Gnocchi with Basil Pesto	Quick & Simple Brownie
13	Bagel with Cheese	Low Carb Broccoli Mash	Mozzarella Cheese Pockets	Summery Bowls with Fresh Vegetables and Protein Quark	Cute Peanut Balls
14	Baked Apples	Roasted Tri-Color Vegetables	No-Bake Coconut Cookies	Beef and Kale Pan	Chocolate Mug Muffins
15	Baked Eggs in the Avocado	Low Carb Broccoli Leek Soup	Cheesy Cauliflower Breadsticks	Salmon and Lemon Relish	Chocolate Spreads with Hazelnuts

16	Banana Pancakes	Turkey & Cream Cheese Sauce	Easy Peanut Butter Cups	Mustard Glazed Salmon	Keto Peanut Butter Cup Style Fudge
17	Breakfast Skillet	Baked Salmon & Pesto	Fried Green Beans Rosemary	Turkey and Tomatoes	Keto and Dairy-Free Vanilla Custard
18	Brunch BLT Wrap	Keto Chicken with Butter & Lemon	Crispy Broccoli Popcorn	Grilled Squid and Tasty Guacamole	Keto Triple Chocolate Mug Cake
19	Cheesy Bacon & Egg Cups	Garlic Chicken	Cheesy Cauliflower Croquettes	Salmon Bowls	Keto Cheesecake Stuffed Brownies
20	Coconut Keto Porridge	Salmon Skewers & Wrapped with Prosciutto	Spinach in Cheese Envelopes	Shrimp & Cauliflower Delight	Keto Raspberry Ice Cream
21	Cream Cheese Eggs	Buffalo Drumsticks & Chili Aioli	Cheesy Mushroom Slices	Scallops and Fennel Sauce	Chocolate Macadamia Nut Fat Bombs
22	Creamy Basil Baked Sausage	Slow Cooked Roasted Pork & Creamy Gravy	Asparagus Fries	Salmon Stuffed with Shrimp	Keto Peanut Butter Chocolate Bars
23	Banana Waffles	Bacon-Wrapped Meatloaf	Kale Chips	Cheesy Pork Casserole	Salted Toffee Nut Cups
24	Keto Cinnamon Coffee	Lamb Chops & Herb Butter	Guacamole	Incredible Salmon Dish	Crisp Meringue Cookies

25	Keto Waffles & Blueberries	Crispy Cuban Pork Roast	Zucchini Noodles	Thai beef salad Tears of the Tiger	Instant Pot Matcha Cookies
26	Baked Avocado Eggs	Keto Barbecued Ribs	Cauliflower Souffle	Stuffed Apples with Shrimp	Matcha Skillet Souffle
27	Mushroom Omelet	Turkey Burgers & Tomato Butter	No-Churn Ice Cream	Grilled Chicken Salad with Oranges	Flourless Keto Brownies
28	Chocolate Sea Salt Smoothie	Keto Hamburger	Cheesecake Cupcakes	Red Curry with Vegetables	Tropical Chocolate Mousse Bites
29	Zucchini Lasagna	Chicken wings & Blue Cheese Dressing	Chocolate Peanut Butter Cups	Baked Turkey Breast with Cranberry Sauce	Coconut Raspberry Slice
30	Vegan Keto Scramble	Salmon Burgers with Lemon Butter & Mash	Low-Carb Almond Coconut Sandies	Italian Keto Casserole	White Chocolate Bark

CONCLUSION

The keto food plan is a low-carb diet designed to place the human frame into a heightened ketogenic state, which might inevitably result in higher pronounced fat burn and weight loss. It is a reasonably accessible food regimen with various keto-friendly meals being readily available in marketplaces at highly low prices. It isn't an eating regimen that is reserved most effectively for the affluent and elite.

Keto diets offer plenty of vitamins per calorie. That is vital because you are older; you need fewer calories. However, you still need an equal number of vitamins as you did in your younger days. You could have a stricter time residing on junk food, not like when you had been younger. This approach is essential to eat foods that guide your health and fight diseases. That can help you live an exciting lifestyle while getting old gracefully. You want to take in more magnificent optimal meals and avoid immoderate and empty calories observed in sugar-wealthy foods like grains. You want to increase the amount of nutrient-wealthy proteins and fat you consume.

Carb-rich ingredients are pushed using society and aren't beneficial to your long-term health. Carb low diets containing excessive quantities of plant and animal fat are way better for increasing insulin sensitivity. It also slows down cognitive decline, making your overall health higher.

It's no longer too late to enhance your possibilities of functioning and feeling as you get older. You can start doing higher and eating higher. Keto for women over 50 years is another danger to repair some of the damage performed in your younger days while you didn't pay attention to what you did eat.

When you begin to make those changes to enhance your weight, immunity, and blood sugar, the better your chances of living better and longer.

All of us get older. However, we will all control our satisfaction with life as we get even older. Keto diets help you enhance your health so that you can thrive instead of being in pains and illness as you get farther away from fifty.

Again, the keto food plan isn't the handiest diet in global health and wellness. You are afforded a wide variety of alternatives and methodologies that you can choose to undertake for yourself. This type of range and diversity inside the enterprise of weight-reduction plan is continually going to be good. This way, people are going with the intention to discover the weight-reduction plan that first-class fits their very own private wishes and their lifestyles. And if you are contemplating adopting the keto food plan for your personal life, then you're going to need to know just how it compares to different options.

It's proper that there are undoubtedly many weight losses plans obtainable at the market, and it'd be too arrogant to say that the keto weight loss plan is high-quality among them all. The keto eating regimen is a high-quality one for you for my part if it takes place to serve your wishes and your goals higher effectively.

As some distance as effectiveness is concerned, there's just no denying how impactful a keto eating regimen maybe for someone who wants to lose a drastic quantity of weight in a wholesome and managed manner. The keto weight-reduction plan also enforces discipline and precision for the agent by incorporating macro counting and meal journaling to ensure accuracy and accountability in the weight-reduction project. There are no external factors that can impact how robust this weight loss plan may be for you. Everything is all within your control.

And lastly, it's a reasonably sustainable weight loss plan because it doesn't merely compromise on taste or range. Sure, there are lots of restrictions. But ultimately, there are lots of alternatives and workarounds that can assist stave off cravings. If these kinds of standards and reasons observe to you and your personal life, then it could genuinely be safe to say that the keto food plan is a high-quality one for you.

Finally, if you enjoyed this book, then I'd like to ask you for a favor, would you be kind enough to leave a review for this book on Amazon? It'd be greatly appreciated!

It would be crucial to help me with this project that I care about a lot. I believe that regardless of the book and the mission that matters. Everybody deserves a healthier and more just life. Maybe people are not aware of it.

Maybe we can help.

With Love,

Jillian Collins

KETO DIET COOKBOOK

for Women after 50

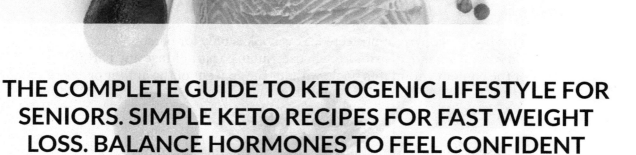

THE COMPLETE GUIDE TO KETOGENIC LIFESTYLE FOR SENIORS. SIMPLE KETO RECIPES FOR FAST WEIGHT LOSS. BALANCE HORMONES TO FEEL CONFIDENT AGAIN. 30-DAY KETO MEAL PLAN

Jillian Collins

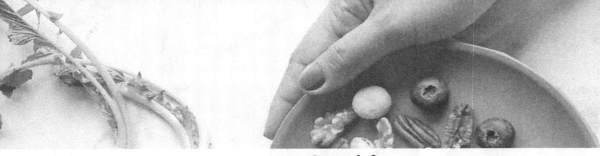

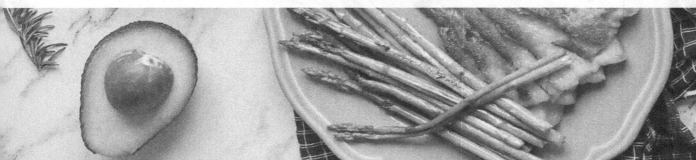

TABLE OF CONTENTS

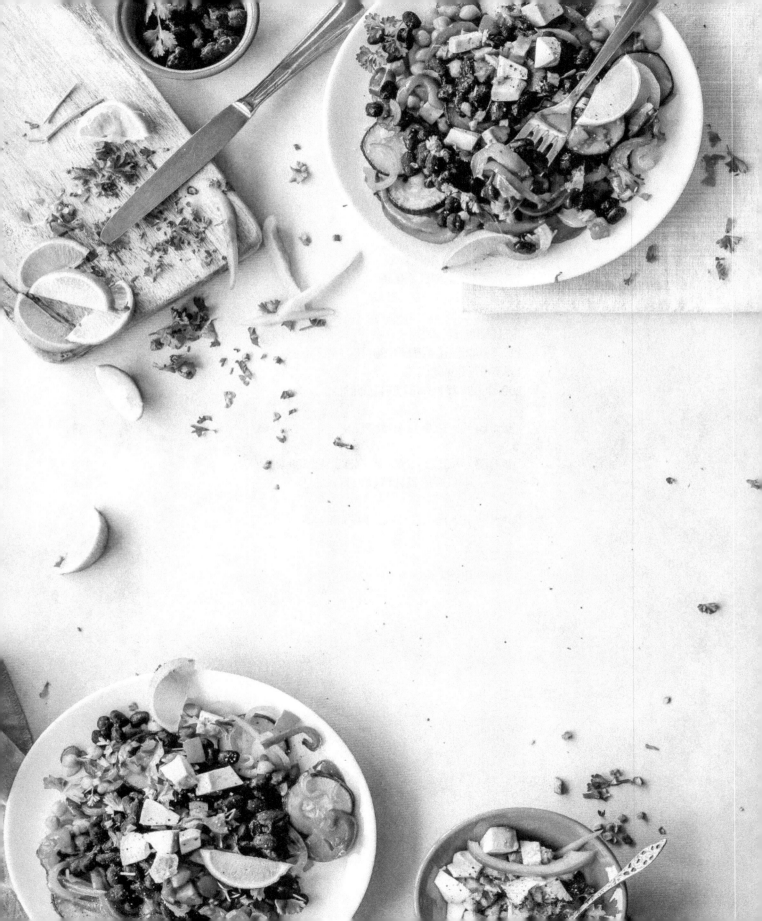

INTRODUCTION

Although I'm 53, I feel fit and super energetic. I eat what I want, I don't deprive myself of my pleasures, and I don't need to spend hours in the gym. I don't feel guilty when I eat ice cream. I go to work and go out with my friends without my menopause, bothering me anymore.

It may seem impossible, but it is.

As women, when our age grows at 50, we are always looking for a quick and effective way to shed our excess weight, get our high blood sugar levels under control, reduce overall inflammation, and improve our physical and mental energy. It's frustrating to have all of these issues, especially the undeniable fats in our belly. Good thing that I found this great solution to all our worries when we reach this age level, and when our body gets weaker as time goes by. The Ketogenic diet plans.

As a woman at this age, we all know that it is much more difficult for us to lose weight than men. I have lived on a starvation level diet and exercise like a triathlete and only lose five pounds. A man will stop putting dressing on his salad and will lose twenty pounds. It just not fair. But we have the fact that we are women to blame. Women naturally have more standing between ourselves and weight loss than men do.

The mere fact that we, women, is the largest single contributor to why we find it difficult to lose weight. Since our bodies always think it needs to be prepared for a possible pregnancy, we will naturally have more body fat and less mass in our muscles than men.

Being in menopause will also cause us to add more pounds to our bodies, especially in the lower half. After menopause, our metabolism naturally slows down. Our hormones levels will decrease. These two factors alone will cause weight gain in the post-menopausal period.

There are numerous diet plan options offered to help shed weight, but the

Ketogenic diet has been the most preferred lately. We've got many concerns around keto's effectiveness and exactly how to follow the diet plan in a healthy and balanced means.

The ketogenic diet for ladies at the age or over 50 is an easy and ideal way to shed extra pounds, stay energetic, and enjoy a healthy life. It does not only balances hormones but also improves our body capabilities without causing any harm to our overall wellness. Thus, if you are fighting with post-menopausal symptoms and other health issues, you should do a Keto diet right away!

A Keto diet is a lifestyle, not a diet so, treat it like the same. The best way to approach keto to gain maximum benefits, especially for women over 50s, is to treat it as a lifestyle. You can't restrict your meal intake through obstructive and strict diets forever, right? It's the fundamental reason fad diets fail — we limit ourselves from too much to get rapid results, then we're are right back again at the weight where we started, or God forbid worse.

Keto is not a kind of diet that can be followed strictly forever — unless you need it as a therapeutic diet (i.e., epilepsy), a very narrow category. In keto diet, we slowly transit into a curative state that we can withstand forever in a healthier way.

So, for me, being on a keto diet does not mean that I will be in ketosis forever. Instead, it means letting myself love consideration, such as a few desserts while vacationing or partying. It does not set me back to enjoy these desserts and let me consider it as the end of the diet. I can wake up the following morning and go back to the keto lifestyle, most suitable for me and my body consistently.

It allows my body to boost its fat loss drastically in many cases, which helps in decreasing pockets of undesirable fat.

With Keto Diet, it's not only giving weight loss assistance to reduce my weight, yet it can likewise ward off yearnings for unhealthy foods and protect me against calories collisions throughout the day. That is why I want it to share with you how promising this Keto diet. As our age grow older, we must not let our body do the same. Focus your mindset on this fantastic diet, read, apply, and enjoy its best benefits.

Within this guide, you will find everything you need to transition to your new lifestyle. You will understand why our body after 50 starts to change and how to manage these changes.I will describe the 2 monsters of Menopause that lurk latent in your body and how to defuse them. We will see how the Ketogenic process will activate fat-burning hormones, activating weight loss regularly, and naturally giving you your perfect shape you desire. To help you, I have included over 200 simple and delicious recipes with ingredients that you can find in your neighborhood.

I know it could be frustrating to choose the dishes, so I have included a 30-day meal plan so you won't waste time. The aim is to leave without getting discouraged!

What I promise you after you read the full guide of Keto Diet for Women after 50 and apply it to your daily lifestyle, especially the 30 days meal plan, you will achieve more than losing weight but also the new and improve healthier

you!

THANK YOU

I hope you'll enjoy these book; is part of the larger labor of love, which led me to create this project. I've put a lot of time, effort, and commitment into providing you with the only guide you'll need to understand how to approach the Ketogenic Diet, start a new lifestyle, and feel happy and Healthy again. All I ask in return is that if you love this book, please leave me an honest review.

I will read all with attention.

Thank you.

CHAPTER 1 - WHY KETO?

The thing about the foods on the Keto Diet is that they deliver a ton of great nutrition and are packed with nutrients. If you have heard of superfoods, well, the Keto Diet is all about leveraging the food you eat for maximum benefit. But even though seniors need fewer calories than their younger counterparts, they do need the same amount of nutrients, and that is a place where the Keto Diet is of great assistance.

IS THE KETOGENIC DIET HEALTHY FOR WOMEN AFTER 50?

The reality is that women aged 50 and older will not have an easy time living on junk food the way they could when they were younger. The body does not snap back the way it once did, and that is why seniors need to be more conscious about the food they are putting in their bodies. The food needs to support their health and fight disease. It is where the quality of life is found and where they can enjoy the years they worked to. Why not spend them in enjoyment instead of being in pain and torment because your diet compromises your ability to enjoy yourself. That is why the Ketogenic diet was built to provide a better and much healthier lifestyle they could ever ask.

When going with the Keto Diet, what ends up happening is that Ketosis helps older people get the nutrition they need to make the most of their senior years instead of suffering through them and lamenting how they can't do what they did when they were younger. It is not how anyone intended to live in their retirement.

WHAT IS KETO?

The ketogenic diet is straightforward in its execution, objective: remain in Ketosis; in any case, the way can be distinctive for every individual. Everybody starts at 20 pure sugars and afterward, after some time, decides what the number of they can expand without being kicked out of Ketosis. I've taken more than 75 net carbs in a day and remained in Ketosis while my significant other, who adhered to his diet and had two chomps, was kicked out of Ketosis. Everybody is different. It's up to each person of us to realize what our own "kick out" point is and remain beneath it.

To figure pure sugars, take the number of starches you devour and subtract the number of fiber grams expended. It is the number you'll use to follow your day by day complete. At the point when nourishment is high in fiber, similar to coconut, you can eat a more significant amount of it regardless of whether the sugar numbers look somewhat terrifying.

When alluding to macros, I'm talking about the equalization of nourishments you eat in a day. They can be categorized as one of the three fundamental macronutrient classes: sugars, proteins, and fat. A few people on the keto diet find that these rates are useful for monitoring their weight reduction and others use them for therapeutic reasons. The off chance that you don't have any therapeutic motivations to adhere to specific rates; at that point, I think a decent day by day beginning stage for the ketogenic diet is 10 percent carbs, 20 percent proteins, and 70 percent fats. If this doesn't keep you in ketosis, attempt 5 percent carbs, 15 percent proteins, and 80 percent fats. At last, it's dependent upon you to discover the parity that works best for you.

There are many number crunchers online that you can use to enter your details, such as weight, stature, sex, weight objective, etc. The adding machine will mention what should be the perfect full scale for you. The measure of carbs (which should, by and large, originate from vegetables) or fats will make Ketosis in the body shifts for various individuals. It is unquestionably not an exact science.

For this guide's plans, the large-scale rates were determined by taking the number of grams of every full scale and duplicating it by the number of calories per gram (9 calories for 1 gram of fat, four calories for 1 gram of carbs or proteins). Afterward, partitioning that by the all outnumber of calories per serving. For instance, envision a dish that has the accompanying nutritional data per serving:

Calories: 184; total fat: 14g; saturated fat: 6g; cholesterol: 224mg.

Sugars: 2g; fiber: 1g; net carbs: 1g; protein: 12g.

To decide the number of a serving's calories originate from fat:

(14 grams of fat) × (9 calories for every gram of fat) = 126 calories from fat

(126 calories from fat for every serving) ÷ (184 complete calories for every serving) = 68.5%

To decide the number of a serving's calories originate from total carbs (not net carbs):

(2 grams of carbs) × (4 calories for every gram of carb) = eight calories from carbs (8 calories from carbs per serving) ÷ (184 all-out calories for each meal) = 4%

To decide the number of a serving's calories originate from protein:

(12 grams of protein) × (4 calories for every gram of protein) = 48 calories from protein

(48 calories from protein for every serving) ÷ (184 all-out calories for each meal) = 26%

Each meal you eat doesn't have to follow these macros; you make a count by the day's end. It enables you to eat a dish of vegetables sautéed in ghee without the need to toss in pancetta.

As you counsel, the macros for every formula in this guide, know that there's a variety among various fixings. For instance, substantial natural cream may have less than one net carb, while a non-natural store-brand may have more. Tomato sauce is another dubious one. Some better assortments of marinara come in as low as four net carbs per ¼ cup since they contain no additional sugar, yet most standard brands have at least 15 net carbs in that equivalent ¼ cup. To appreciate an Italian fix every so often, I suggest spending too much on the great stuff or making your very own sauce.

Even though the ketogenic diet isn't intended to be exclusionary, and you could surely get your 20 net carbs every day from a solitary cut of bread, you presumably won't make it far in a ketogenic way of life. Your glucose will spike and probably show you out of Ketosis, and it won't be any good times. Attempt instead of some rich veggies and obey-gooey fondue, and that cut of bread won't be vital. Keep a watch out: Before long, you will lose your desires for bread!

GETTING INTO KETOSIS

Achieving Ketosis is not as simple as it may sound. Ketosis is achieved when your body starts using ketones instead of glucose as fuel. The liver breaks down excess fats stored in the body to produce ketones. This metabolic condition comes about when carbohydrates in the body are low and instead are replaced by fats. As an older woman on a keto diet, you will realize that your appetite tends to be suppressed because of the foods you consume, and this sense of fullness makes you eat less, making you lose weight when the fats are broken down.

Ketosis not only benefits your body by making you shed some weight, but it also reduces the risk of diseases such as diabetes and blood pressure. Your question now is how to achieve this state of Ketosis to enjoy all its benefits fully. Follow the following simple steps to get into Ketosis quickly:

Fasting

A keto diet's main aim is to lower your carb intake by replacing it with high fat intake. Before you start practicing your keto diet, you need first to detox your body through fasting. Fasting helps remove any carbs present in your body. Lowering the carbs' level makes your transition from the ordinary diet to a keto diet much more manageable. Based on your past eating habits, you may decide to fast for 24, 48, or 72 hours. Therefore, fasting forms the first step that helps you get to Ketosis much faster.

LIMIT YOUR CARB INTAKE

A keto diet is simply a low carb diet where you increase your fat intake, moderate protein intake, and lower carb intake. As a woman at 50 years of age or older, you should look forward to reducing your daily carb intake by consuming foods and drinks that are keto-friendly. For you to achieve Ketosis, your daily carb intake should fall to as low as between 5-10% of your entire diet.

Upon lowering your carb intake, your body will be left with minimal carbs to convert into glucose, and it will have no other option than to break down the excess fats to produce ketones through Ketosis.

INCREASE YOUR INTAKE OF HEALTHY FATS

After lowering your carb intake, your body may become weak if the necessary alternative measures are not taken. That's why you need to ensure you consume enough food, eating enough healthy fats to substitute for the missing carbs.

Consuming the right fatty foods helps regulate your appetite by giving you a feeling of fullness. With a controlled appetite, now and then, you will not need to eat. It gives your body a favorable environment to break down excess fats, making you shed some weight.

MODERATE YOUR INTAKE OF PROTEINS

Having achieved a low-carb intake and an increased fat intake, you now need to check your protein intake. Proteins are essential components of your body since they help in the growth and repair of body tissues. In the absence of proteins, your body muscles will be weak, and this may affect your health at large.

ENGAGE IN PHYSICAL EXERCISE

When your body has a low number of carbs and eventually initiates Ketosis, you will find it that you will have a sluggish feeling anytime you exercise. To prevent your body from becoming lazy during Ketosis, you should incorporate a daily workout routine as you start your keto diet.

SIGNS YOU ARE INTO KETOSIS

You can likewise evaluate how you are feeling to identify whether your body is into Ketosis.

Some individuals might experience "keto influenza." That can last for merely a couple of days or as much as a couple of weeks. It generally consists of signs consisting of headache, nausea, tiredness, sleeping disorders, irregularity, and irritation. Ensuring you remain consuming and hydrated lots of electrolytes can assist in treating these signs quicker.

Other typical symptoms and signs to keep an eye out for consist of:

- Increased thirst and more regular urination

- Keto breathes or fruity-smelling breath

- Dry mouth

- A decline in cravings

- Weight reduction

- Preliminary weak point and tiredness (this must ultimately decrease)

- Insufficient sleep disturbances (this need to likewise diminish)

- Increased energy, psychological clearness, and focus

CHAPTER 2 - KETOGENIC DIET FOR WOMEN AFTER 50

CHANGES IN YOUR BODY AFTER 50

There are many changes in your physical body as you age, and it is not in your hands and not due to any single factor. Many things are working behind the scenes like your lifestyle choices that you make daily or even your genetics. Some factors are genuinely not in your control, but others —like the choices you make— can be altered. So, the decisions you make can literally either make your health or break it.

Some of the changes that occur in a woman's body after the age of 50 are as follows:

MENOPAUSE

The most significant change is menopause, and there is no denying it. Menopause can drastically change the body of a woman. But as the term suggests, menopause does not pause anything but instead causes a shift towards a different hormonal scenario. Your body then learns to strike a new kind of balance after considering its present situation of hormones. But what is more of a rollercoaster ride is not menopause itself but the symptoms that come before it. There are night sweats and hot flashes and drastic mood swings. Some women even face troubles in sleeping, and some can even go into depression.

After menopause, women also face urinary incontinence issues because their muscles in the pelvic region start weakening. Some women face this problem, known as pelvic prolapse, which is a significant reason behind urinary incontinence. If you have had children or are obese, then your risk of urinary incontinence increases further. The weight, in turn, also enhances the chances of developing fibroids in the uterus. These, in the years, can either shrink or develop into more giant tumors. Some of the symptoms that signify that you have fibroids in your uterus are pelvic fullness, frequent urination, painful intercourse, and heavy bleeding.

REDUCTION IN BONE DENSITY

Several studies have proved that osteoporosis is a problem present in greater frequencies in women than in men. It is a condition where your bone density becomes less, rendering your bones weak and thin. And thus, then tend to break very easily. Every woman in her 50s is likely to experience a reduction in their bone density. Also, after menopause, 30% of the bone mass in women is lost. Moreover, if a woman has early menopause, that can cause an even more significant amount of bone loss by the time they reach 55.

Whenever you are in your 50s or have got your menopause before that, get a bone density test done. In case you are already in the risk category of being inflicted by a reduced bone density, you should get tested more. You must also know that certain medications are not particularly good for your bone density and might compromise it. So, getting tried is essential.

LOSS OF MUSCLES

After you turn 50, there is a gradual decrease in muscle mass, and some think this happens in men only. But this is not true. Loss of muscle mass is something that affects everyone, including women. And with this, there is a decrease in your physical strength as well. The best method to avoid this is by engaging in exercises that are all about strength training. It will neutralize the effect a bit. Or, you can practice doing squats and lunges twice or thrice a week in your house itself. There is another benefit that you will derive from these exercises, and that is, you will be able to regain a better sense of balance.

WEAKER JOINTS

With age, your joints will start becoming more fragile, and this is not because of a reduction in bone density, but because the cartilage present around your joints begins to wear down. The effects of these are felt even more when you are over 50. You'll start developing arthritis and joint pain problems, and your posture is also gets affected. Avoid slouching because the more slouch, the more your body lays stress on your joints, and they become weaker. Moreover, you need to keep a check on your weight too. When your body weight increases, your body has to carry that extra weight around even when the joints become weak, making it even more difficult.

SIGNS OF AGING ON SKIN

One of the obvious signs of aging is seen on your skin. There will be spots and fine lines and also a bit of sagging. Even if you maintain your skin a lot, there will be some signs of aging that you cannot avoid. The symptoms will become worse, especially if you were not caring about your skin during your younger years. You might have skipped sunscreen then, but now, doing that will wreak havoc on your skin. Moreover, your skin will get irritated very quickly, and, in some women, it also feels very dry.

The best way to deal with all these changes is to go for regular health screenings to be aware of what is happening in your body.

MENOPAUSE AND KETO DIET

A woman that uses up such a multitude of carbohydrates can begin menopause indications. Let's see how a ketogenic diet plan can assist with the signs and negative effects of this menopause.

CONTROLLING INSULIN LEVELS

By taking place a ketogenic diet plan, females with PCOS (polycystic-over-the-air problem) can help prevent their hormones. Exploration concentrated on the impact of low-glycemic diet plans has shown this influence. PCOS causes insulin affectability fears, to be aided by insulin-decreasing homes of low-glycemic carbohydrates.

FAT LOSS

Menopause can trigger metabolic treatment to alter and also reduce. One of the most widely known complaints of menopause is an increase in body weight and belly fat. A reduced level of estrogen commonly causes weight gain. A diet plan with virtually no carbohydrates is beneficial for decreasing muscle to fat ratio. Ketosis reduces hunger by controlling the development of the 'food cravings hormonal agent' called ghrelin. You are much less ravenous while in ketosis.

A DECREASE IN HOT FLASHES

No person extensively comprehends hot flashes, as well as why they happen. Hormonal adjustments that affect the command post, in all probability, have something to do with this. The switchboard deals with the internal heat's degree. Adjustments in hormonal representatives can also disrupt this indoor regulatory authority. It winds up being significantly sensitive to adjustments in interior warm level levels.

Ketones, in which its creation stimulates all through a ketogenic diet, make a solid wellspring of energy for the mind. Scientists have shown that ketones demo to support the nerve center. The body will handle its temperature degree much better. The proximity of ketones attempts to improve your body's indoor regulator.

EXCELLENT NIGHT'S REST

You will enhance lay while on a ketogenic diet on account of a great deal steadier sugar degree. With substantially increasingly modified hormones and also significantly fewer warm flashes, you will relax much better. Reduced pressure and boosted success are 2 of the advantages of better rest.

THE 2 MONSTERS OF THE MENOPAUSE

Few people know the true symptoms of Menopause, hot flashes are certainly one of them, but none (or almost) remember the following:

- Chronic inflammation

- Chronic stress

These two shadows that lurk in one of the most delicate phases of a woman's life are the ones that must be made beforehand to reduce their physical and emotional impact.

A diction says ...

"Prevention is better than cure."

And in your case, it has never been so true!

But let's go in order ...

CHRONIC INFLAMMATION

Inflammation is one of Mother Nature's most ingenious ploys to regulate toxicity in our body.

This happens when tissue is damaged and congested and loaded with toxins.

It consists of the tissues' vasodilation to ensure that the flow of blood and, therefore, all the repairing elements act on the inflamed area.

So ensure that the influx of these elements is maximal.

Therefore, vasodilation, global dilation of the entire circulatory system to ensure that the influx of repairing and cleaning elements is maximal.

The inflammation also accelerates the metabolism and a rise in temperature so that the process is faster.

Is the inflammatory reaction a very positive thing then?

Of course, yes.

So why is it even so dangerous?

Now imagine ...

this process is managed by our body as there were two pedals:

that of the accelerator and that of the brake.

These two pedals are used to balance the organism and ensure that the process does not pack.

But you don't feel well.

This means that the body no longer regulates the process.

It no longer has the brake and packs up.

The inflammatory reaction becomes too important.

The amount of toxins has become too important, and your body can no longer tolerate it.

The game of inflammation is to bring balance to regulate the process of cleansing from toxins.

It must be tolerated ...

If you pass the maximum limit that the body can tolerate then, you go into chronic inflammation.

This is the reason for many of your problems.

Now,

surely you have already heard about it somewhere

Unfortunately, it is not a topic that is often talked about ...

Nobody tells you:

"Be careful, take care of yourself, your body, and perpetually inflamed, don't wait!"

You simply return to your life bombarded with other news.

The result of such a life without awareness?

Confusion".

You eat what happens at the supermarket, you drink what is on the shelves and give it to your children.

You've been doing it for years now; what will it ever be.

Have you ever wondered why TV or movie stars are always beautiful and happy even during their menopause period?

You may be thinking that they have a lot of money and can get everything!

Believe me, no.

Money cannot buy health.

They've just been aware of these monsters for a long time, and their coaches teach them the right lifestyle.

They are not aliens. They are just charismatic people with a strong mindset.

They want to achieve their goals.

This is the secret of their success.

Not magic.

I want to tell you an anecdote about technology.

There has been news about this disease developed by the excessive use of Social Networks, called "Attention Deficit Disorder" in short ADHAD.

I tell you this because you are aware of a very curious fact ..

The creators of these addictive tools themselves have categorically prohibited the use of their children.

Mmmm ???

Did you turn on the light bulb?

Of course, they know very well what the excessive use of social media entails, and their primary purpose is to keep you attacked as much as possible.

So I want to protect their children from these diseases.

Here this also happens with chronic inflammation.

All doctors know it's there.

But no major media talks about it.

They don't teach it in school.

Can you imagine a world without pharmacies?

A few years ago, inflammation was a problem like any other, a symptom to "extinguish" with the right medicines but not to worry too much.

Although the role of chronic inflammation in diseases has been known for some time, research has brought to light surprising and highly important information about its origins in more recent years.

I invite you to check on google Scholar and inform yourself.

Research continues.

But something can be done right away and is under our control:

Nutrition.

The Ketogenic lifestyle will be your best ally.

Let's look at some causes of chronic inflammation:

1. YOU ARE OVERWEIGHT

If your body has a few extra pounds, it can generate an inflammatory response in the fat cells.

As we age, fatty tissue affects some cells in our body. When this happens, the inflammation is more prone to develop.

Obesity in young people can cause warning signs in fat cells.

What happens is that the immune system starts acting to defend the body, while nothing is harming it.

2. YOU DRINK TOO MUCH ALCOHOL AND CARBONATED DRINKS.

Alcohol = inflammation.

Physiologically, alcohol breaks down in the body. This reaction produces toxic by-products that promote inflammation.

We all know that the liver is the main one involved in any process of decomposition and transformation of alcohol.

This means that when we drink too much alcohol, the liver is the first to have inflammation.

If we do not stop drinking such drinks, we prevent the liver from resting, which will inevitably become toxic.

Finally, we can cause serious problems such as steatosis or fatty liver.

If you build up a lot of fat in addition to consuming a lot of alcohol, you can develop cirrhosis or hepatitis.

3. YOUR CONTRACEPTIVE METHOD

Contraception = inflammation.

During the pre-menopausal period, women tend to control their births in many ways.

Some of them take the birth control pill.

This way, they avoid conceiving in old age but could also promote the causes of inflammation. Pre-menopausal women who take oral contraceptives appear to be more at risk than those who opt-out of the pill.

In 2014, the US magazine PLoS One published preliminary research on this topic.

The study showed that inflammation in women who don't take the pill is minimal.

This does not mean that contraceptives should not be consumed.

Your body needs a cleansing a shower.

He, too, deserves to feel good.

For years he has been at the mercy of an uncontrolled diet of drugs taken as if they were candy and a polluted environment.

Your body is tired.

CHRONIC STRESS

As mentioned above, you and I have grown up in a world where we are continually bombarded with information and consequently, a significant overabundance of "knowledge."

Today everyone knows that if we eat fish, it will provide us with a lot of phosphorus, but why?

We know a lot, and with the advent of the internet and smartphones, this has only made things worse.

Social, blogs, and sites of all kinds are there to create content to let you know something every day.

A continuous bombardment.

This confuses.

But it also causes another thing that leads us to ruin ….

Stress.

This is the second monster.

We are here to try to give you the means to gain control.

Surely on menopause, you will have heard everything about, you will know many things and have sold all kinds of solutions.

Nutrition is, of course, essential, but something is missing …

We must question ourselves and understand how it is that we must live.

I want to tell you a short story.

The story of a GoldFish.

"A goldfish named Pepe lives in the home of a beautiful family.

One day the father who took care of the little fish leaves for work.

A few days later, he receives a call from his son -

"Dad, Pepe is not feeling well!"

Dad: - "What do you mean by not feeling well?"

Son: - "She's swimming on her stomach."

Dad takes his things and goes home.

Arriving home, he goes to the aquarium and immediately notices what was wrong.

The fish didn't feel well because the water was dirty and rotten. "

Nobody had taken care of the little fish.

Now,

There would be two solutions; one is to take Pepe to the Doctor and have him prescribe some medicine, or remove Pepe from that dirty water and clean the aquarium.

Dad chose the second one, and Pepe went back to swimming happily.

Taking inspiration from this story, it is clear that one of the main problems in your life is the environment around you.

A busy life surrounds you with a lifestyle that creates your stress.

Rotten water could be your work environment, the situation at home with your husband, whatever.

Everything out there leads to stress.

Drive a car.

Pay your bills.

Take the children to school.

Prepare dinner.

Listen to your boss giving you orders.

We are constantly seeking solutions for everything.

If you've had a SHIT day, you get home, and your partner has had the same day.

Imagine two atomic bombs meeting. BOOM!

So, you can do all the diets in the world do all the treatments you want, but if you don't change your mental state, it won't change much.

The message is this; everything starts from within into your head.

The real healer is you.

Mind, nature, and time are your best allies.

Ten years of inadequate nutrition and stress don't go away in two days.

Imagine your organs as sponges full of toxins and mucus. Years of foods like cereals, bread, and pasta are like carpet glue.

Now, imagine a kitchen pot full of pasta left there and try to wash it without using your hands or using sponges to scratch or water to rinse?

This is kind of what happens in your body.

It takes time and education to reshape your body.

BENEFITS OF KETO DIET FOR WOMEN AFTER 50
LOSS AND MAINTENANCE OF WEIGHT

Gaining extra pounds (especially around the abdomen) and struggling with controlling the weight are common nuisances that menopausal and post-menopausal women have to deal with. As you can already imagine, this age-related problem is also a result of the decline in estrogen levels.

Going Keto can help you lose weight and burn fat in a couple of ways

Going Keto Decreases Your Appetite

Going Keto Leads to Rapid Weight Loss

Control of Glucose in the Body

Science has found out that decreased estrogen levels can promote insulin resistance, and in turn, increase the blood sugar. Having an insulin resistance, your body is practically immune to the effects of insulin. When that happens, your cells do not open up for glucose to enter, which leaves the blood sugar endlessly traveling in the bloodstream.

A REDUCTION IN RELIANCE ON THE MEDICATIONS-RELATED TO DIABETES

With Keto, you drastically limit your carbs and sugars consumption. With little blood sugar, your body does not need to release insulin to manage it. Thus, you prevent developing diabetes symptoms. If you already have it, the diet helps you to order it.

CONTROL OF HIGH BLOOD PRESSURE

Once you attain 50, you must monitor your blood pressure rates. Reduction in the intake of carbohydrates is a proven way to lower your blood pressure. When you cut down on your carbs and lower your blood sugar levels, you significantly reduce your chances of getting other diseases.

AN IMPROVED MENTAL PERFORMANCE

The keto diet provides your body and brain with a stable fuel source — ketones. The diet prevents sugar swings that are associated with a carb-rich diet. That allows you to avoid brain fog, improves your focus, concentration, and mental clarity.

RESTORATION OF INSULIN SENSITIVITY

That is the first objective of a keto diet. It helps stabilize the insulin levels and thereby improve fat burning. Using a keto diet helps preserve your muscles while burning fat in your body.

IMPROVE CHOLESTEROL LEVELS

It will help reduce blood cholesterol levels by consuming fewer carbohydrates while on the keto diet. That is due to the increased lipolysis condition. That leads to lower levels of LDL cholesterol and higher levels of HDL cholesterol.

SATIETY

Eating protein reduces the ghrelin (the hunger hormone) and stimulates the production of the satiety hormones. When you eat protein, it's transformed into amino acids, which help your body with various processes such as building muscle and regulating immune function

MOST COMMON MISTAKE

Getting energy from fat, not sugar, is a very good approach and, as we have seen, can bring various health benefits. However, if you keep on the ketogenic diet every day, you can make some mistakes. If you know them, you can avoid them and realize their full potential:

Give up before you stop ketosis

Lack of salt and minerals

Consume too much protein

Insufficient fat consumption

Consume bad quality food

Do not introduce the right amount of fiber

Eat raw vegetables

Consume the highest protein load at dinner

Not drinking enough

BENEFITS OF KETO DIET FOR WOMEN AFTER 50
LOSS AND MAINTENANCE OF WEIGHT

Gaining extra pounds (especially around the abdomen) and struggling with controlling the weight are common nuisances that menopausal and post-menopausal women have to deal with. As you can already imagine, this age-related problem is also a result of the decline in estrogen levels.

Going Keto can help you lose weight and burn fat in a couple of ways:

- Decreases appetite

- Leads to rapid weight loss

- Controls glucose in the body

Science has found out that decreased estrogen levels can promote insulin resistance, and in turn, increase the blood sugar. Having an insulin resistance makes your body practically immune to the effects of insulin. When that happens, your cells do not open up for glucose to enter, which leaves the blood sugar endlessly traveling in the bloodstream.

A REDUCTION IN RELIANCE ON THE MEDICATIONS RELATED TO DIABETES

With Keto, you drastically limit your carbs and sugars consumption. With little blood sugar, your body does not need to release insulin to manage it. Thus, you prevent developing diabetes symptoms. If you already have it, the diet helps you to order it.

CONTROL OF HIGH BLOOD PRESSURE

Once you attain 50, you must monitor your blood pressure rates. Reduction in the intake of carbohydrates is a proven way to lower your blood pressure. When you cut down on your carbs and lower your blood sugar levels, you significantly reduce your chances of getting other diseases.

AN IMPROVED MENTAL PERFORMANCE

The keto diet provides your body and brain with a stable fuel source — ketones. The diet prevents sugar swings that are associated with a carb-rich diet. That allows you to avoid brain fog, improves your focus, concentration, and mental clarity.

RESTORATION OF INSULIN SENSITIVITY

That is the first objective of a keto diet. It helps stabilize the insulin levels and thereby improve fat burning. Using a keto diet helps preserve your muscles while burning fat in your body.

IMPROVE CHOLESTEROL LEVELS

It will help reduce blood cholesterol levels by consuming fewer carbohydrates while on the keto diet. That is due to the increased lipolysis condition. That leads to lower levels of LDL cholesterol and higher levels of HDL cholesterol.

SATIETY

Eating protein reduces the ghrelin (the hunger hormone) and stimulates the production of the satiety hormones. When you eat protein, it's transformed into amino acids, which help your body with various processes such as building muscle and regulating immune function

MOST COMMON MISTAKES

Getting energy from fat, not sugar, is a very good approach and, as we have seen, can bring various health benefits. However, if you keep on the ketogenic diet every day, you can make some mistakes. If you know them, you can avoid them and realize their full potential:

- Give up before you stop ketosis

- Lack of salt and minerals

- Consume too much protein

- Insufficient fat consumption

- Consume bad quality food

- Do not introduce the right amount of fiber

- Eat raw vegetables

- Consume the highest protein load at dinner

- Not drinking enough water

CHAPTER 3 - INTERMITTENT FASTING AND KETO DIET

WHAT IS INTERMITTENT FASTING?

Intermittent fasting is fasting when you keep away any foodstuff involving calories among ordinary nutritious ingredients. It is not starvation or a way for you to eat junk food with no consequences. There are various methods used to practice IF; they divide time into hours or divide time into days. Since the regiment's response varies from person to person, no process can be called the best.

Knowing that intermittent fasting cannot make you lose the additional pounds you may have instantaneously is essential, but it can prevent unhealthy addictions to meals. It's a nutritional practice that requires you to be determined to follow to get the maximum gain. If you already have a minimum duration to eat due to your schedule, this regiment will suit you like a duck to water, but you will always need to be conscious of what you are eating if you are a foodie. Choose the appropriate regiment after expert guidance. You should see it as a segment of your schedule to get healthy, but not the only component.

Intermittent fasting is for those who want to regulate their hormones and burn surplus body fat. This diet allows for healthier whole foods and an all-round diet, which is better than living off processed foods and sugars, which are unhealthy. It can also benefit individuals who are sugar-addicted or those who ate empty calories. Drinks and sodas with very few nutrients, but full of calories, are included in these products. Finally, people generally want to do better in life and enjoy a food plan that doesn't require too much planning or maintenance.

Even if intermittent fasting may not be for you reading this book will equip you with the necessary information required to help another person or to use it eventually in life.

DIFFERENT METHODS

IF regiments are numerous to the point that you can choose from any that you like. Always make sure to select a regimen that will fit in your schedule so that it is possible to maintain it.

There are several short methods for fasting, including:

THE 12-HOUR FAST

That's what the regular living routine is called as you eat three meals a day and fast at night as you sleep. The generally small breakfast would break the fast. It is called the traditional method. Any regiment can help you lose weight only if you follow it correctly.

The higher the levels of insulin are as a result of more people adding regular eating and snacking. It can cause resistance to insulin and, ultimately, obesity. This fasting technique sets aside twelve hours in which the body has low insulin levels, reducing the likelihood of insulin resistance. It can't help you lose excess fat, but it can help prevent obesity.

THE 16-HOUR FAST

This fasting for 16 hours is followed by an 8-hour window where you can eat what you like. Luckily you can sleep through most of it, so it's not difficult to keep doing it. Because it requires only small changes like just skipping your lunch, it has an enormous advantage over others, such as the 12 hours fast.

THE 20-HOUR FAST

It's called the "warrior diet." It includes fasting all day long and eating a lot of calories at night. It's meant to keep you from having breakfast, lunch, and other meals for most of the day, so you're getting all your nutrients from dinner. It is a division scheme of 20:4 with four hours of food followed by twenty hours of fasting. It's one of the easiest to do as you're allowed to eat a huge meal of calorific value, so you're going to feel fuller for longer. Start your daytime calories and have a big evening dinner to relax in this diet. You're going to gradually reduce what you're eating during the day and eventually leave dinner as your only meal.

The longer you do these fasting regiments, the more you will be able to maintain a fast. You will come to find out that you will not always feel hungry. The excitement of benefits will make you increase your period of fasting by a couple of hours. Unknowingly, therefore, you are plunging into longer stages of fasting. You can adhere to your regiment religiously, but eating an extra hour will not ruin your fasting or fat burning.

The easiest way to track your feeding is to do it once a day is because it doesn't require a lot of thought. It's just eating at that moment every day on one dinner so that you can use your mental energy on the more important stuff. Unfortunately, it can cause a plateau of weight loss, where you are not losing or gaining weight. That's because you're going to consume the same number of calories every day and significantly less on a typical working day than you would eat. That's the best way to maintain your weight. You will have to change your fasting regiment to lose fat after a while. Timing your meals and fasting windows will lead to optimal loss of fat instead of random fasting. Choose one that can be maintained and modified if necessary.

There are longer fasting regiments, these include:

THE 24-HOUR FAST

It's a scheme of eating breakfast, lunch, or dinner in a day and then eating the following day at the same time. If you decide to eat lunch, then it only involves skipping breakfast and dinner, so nothing is disrupted in your life. It saves time and money because you're not going to eat as much, and piling up dishes will not be a worry of yours. Knowing that you are fasting will be a task for people unless they are very interested in eating methods. By eating unprocessed natural foods, you should have enough vitamins, minerals, and oxygen to avoid nutrient deficiencies. You can do this weekly, but twice or three times a week, it is suggested.

During such long fasts, you should not knowingly avoid eating calories. What you are taking should be high in fat, low in carbohydrates, and unprocessed; there's nothing you shouldn't eat. It would be best if you consumed until you are adequately fed as the duration of fasting lets you burn a bunch of fat, and it will be difficult over time to try to cut more purposefully.

THE 36-HOUR FAST

You retain in this fast for one and a half days without eating. For instance, if you eat lunch today, you consume no meal until the day's breakfast after the following day. This fast should be done about three times a week for people with type 2 diabetes. After the person reaches the desired weight and all diabetes medications are successfully removed, they can reduce the number of days of fasting to a level that will make it easier for them to do while maintaining their gains. Blood sugar should usually be checked as small or high.

THE 42-HOUR FAST

It is adding six hours to the 36 hours fast, resulting in a fast of forty-two hours carried out about two times a week.

THE 5:2 FAST

This technique is conducted to prevent you from totally abstaining from meals and have cycles of calorie consumption. These calories are reduced to a rate that leads to many hormonal advantages of fasting. It consists of five days of regular feeding with two days of fasting. With some protein and oil-based sauce or green vegetables and half an avocado, you can eat some vegetable salad during these fasting days; furthermore, do not eat any dinner. These days of fasting can be placed randomly or following each other in a week at specific times. This method is designed to create faster for more people, as many find it challenging to avoid eating altogether. There's no exact time to follow; as soon as you want, you can follow it.

THE ALTERNATE-DAY FAST

It may seem similar to the 5:2 fasting regimen, but it is not. It's fasting every day. This technique can be followed until you lose as much weight as you want, then you can reduce days of fasting. It allows weight loss to be maintained.

It is possible to move to different fasting regiments as your schedule can change. Intermittent fasting is not about a time-limiting eating window; it is flexible, so you can move your eating and fasting time to suit you, but don't keep changing them all the time; this reduces the effect of fasting on your body. You can even combine some fasting regiments like the 5:2 technique and the 24-hour fasting by having lunch before your fasting day at a particular moment and adding only lunch at the fasting lunch and doing the same for the following fasting day. With this, for twenty-four hours, you could not eat any calories and set your days of fasting as in the 5:2 method of fasting. Choose the fasting day technique that works well with you and can synchronize with your life.

A schedule allows you to create a routine after frequent fasting that makes it easier to integrate into your life. You can plan, but there's no problem if you can't. Even if you can't plan to fast, you should be open-minded fasting to opportunities. You can fast every month or every year. Frankly, you won't lose weight on losing annual fasts.

INTERMITTENT AND KETO DIET

You know all of the different ways to fast, and you know what the ketogenic diet is. The primary purpose of intermittent fasting is to not eat as much during the day. Intermittent fasting can boost your fat burning. When your body is a fasted state, your body will turn to your fat stores for energy. It is when the body starts forming ketones to fuel you and your brain. Now, the ketogenic diet does the same thing without any fasting. However, many people find they don't feel as hungry when following a keto diet. It means that they start fasting simply because they don't feel like they need to eat.

You don't have to fast when on keto, and you don't have to follow keto when fasting. You can choose whichever method, but some people will find that fasting becomes easier on a ketogenic diet.

People who follow a ketogenic diet will have lower insulin levels and blood glucose levels. They have a reduced appetite because of the effects of the ketogenic diet. It means that they won't have any sugar crashes, and they won't feel as hungry.

If you maintain a regular diet, high in carbs, and fasting, you may experience an increase in hunger hormones, and your blood glucose may drop quickly. It could end up causing you to feel irritable, shaky, and weak. It could mean that you feel hungry all of the time. It doesn't always happen, though.

Using both ketogenic diet and intermittent fasting for weight loss is a great idea, but remember, you can use them separately.

CHAPTER 4 - THE KETO SOLUTION TO WEIGHT PROBLEMS FOR WOMEN AFTER 50

Routines are essential on this diet, and it's something that will help you stay healthy as you age and become lost in your average weight. In this phase, we will be giving you tips and tricks to make this diet work better for you and help you get an idea of routines that you can put in place for yourself.

TIP NUMBER ONE

DRINK WATER! That is vital for any diet that you're on, and you need it if not on one as well. However, this essential tip is crucial on a keto diet because when you are eating fewer carbs, you are storing less water, meaning that you will get dehydrated very quickly. Please aim for more than the daily amount of water; however, think back that drinking too much water can be fatal as your kidneys can only handle so much as once. It has mostly happened to soldiers in the military, it does happen to dieters, so it is something to be aware of.

TIP NUMBER TWO

Do it as a daily routine to try and lower your stress. Stress will not allow you to get into ketosis, which states that keto wants to put you in. The reason for this being that stress increases the hormone known as cortisol in your blood. That is because your body has too much sugar in your blood. If you're handling a high level of stress right now, this diet is not a great idea. Some great ideas for this would be getting into the habit or routine of taking the time to do relaxing activities, such as walking and making sure that sleep well, which leads to another exercise that you need to do.

TIP NUMBER THREE

Staying consistent is another routine that you need to get yourself into. No matter what you are choosing to do, make sure it's something that you can do. Try a routine for a couple of weeks and make serious notes of mental and physical problems you're going through and any emotional issues that come your way. Make changes as necessary until you find something that works well for you and stick to it. Remember that you need to give yourself time to get used to this and time to get used to changes before giving up.

TIP NUMBER FOUR

Be honest with yourself as well. That is another big tip for this diet. If you're not honest with yourself, this isn't going to work. If something isn't working, you need to understand that and change it. Are you giving yourself enough time to make changes? Are you pushing too hard? If yes, you need to understand what is going on with yourself and how you need to deal with the changes you're going through. Remember not to get upset or frustrated. This diet takes time, and you need to be a little more patient to make this work effectively.

TIP NUMBER FIVE

Doing a routine of cooking for yourself will also help you so much on this diet. Eating out is fun, but honestly, it can be hard to eat out on this diet. It is practicable to do so with a little bit of special ordering and creativity, but you can avoid all the trouble by only cooking for yourself. It saves time, and it saves a lot of cash.

Get into the habit of cleaning your kitchen. It's tough to stick to a diet if your kitchen is dirty and full of junk food. Clear out the junk and replace all of the wrong food with healthy keto food instead. Remember, with this diet, no soda, pasta, bread, candy, and things. Replacing your food with healthy food and making a routine of cleaning your kitchen and keeping the bad food out will help you be more successful with your diet, which is what you want here.

TIP NUMBER SIX

Another tip is to make sure that you're improving your gut health. That is so important. Your gut is pretty much linked to every other system in your body, so make sure that this something that you want to take seriously.

TIP NUMBER EIGHT

The last tip is to mention exercise again. Getting into the exercise routine can boost your ketone levels, and it can help you with your issues on transitioning to keto. Exercises also use different types of energy for your fuel that you need. When your body gets rid of the glycogen storages, it needs other forms of power, and it will turn into that energy that you need. Just remember to avoid exercises that are going to hurt you. Stay in the smaller activities and lower intensity.

Following these tips and getting into these routines will keep you stay on track and ensure that your diet will go as smoothly as possible.

CHAPTER 5 - KETO IN CONTROLLING BLOOD SUGAR

There is an association between inadequate glucose and cerebrum related conditions like Alzheimer's sickness, dementia, and Parkinson's Disease when you aged. A few factors that may add to Alzheimer's infection incorporate:

- An abundance of carbohydrates admission, mainly from fructose, is radically decreased in the ketogenic keto diet.

- An absence of keto dietary fats and cholesterol, which are limitless and sound on the ketogenic keto diet.

- Oxidative pressure, which being in ketosis ensures against.

- Utilizing a ketogenic keto diet to assist control with blooding sugar and improve sustenance may help enhance insulin reaction and secure against memory issues that regularly happened with age.

SIGNIFICANCE OF KETO FOR AGEING

Keto nourishments convey a high measure of sustenance per calorie. That is significant because the basal metabolic rate (the ratio of calories required every day to endure) is less for seniors. Yet, they despise everything that needs an equal measure of supplements from more youthful individuals.

A woman aged 50 plus will have a lot harder time living on lousy nourishments than a high schooler or 20-something whose body is as yet flexible. That makes it much increasingly vital for seniors to eat nourishments that are well-being supporting and infection battling. It can indeed mean the distinction between appreciating the brilliant years without limit or spending them in torment and misery.

Subsequently, seniors need to eat a progressively ideal eating routine by keeping away from "void calories" from sugars or nourishments wealthy in enemies of supplements, such as entire grains, and expanding their measure of supplement rich fats and proteins.

Likewise, a significant part of the nourishment picked by older individuals (or given in an emergency clinic or clinical settings) will, in general, be vigorously prepared and extremely poor in supplements, for example, white bread, pasta, prunes, pureed potatoes, and puddings.

The high-carb keto diet so broadly pushed by the legislature isn't best for supporting our senior residents and their long-haul well-being. An eating regimen low in carbohydrates and wealthy in creature and plant fats are obviously better for advancing better insulin affectability, fewer occurrences of subjective decay, and generally speaking, better well-being.

In a Keto Talk web recording with Jimmy Moore, Dr. Adam Nally talk about how he has numerous older patients excelling on a keto diet. In light of the data talked about over, this bodes well.

KETOSIS FOR LONGEVITY

Regardless of our age, it's never an impractical notion to improve your odds of feeling and work great for an excellent remainder. It's never the point where it's possible to begin growing, although the sooner we start, the better our odds of maintaining a strategic distance from the ailment. In any event, for the individuals who have spent numerous years not regarding their bodies just as they should, ketosis for seniors can fix a portion of the harm.

We're all getting older, and demise is, obviously, unavoidable. In any case, what we CAN control to a degree is the personal satisfaction end route. Individuals are presently living longer, but at the same time, we're getting more broken down by following the standard eating routine of the more significant part. The ketogenic keto diet can help seniors improve their well-being body to flourish instead of being wiped out or in torment during the latter, long periods of life.

CHAPTER 6 - HELPFUL SHOPPING LIST TIPS FOR KETO MEALS

Going shopping for your keto meals can be a bit demanding. The market is full of many processed and packaged foods that are not keto-friendly.

You will also need to keep an eye out for individual whole grains as they can be too starchy, for instance, potatoes.

Always remember that every item on your grocery cart should be low in carbs and rich in fat, and finally, the amount of protein intake in each meal should be moderate.

To help you, here is a list of items to get when grocery-shopping on the keto diet. Each product on the list is perfectly healthy and beneficial for a woman of 50 years who is on a keto diet.

SEAFOOD

Seafood, which includes sardines, wild salmon, mackerel, tuna, cod, mussels, crab, and shrimp, are all keto-friendly and should be part of your grocery shopping list. They are uniquely high in omega-3 fatty acids and have a high-quality source of protein; they also provide a healthy dose of fat and contain other excellent nutrients such as selenium and other vitamins and minerals. Besides, recent studies have shown that eating seafood can decrease the risk of heart attack, stroke, obesity, and hypertension.

LOW-CARB VEGETABLES

Your shopping list should have vegetables that have low carb content and are rich in minerals, vitamins, fiber, and antioxidants. Vegetables rich in fiber serve as an excellent vehicle to fatty diet, helping prevent constipation. Low-carb vegetables such as spinach, mushrooms, cauliflower, bell peppers, cabbage, brussels sprouts, arugula, eggplant broccoli, zucchini, fennel, celery, and kale are excellent for keto diets.

LOW-SUGAR FRUITS

You will have to be cautious about the type of fruits you take if you don't want to make your body out of ketosis, although some categories of fruits are still okay. You should add low-sugar fruits like avocado, blueberries, coconut, limes, tomatoes, blackberries, raspberries, strawberries, rhubarbs, cantaloupes, watermelons, and lemons to your shopping cart. The fruits expected to be on your list should contain low-carb content.

MEAT AND POULTRY

Meat products such as turkey, beef, pork, venison, chicken, and lamb are excellent on the keto diet and play a large part in it; however, it is essential to pick quality over quantity. Keto diet depends on animal protein, so it is necessary to buy grass-fed organic beef and organic protein. Going with natural picks reduces environmental toxins, while red meats from grass-fed animals have the proper and healthy composition of fat your body can easily absorb.

NUTS AND SEEDS

Nuts and seeds should be a must in your grocery shopping list. They are rich in protein to keep you filled in between meals, as well as a rich source of healthy fats. Some excellent nuts and seeds include flaxseed, chia seed, pecan, pistachios, almonds, hazelnuts, sesame, pumpkin seeds, cashews, macadamia nuts, brazil nuts, walnuts, hemp seed, sunflower seeds, and almonds.

Moreover, seeds contain polyunsaturated fats, which have the best ratio of Omega-6 and Omega-3, such as chia seeds, flaxseeds, and hemp seeds.

DAIRY PRODUCTS

It is essential to think twice that dairy has no carbs, so try to limit your consumption to not more than 3-4 ounces per day. Some excellent dairy products are hard cheese, cream, Greek yogurt, butter, and soft cheese. These are the excellent pedigree of protein, calcium, plus healthy fats.

OILS

As expected, oils are a vital part of your shopping list. Oils could be from nuts like walnuts or fruits such as olives, as they are both excellent sources of healthy fats. Different oils give different flavors; you might want to mix your buys. Some keto-friendly oils include coconut oil, nut oils, MCT oils, extra-virgin olive oil, and avocado oil.

KETO-FRIENDLY CONDIMENTS

Mustard, oil-based salad dressing, unsweetened ketchup, and olive oil mayonnaise are good examples of keto-friendly condiments. These condiments add flavor to several dishes. Keto-friendly sauces are hard to find as there are many highly-processed ones out there. If you are doubtful of added information, you should check the nutritional info.

EGGS

Similar to meat and poultry, another excellent source of animal protein are eggs. You can also grab a hard-boiled egg for a quick snack.

OLIVES

Olive fruits are one of the few packaged foods that are keto-approved. They are also rich in antioxidants and offer a healthy monounsaturated source of fat; They are a viable option if you are craving something salty, and they have a low carb content. That is seen in the 3 grams of net carbs in a handful.

KETO-APPROVED SNACKS

Keto-friendly snacks include sugar-free jerky, nut, low-carb crackers, nut butter, and dried seaweed. Although it's best to take whole foods, you might need some convenience to seek some already packaged snacks from the store.

COFFEE AND TEA

You can add unsweetened tea and coffee to your grocery list. Even though you are on a keto diet, it does not mean you have to forget about caffeine, as unsweetened coffee is great while on the keto diet.

CHOCOLATE

Chocolate lovers, you're in luck. Dark chocolate is the perfect ketogenic dessert after a long day. Not all chocolate is equal; check that it contains at least 70% of cacao.

CHAPTER 7 - FOODS TO AVOID

For us women over 50 who want to get into Keto diet, it is good to know the foods that we should avoid like grains, fruits with high sugar content, starchy vegetables, fruit juice and carrot juice, sugar (including honey and syrup), chips, crackers, and baked goods.

These items are high in sugar and carbohydrates and will not be useful in a low-carbohydrate Keto diet.

FRUITS AND STARCHY VEGETABLES.

Juice, fruit, and sugar are definite no-no's on the keto diet. The excess sugars will not only spike your carbohydrates, but they will also cause insulin to be released in response to the spike in blood sugar. It is all the opposite of the goal of ketosis. There will be too many carbohydrates available for the body to convert to energy. It will make it impossible for the body to be starved of carbs and glucose, and the body will not switch to using fat as energy. Starchy vegetables like corn and beets have high sugar content. Bananas, apples, raisins, and mangoes are too high in sugar content to include on the keto diet. Fruit and sugar will have to be avoided to reach ketosis.

GRAINS, BREAD, AND PASTA.

Grains are high in carbohydrates. Don't try to substitute grains with gluten-free bread and pasta. Even the gluten-free items tend to replace the grains with other foods that are also high in carbohydrates like chickpea flour.

To replace pasta, try the zucchini spirals or shirataki noodles. These noodles are very low in carbohydrates and may be an alternative to high carb grain pasta that meets your needs. Butternut squash spirals are also readily available, but winter squash is high in carbohydrates. Quinoa is a protein-rich grain; there are too many carbohydrates for this grain to be included in the keto food list. Rice and potatoes, brown rice, and sweet potatoes have too many carbs for even the healthy alternatives to be included in your food plan.

LEGUMES.

Avoid beans and legumes like lentils, pinto, black beans, and chickpeas. Though they happen to be high in fiber, they unfortunately also are high in carbohydrates. That makes beans a poor addition to the ketogenic diet. They can be used sparingly when added in small amounts to recipes like soups and stews.

They are nutritious, but like starchy vegetables, they do not fit well in the keto lifestyle.

COATED MEAT.

Meats with added sugar such as flavored maple sausage and bacon should be avoided. Also, breaded chicken and fish are not allowed on the keto diet. These foods have carbohydrates and are not options on the diet. It is better to eat less processed food, and if there are any added flavorings, you should add them yourself to maintain control of the additions.

LOW FAT.

Foods labeled as low fat often contain sugar or unapproved sugar substitutes, which act like sugar and trick your body into a spike in blood sugar and short-term satisfaction. It is right for items you may not associate with sweet flavors like salad dressing and mayonnaise. In these instances, full-fat options are included on the keto diet, so it's okay to eat the real food and avoid processed imitation.

VEGETABLE OILS.

The nutritional value of vegetables, canola, and corn oils is not ideal for the keto diet since they are high in polyunsaturated fatty acids (PUFA). These PUFAs are bad for your heart as they release plaque into arteries. They also cause inflammation in the liver and may promote liver disease. Vegetable oils may be a cause of obesity. Vegetable oil is unhealthy.

Of course, most foods are technically allowed on the ketogenic diet. To include some of these forbidden foods in your diet and remain in ketosis, measure your foods and flavorings and know what you are consuming when it comes to carbohydrates and overall calories. Because carbohydrates' consumption spikes blood sugar levels, when blood sugar drops, there will be a feeling of malaise and hunger when the carbohydrates wear off. It is better to eat more calories from foods that will sustain a constant blood sugar level and foods to help keep your stomach feeling full.

CHAPTER 8 - HOW TO PREPARE YOUR KITCHEN

Before I move on to the recipes, I want to list some of the most-used gadgets to cook keto-friendly meals. I'm not proposing that you have to have all of this in your Kitchen to follow the ketogenic diet successfully, so please don't go out and buy anything you won't use.

You'll see I'm not listing cutlery and crockery and other items commonly found in a kitchen. I think in your 50 years on earth; you've spent enough time in a kitchen to know the basics required to cook food.

KITCHEN SCALES

Out of all the things on the list, this is one I would highly recommend buying. In the beginning, you won't be able to eyeball your macros as the more experienced keto dieters can. You will have to use a kitchen scale to weigh your food to know how much you are eating. You can then punch these numbers into a Carb and calorie tracker app, and it will let you know if you're on track.

STORAGE AND FOOD PREP CONTAINERS

Essential for meal prepping and storing leftovers.

SLOW COOKER

If you plan on prepping your meals in advance, I suggest investing in a slow cooker. Cook a large amount of food right away and then divide it into portions for the week. If meal prepping is not your thing, you can still use the slow cooker to prepare a keto-friendly meal in a fraction of the time.

SPIRALIZERS

It is a nifty little gadget if you want to fool your eyes into thinking you're eating pasta. You can spiral different veggies into forms and sizes that resemble spaghetti, fettuccine, or other shapes.

EGG COOKER

Okay, you'll soon come to find that you'll be eating more eggs than usual. They're high in fat and protein and low in carbs, and that makes eggs a great snack. Boil a few eggs, pop them in the fridge and enjoy when you're feeling a little hungry.

IMMERSION BLENDER

This is a baby food processor that you can hold in your hands to blitz up smoothies, make your Hollandaise sauce, ground nuts, or whip some cream to add to your coffee. Just make sure you buy one with multiple attachments.

FRYING PAN/SKILLET

You'll be eating a lot of steaks, so why not get a frying pan or skillet to cook it in?

ROASTING PAN

A whole chicken or beef roast surrounded by veggies, roasted in the oven, and then covered in a creamy cheese sauce. It doesn't sound like you're on a diet. A roasting pan is a perfect container to make delicious meals in the oven.

SAFETY FIRST

As this guide ends and you get ready to try out some top keto recipes, just a reminder to put your safety first. It's possible to get so carried away in what you're doing to forget some standard safety rules. It is dangerous when you're working with open flames, boiling water, steam, and knives.

I think many people don't know how to handle knives safely because they try to mimic cutting techniques they see on TV. I remember I once showed off my non-existent chopping skills and almost lost a finger.

So, allow me to talk about a quick crash course in knife safety:

- Always use a cutting board. Don't cut anything while holding it in your hand.

- Do not leave knives lying around in the sink. Clean them as soon as possible and put them away.

- Don't store knives loose in a drawer. You may be reaching for something else and then get a nasty surprise.

- Dull knives cause more injuries. Always use a sharp knife.

- On the hand that's holding the item that is being cut, curl your fingers under. If you keep them straight, they'll be in the way.

- Always point the knife away from you; blade facing down. Don't run or fool around with a knife in your hand.

- Keep your focus while you're chopping, dicing, or mincing.

- If you drop a knife, don't try to catch it. Please step back and let it fall.

Okay, for you to look through the recipes, find one you like, and head to the Kitchen! I hope you found the Keto knowledge in this guide helpful and feel that you now know enough to start the ketogenic diet confidently. I promise you—speaking as a woman over 50—this diet will change your life for the better.

CHAPTER 9 - BREAKFAST

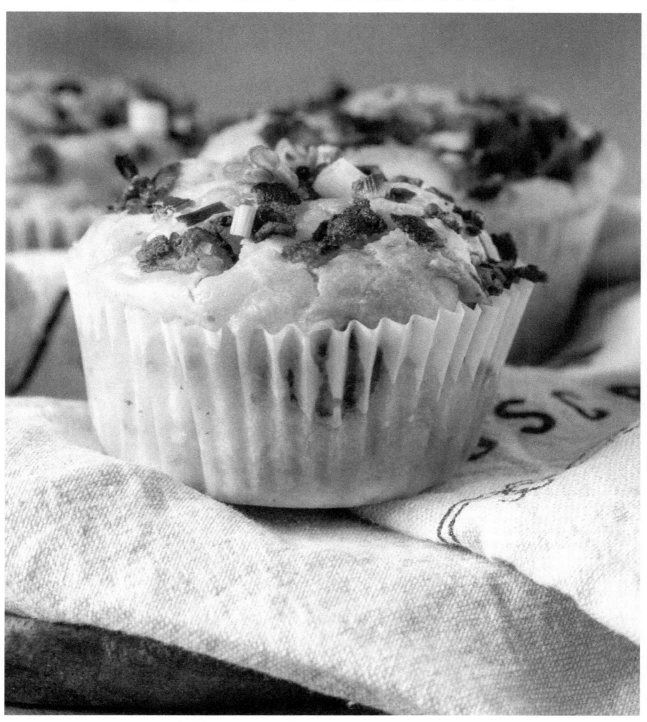

1. CHEESE CREPES

COOKING: 20' **PREPARATION: 15'** **SERVINGS: 5**

INGREDIENTS

- » 6 ounces cream cheese
- » 1/3 cup Parmesan cheese
- » 6 large organic eggs
- » 1 teaspoon granulated erythritol
- » 1½ tablespoon coconut flour
- » 1/8 teaspoon xanthan gum
- » 2 tablespoons unsalted butter

DIRECTIONS

1. Pulse the cream cheese, Parmesan cheese, eggs, and erythritol using a blender.
2. Place the coconut flour and xanthan gum and pulse again.
3. Now, pulse at medium speed. Transfer and put aside within 5 minutes.
4. Melt butter over medium-low heat.
5. Place 1 portion of the mixture and tilt the pan to spread into a thin layer.
6. Cook within 1½ minutes.
7. Flip the crepe and cook within 15-20 seconds more. Serve.

NUTRITION:

Calories 297, Net Carbs 1.9 g , Total Fat 25.1 g, Cholesterol 281 mg, Total Carbs 3.5 g , Protein 13.7 g

2. RICOTTA PANCAKES

COOKING: 20' **PREPARATION: 10'** **SERVINGS: 4**

INGREDIENTS

- » 4 organic eggs
- » ½ cup ricotta cheese
- » ¼ cup vanilla whey protein powder
- » ½ teaspoon organic baking powder
- » Salt
- » ½ teaspoon liquid stevia
- » 2 tablespoons unsalted butter

DIRECTIONS

1. Pulse all the fixing in the blender. Warm-up butter over medium heat. Put the batter and spread it evenly. Cook within 2 minutes. Flip and cook again within 1–2 minutes. Serve.

NUTRITION:

Calories 184, Net Carbs 2.7 g, Total Fat 12.9 g, Total Carbs 2.7 g, Sugar 0.8 g, Protein 14.6 g

3. YOGURT WAFFLES

COOKING: 25'　　　**PREPARATION: 15'**　　　**SERVINGS: 5**

INGREDIENTS

- » ½ cup golden flax seeds meal
- » ½ cup plus 3 tablespoons almond flour
- » 1-1½ tablespoons granulated erythritol
- » 1 tablespoon vanilla whey protein powder
- » ¼ teaspoon baking soda
- » ½ teaspoon organic baking powder
- » ¼ teaspoon xanthan gum
- » Salt
- » 1 large organic egg
- » 1 organic egg
- » 2 tablespoons unsweetened almond milk
- » 1½ tablespoons unsalted butter
- » 3 ounces plain Greek yogurt

DIRECTIONS

1. Preheat the waffle iron and then grease it.
2. Mix add the flour, erythritol, protein powder, baking soda, baking powder, xanthan gum, and salt.
3. Beat the egg white until stiff peaks. In a third bowl, add 2 egg yolks, whole egg, almond milk, butter, yogurt, and beat.
4. Put egg mixture into the bowl of the flour mixture and mix.
5. Gently, fold in the beaten egg whites. Place ¼ cup of the mixture into preheated waffle iron and cook for about 4–5 minutes. Serve.

NUTRITION:

Calories 250, Net Carbs 3.2 g , Total Fat 18.7 g, Protein 8.4 g

4. BROCCOLI MUFFINS

COOKING: 20'　　　**PREPARATION: 15'**　　　**SERVINGS: 6**

INGREDIENTS

- » 2 tablespoons unsalted butter
- » 6 large organic eggs
- » ½ cup heavy whipping cream
- » ½ cup Parmesan cheese
- » Salt & ground black pepper
- » 1¼ cups broccoli
- » 2 tablespoons parsley
- » ½ cup Swiss cheese

DIRECTIONS

1. Warm-up oven to 350°F, then grease a 12-cup muffin tin.

2. Mix the eggs, cream, Parmesan cheese, salt, and black pepper.

3. Divide the broccoli and parsley in the muffin cup.

4. Top with the egg mixture, with Swiss cheese.

5. Bake within 20 minutes. Cool for about 5 minutes. Serve.

NUTRITION:

Calories 231, Net Carbs 2 g, Total Fat 18.1 g, Cholesterol 228 mg , Sodium 352 mg, Protein 13.5 g

5. PUMPKIN BREAD

COOKING: 1 HOUR   **PREPARATION: 15'**   **SERVINGS: 16**

INGREDIENTS

- » 1 2/3 cups almond flour
- » 1½ teaspoons organic baking powder
- » ½ teaspoon pumpkin pie spice
- » ½ teaspoon cinnamon
- » ½ teaspoon cloves
- » ½ teaspoon salt
- » 8 ounces cream cheese
- » 6 organic eggs
- » 1 tablespoon coconut flour
- » 1 cup powdered erythritol
- » 1 teaspoon stevia powder
- » 1 teaspoon organic lemon extract
- » 1 cup pumpkin puree
- » ½ cup of coconut oil

DIRECTIONS

1. Warm-up oven to 325°F. Grease 2 bread loaf pans.
2. Mix almond flour, baking powder, spices, and salt in a small bowl.
3. In a second bowl, add the cream cheese, 1 egg, coconut flour, ¼ cup of erythritol, and ¼ teaspoon of the stevia, and beat.
4. In a third bowl, add the pumpkin puree, oil, 5 eggs, ¾ cup of the erythritol, and ¾ teaspoon of the stevia and mix.
5. Mix the pumpkin mixture into the bowl of the flour mixture.
6. Place about ¼ of the pumpkin mixture into each loaf pan.
7. Top each pan with the cream cheese mixture, plus the rest pumpkin mixture.
8. Bake within 50–60 minutes. Cold within 10 minutes. Slice and serve.

NUTRITION:

Calories 216, Net Carbs 2.5 g, Total Fat 19.8 g, Cholesterol 77 mg, Sodium 140 mg, Protein 3.4 g

6. EGGS IN AVOCADO CUPS

COOKING: 20'   **PREPARATION: 10'**   **SERVINGS: 4**

INGREDIENTS

- » 2 avocados
- » 4 organic eggs
- » Salt
- » Ground black pepper
- » 4 tablespoons cheddar cheese
- » 2 cooked bacon
- » 1 tablespoon scallion greens

DIRECTIONS

1. Warm-up oven to 400°F. Remove 2 tablespoons of flesh from the avocado.
2. Place avocado halves into a small baking dish.
3. Crack an egg in each avocado half and sprinkle with salt plus black pepper.
4. Top each egg with cheddar cheese evenly.
5. Bake within 20 minutes. Serve with bacon and chives.

NUTRITION:

Calories 343, Net Carbs 2.2 g, Total Fat 29.1 g, Cholesterol 186 mg, Sodium 372 mg, Protein 13.8 g

7. CHEDDAR SCRAMBLE

COOKING: 8'   **PREPARATION: 10'**   **SERVINGS: 6**

INGREDIENTS

» 2 tablespoons olive oil
» 1 small yellow onion
» 12 large organic eggs
» Salt and ground black pepper
» 4 ounces cheddar cheese

DIRECTIONS

1. Warm-up oil over medium heat.
2. Sauté the onion within 4–5 minutes.
3. Add the eggs, salt, and black pepper and cook within 3 minutes.
4. Remove then stir in the cheese. Serve.

NUTRITION:

Calories 264, Net Carbs 1.8 g, Total Fat 20.9 g, Cholesterol 392 mg, Sodium 285 mg, Protein 17.4 g

8. BACON OMELET

COOKING: 15'   **PREPARATION: 10'**   **SERVINGS: 2**

INGREDIENTS

» 4 organic eggs
» 1 tablespoon chives
» Salt
» ground black pepper
» 4 bacon slices
» 1 tablespoon unsalted butter
» 2 ounces cheddar cheese

DIRECTIONS

1. Beat the eggs, chives, salt, and black pepper in a bowl.

2. Warm-up a pan over medium-high heat then cooks the bacon slices within 8–10 minutes.

3. Chop the bacon slices. Melt butter and cook the egg mixture within 2 minutes.

4. Flip the omelet and top with chopped bacon. Cook within 1–2 minutes.

5. Remove then put the cheese in the center of the omelet. Serve.

NUTRITION:

Calories 427, Net Carbs 1.2 g, Total Fat 28.2 g, Cholesterol 469 mg, Sodium 668 mg, Sugar 1 g, Protein 29.1g

9. GREEN VEGGIES QUICHE

COOKING: 20'   **PREPARATION: 20'**   **SERVINGS: 4**

INGREDIENTS

- » 6 organic eggs
- » ½ cup unsweetened almond milk
- » Salt and ground black pepper
- » 2 cups baby spinach
- » ½ cup green bell pepper
- » 1 scallion
- » ¼ cup cilantro
- » 1 tablespoon chives,
- » 3 tablespoons mozzarella cheese

DIRECTIONS

1. Warm-up broiler of the oven, then mix Parmesan cheese, eggs, salt, and black pepper in a bowl.
2. Melt butter, then cook the chicken and asparagus within 2–3 minutes.
3. Add the egg mixture and tomatoes and mix. Cook within 4–5 minutes.
4. Remove then sprinkle with the Parmesan cheese.
5. Transfer the wok under the broiler and broil within 3–4 minutes. Slice and serve.

NUTRITION:

Calories 158, Net Carbs 1.3 g, Total Fat 9.3 g, Cholesterol 265 mg, Sodium 267 mg, Sugar 1 g

11. SOUTHWEST SCRAMBLED EGG BITES

COOKING: 23'   **PREPARATION: 10'**   **SERVINGS: 4**

INGREDIENTS

- » 5 eggs
- » 1/2 teaspoon hot pepper sauce
- » 1/3 cup tomatoes
- » 3 tablespoons green chilies
- » 1 teaspoon black pepper
- » 1/2 teaspoon salt
- » 2 tablespoons nondairy milk

DIRECTIONS

1. Mix both the eggs and milk in a large cup. Add the hot sauce, pepper, and salt. Put a small diced chilies and diced tomatoes in silicone cups. Fill each with 3/4 full with the egg mixture. Put the trivet in the pot and pour 1 cup water. Put the mold on the trivet. Set to high for 8 minutes. Cooldown before serving.

NUTRITION:

Calories: 106, Carbs: 2g, Protein: 7.5g, Fats: 7.4g

12. BACON EGG BITES

COOKING: 22'   **PREPARATION: 10'**   **SERVINGS: 9**

INGREDIENTS

» 1 cup cheese
» 1/2 green pepper
» 1/2 cup cottage cheese
» 4 slices bacon
» Pepper
» Salt
» 1 cup red onion
» 1 cup of water
» 1/4 cup whip cream
» 1/4 cup egg whites
» 4 eggs

DIRECTIONS

1. Blend egg whites, eggs, cream, cheese (cottage), shredded cheese, pepper, and salt within 30 to 45 seconds in a blender. Put the egg mixture into mini muffin cups. Top each with bacon, peppers, and onion. Cover the muffin cups tightly with foil. Place the trivet in the pot and pour 1 cup water. Put the cups on the trivet. Set to steam for 12 minutes. Cooldown before serving.

NUTRITION:

Calories: 124, Carbs: 3g, Protein: 9g, Fats: 8

13. OMELET BITES

COOKING: 8'   **PREPARATION: 5'**   **SERVINGS: 3**

INGREDIENTS

» 1 handful mushrooms
» Green onion
» Green peppers
» 1/8 teaspoon hot sauce
» Pepper, salt, mustard, garlic powder
» 1/2 cup cheese cheddar
» 1/2 cup cheese cottage
» 2 deli ham slices
» 4 eggs

DIRECTIONS

1. Whisk eggs, then the cheddar and cottage. Put the ham, veggies, and seasonings; mix. Pour the mixture into greased silicone molds. Put the trivet with the molds in the pot then fill with 2 cups water. Steam for about 8 minutes. Transfer, cooldown before serving.

NUTRITION:

Calories: 260, Carbs: 6g, Protein: 22g, Fats: 16g

14. CHEDDAR & BACON EGG BITES

COOKING: 8'   **PREPARATION: 10'**   **SERVINGS: 7**

INGREDIENTS

- » 1 cup sharp cheddar cheese
- » 1 tablespoon parsley flakes
- » 4 eggs
- » 4 tablespoons cream
- » Hot sauce
- » 1 cup of water
- » 1/2 cup cheese
- » 4 slices bacon

DIRECTIONS

1. Blend the cream, cheddar, cottage, and egg in the blender; 30 seconds. Stir in the parsley. Grease silicone egg bite molds. Divide the crumbled bacon between them. Put the egg batter into each cup. With a piece of foil, cover each mold. Place the trivet with the molds in the pot then fill with 1 cup water. Steam for 8 minutes. Remove, let rest for 5 minutes. Serve, sprinkled with black pepper, and optional hot sauce.

NUTRITION:

Calories: 167, Carbs: 1.5g, Protein: 13.5g, Fats: 11.7g

15. AVOCADO PICO EGG BITES

COOKING: 10'   **PREPARATION: 15'**   **SERVINGS: 7**

INGREDIENTS

Egg bites:
- » 1/ cup cheese cottage
- » 1/2 cup cheese Mexican blend
- » 1/4 cup cream heavy cream
- » 1/4 teaspoon chili powder
- » 1/4 teaspoon cumin
- » 1/4 teaspoon garlic powder
- » 4 eggs
- » Pepper
- » Salt

Pico de Gallo:
- » 1 avocado
- » 1 jalapeno
- » 1/2 teaspoon salt
- » 1/4 onion
- » 2 tablespoons cilantro
- » 2 teaspoons lime juice
- » 4 Roma tomatoes

DIRECTIONS

1. Mix all of the Pico de Gallo fixing except for the avocado. Gently fold in the avocado.

2. Blend all the egg bites ingredients in a blender. Spoon 1 tablespoon of Pico de Gallo into each egg bite silicone mold. Place the trivet in the pot then fill with 1 cup water. Put the molds in the trivet. Set to high within 10 minutes. Remove. Serve topped with cheese and Pico de Gallo.

NUTRITION:

Calories: 118, Carbs: 1g, Protein: 7g, Fats: 9g

16. SALMON SCRAMBLE

COOKING: 5'　　**PREPARATION: 10'**　　**SERVINGS: 1**

INGREDIENTS

- » 2 smoked salmon pieces
- » 1 organic egg yolk
- » 1/8 tsp. red pepper flakes
- » Black pepper
- » 2 organic eggs
- » 1 tbsp. dill
- » 1/8 tsp. garlic powder
- » 1 tbsp. olive oil

DIRECTIONS

1. Beat all items except salmon and oil. Stir in chopped salmon. Warm-up oil over medium-low heat in a frying pan. Add the egg mixture and cook within 3-5 minutes. Serve.

NUTRITION:

Calories: 376, Carbs: 3.4g, Protein: 24g, Fats: 24.8g

17. MEXICAN SCRAMBLED EGGS

COOKING: 10'　　**PREPARATION: 5'**　　**SERVINGS: 6**

INGREDIENTS

- » 6 eggs
- » 2 jalapeños
- » 1 tomato
- » 3 oz. cheese
- » 2 tbsp. butter

DIRECTIONS

1. Warm-up butter over medium heat in a large pan. Add tomatoes, jalapeños, and green onions then cook within 3 minutes. Add eggs, and continue within 2 minutes. Add cheese and season to taste. Serve.

NUTRITION:

Calories: 239, Carbs: 2.38g, Protein: 13.92g, Fats: 19.32g

18. CAPRESE OMELET

COOKING: 10'   **PREPARATION: 10'**   **SERVINGS: 2**

INGREDIENTS

- » 6 eggs
- » 2 tbsp. olive oil
- » 3½ oz. halved cherry tomatoes
- » Dried basil 1 tbsp. dried basil
- » 5 1/3 oz. mozzarella cheese

DIRECTIONS

1. Mix the basil, eggs, salt, and black pepper in a bowl. Place a large skillet with oil over medium heat. Once hot, add tomatoes and cook. Top with egg and cook. Add cheese, adjust heat to low, and allow to fully set before serving.

NUTRITION:

Calories: 423, Carbs: 6.81g, Protein: 43.08g, Fats: 60.44g

19. SAUSAGE OMELET

COOKING: 15'   **PREPARATION: 10'**   **SERVINGS: 2**

INGREDIENTS

- » ½ pound gluten-free sausage links
- » ½ cup heavy whipping cream
- » Salt
- » Black pepper
- » 8 large organic eggs
- » 1 cup cheddar cheese
- » ¼ tsp. red pepper flakes

DIRECTIONS

1. Warm-up oven to 350°F. Grease a baking dish. Cook the sausage within 8–10 minutes.

2. Put the rest of the fixing in a bowl and beat. Remove sausage from the heat. Place cooked sausage in the baking dish then top with the egg mixture. Bake within 30 minutes. Slice and serve.

NUTRITION:

Calories: 334, Carbs: 1.1g, Protein: 20.6g, Fats: 27.3g

20. BROWN HASH WITH ZUCCHINI

COOKING: 20'   **PREPARATION: 10'**   **SERVINGS: 2**

INGREDIENTS

- » 1 small onion
- » 6 to 8 mushrooms
- » 2 cups grass-fed ground beef
- » 1 pinch salt
- » 1 pinch ground black pepper
- » ½ tsp smoked paprika
- » 2 eggs
- » 1 avocado
- » 10 black olives

DIRECTIONS

1. Warm-up air fryer for 350° F. Grease a pan with coconut oil. Add the onions, the mushrooms, the salt plus pepper to the pan. Add the ground beef and the smoked paprika and eggs. Mix, then place the pan in Air Fryer. Set to cook within 18 to 20 minutes with a temperature, 375° F. Serve with chopped parsley and diced avocado!

NUTRITION:

Calories: 290, Carbs: 15g, Protein: 20g, Fats: 23g

21. CRUNCHY RADISH & ZUCCHINI HASH BROWNS

COOKING: 10'   **PREPARATION: 10'**   **SERVINGS: 6**

INGREDIENTS

- » 1 teaspoon onion powder
- » 1/2 cup zucchini
- » 1/ cup cheddar cheese
- » 1/2 cup radishes
- » 3 egg whites
- » Pepper
- » Salt

DIRECTIONS

1. Mix the egg whites in a bowl. Stir in the radishes, zucchini, seasonings, and cheese. Shape into 6 patties. Warm-up skillet over the medium-high setting. Grease. Cook the patties. Adjust to medium-low; cook for 3 to 5 minutes more. Serve.

NUTRITION:

Calories: 70, Carbs: 1g, Protein: 5.5g, Fats: 4.7g

22. FENNEL QUICHE

COOKING: 18'   **PREPARATION: 15'**   **SERVINGS: 4**

INGREDIENTS

- » 10 oz. fennel
- » 1 cup spinach
- » 5 eggs
- » ½ cup almond flour
- » 1 teaspoon olive oil
- » 1 tablespoon butter
- » 1 teaspoon salt
- » ¼ cup heavy cream
- » 1 teaspoon ground black pepper

DIRECTIONS

1. Combine the chopped spinach and chopped fennel in the big bowl. Whisk the egg in the separate bowl. Combine the whisked eggs with the almond flour, butter, salt, heavy cream, and ground black pepper. Warm-up air fryer to 360 F. Grease. Then add the spinach-fennel mixture and pour the whisked egg mixture. Cook within 18 minutes. Remove then chill. Slice and serve.

NUTRITION:

Calories: 249, Carbs: 9.4g, Protein: 11.3g, Fats: 19.1g

23. TURKEY HASH

COOKING: 25'   **PREPARATION: 10'**   **SERVINGS: 5**

INGREDIENTS

- » 3 cups cauliflower florets
- » 1 small yellow onion
- » Salt
- » Ground black pepper
- » 1/4 cup heavy cream
- » 2 tbsp. unsalted butter
- » 1 tsp. dried thyme
- » 1-pound cooked turkey meat

DIRECTIONS

1. Put the cauliflower in a salt boiling water and cook within 4 minutes. Then chop the cauliflower and set aside. Dissolve the butter over medium heat in a large skillet and sauté onion within 4-5 minutes. Add thyme, salt, and black pepper and sauté again within 1 minute. Stir in cauliflower and cook within 2 minutes. Stir in turkey and cook within 5-6 minutes. Stir in the cream and cook within 2 minutes more. Serve.

NUTRITION:

Calories: 237, Carbs: 4.8g, Protein: 28.1g, Fats: 11.5g

24. CRUSTLESS VEGGIE QUICHE

COOKING: 30'　　　**PREPARATION: 10'**　　　**SERVINGS: 6**

INGREDIENTS

- » 1 & 1/2 cups Colby Jack cheese
- » 1 red pepper
- » 1/2 cup coconut milk
- » 1/4 teaspoon salt
- » Additional low-carb veggies
- » 1 cup tomatoes
- » 1/2 cup arrowroot flour
- » 1 teaspoon black pepper
- » 2 green onions
- » 8 eggs

DIRECTIONS

1. Whisk the milk, egg, flour, pepper, and salt in a large bowl. Mix in the veggies and 1 cup cheese. Pour the mixture into a heatproof container. Cover it with foil. Place the trivet in the pot then fill with 1 cup water. Cook high within 30 minutes. Remove and uncover. Top with the rest of the cheese. Cover then let sit for 2 minutes. Serve!

NUTRITION:

Calories: 244, Carbs: 6.4g, Protein: 14.6g, Fats: 17.7g

25. CRUSTLESS BROCCOLI & CHEDDAR QUICHE

COOKING: 25'　　　**PREPARATION: 10'**　　　**SERVINGS: 4**

INGREDIENTS

- » 1 cup cheddar cheese
- » 1/2 cup nondairy milk
- » 1/4 teaspoon black pepper
- » 6 eggs
- » 1 head broccoli
- » 1/ teaspoon kosher salt
- » 3 green onions

DIRECTIONS

1. Grease a 1 1/2-quart soufflé dish. In a bowl, whisk the milk, eggs, pepper, and salt. Stir in the cheese, broccoli, and green onions. Pour the mixture into the greased dish. Place the trivet in the pot then fill with 1 1/2 cups water. Set to high for 25 minutes. Slice and serve.

NUTRITION:

Calories: 301, Carbs: 4.7g, Protein: 17.9g, Fats: 23.3g

26. KETO ZUCCHINI BREAD

COOKING: 50'   **PREPARATION: 10'**   **SERVINGS: 4**

INGREDIENTS

- » 4 medium eggs
- » 1 large zucchini
- » 2 cups of almond flour
- » Quarter cup coconut flour
- » 8 tablespoons coconut oil
- » 1 teaspoon baking powder
- » 1 teaspoon vanilla extract
- » A pinch of salt

DIRECTIONS

1. Warm-up, the oven to 350 F., combine all the components in a large bowl. Squeeze out all the moisture from the zucchini. Pour into a bread pot and bake for 50 minutes. Serve.

NUTRITION:

Calories: 267, Carbs: 11g, Fat: 23g, Protein: 0g

27. KETO ALMOND BREAD RECIPE

COOKING: 30'   **PREPARATION: 10'**   **SERVINGS: 6**

INGREDIENTS

- » 2 eggs
- » 1 cup almond flour
- » 1/5 teaspoons baking powder
- » 3 tablespoons olive oil
- » 1 teaspoon powdered mustard
- » Spices
- » 1 teaspoon coarse salt
- » 1 teaspoon immediate gluten-free yeast

DIRECTIONS

1. Warm-up oven to 350 F. Combine eggs, almond flour, baking powder, mustard powder, salt, and olive oil. Place the mixture on a small greased baking sheet—Bake within 30 minutes. Slice and serve.

NUTRITION:

Calories: 270, Carbs: 3g, Fat: 27g, Protein: 6g

28. QUICK KETO TOAST

COOKING: 5'   PREPARATION: 10'   SERVINGS: 4

INGREDIENTS

- » 1/3 cup almond flour
- » 1/2 teaspoon baking powder
- » 1/8 teaspoon salt
- » 1 egg
- » 1 tablespoon ghee

DIRECTIONS

1. Warm-up oven to 200 F.
2. Put all the bread components in a container and mix well.
3. Microwave the mixture within 90 seconds.
4. Cooldown and cut it into four slices.
5. Bake within 4 minutes.
6. Serve with additional ghee.

NUTRITION:

Calories: 270, Carbs: 3g, Fat: 27g, Protein: 6g

29. KETO LOAF OF BREAD

COOKING: 60'   PREPARATION: 10'   SERVINGS: 6

INGREDIENTS

- » 3 cups almond flour
- » 3 tablespoons whey protein powder
- » 2 tbsp. & 1/2 cup coconut oil
- » 1/4 cup coconut milk
- » 3 beaten eggs
- » 2 teaspoons baking powder
- » 1 teaspoon baking soda
- » 1 tablespoon Italian flavor
- » 1/4 teaspoon salt

DIRECTIONS

1. Warm-up the oven to 150 F. Grease a bread pan.
2. Combine all items in a large bowl. Pour the dough into the pan and roll it out to fill as well.
3. Bake for 60 minutes. Slice and serve.

NUTRITION:

Calories: 117, Carbs: 5g, Fat: 15g, Protein: 4g

30. BLUEBERRY LOAF

COOKING: 70'   **PREPARATION: 10'**   **SERVINGS: 6**

INGREDIENTS

- » 1 1/2 cups Almond Flour
- » 1 tablespoon Coconut Flour
- » 1 1/2 teaspoons baking powder
- » 7 tbsp Truvia
- » 3 tablespoon oil
- » 4 tablespoons heavy cream
- » 1 teaspoon vanilla
- » 2 eggs
- » 100 grams' wild blueberries

DIRECTIONS

1. Warm-up oven to 300 degrees.
2. Combine almond flour, coconut flour, baking powder, and six tablespoons Truvia.
3. Mix oil, whipping cream, and vanilla. Mix damp and dry ingredients
4. Wash off blueberries and include 1 tbsp. of Truvia and stir.
5. Put blueberries on top of the batter. Bake within 1 hour and 10 minutes, turning the loaf pan within 30 minutes. Cool before serving.

NUTRITION:

Calories: 170, Carbs: 21g, Protein: 2g

31. SIMPLE LOAF OF BREAD

COOKING: 60'   **PREPARATION: 10'**   **SERVINGS: 6**

INGREDIENTS

- » 3 cups almond flour
- » 1/2 cup + 2 tablespoons olive oil
- » Quarter cup almond milk
- » 3 eggs
- » 2 teaspoons baking powder.
- » 1 teaspoon baking soda.
- » 1/4 teaspoon salt

DIRECTIONS

1. Warm-up oven to 300F. Grease the bread. Mix all the items. Bake for 60 minutes. Leave to cool. Serve.

NUTRITION:

Calories: 250, Carbs: 52g, Fat: 2g, Protein: 7g

69

32. KETO AVOCADO CHOCOLATE BREAD

COOKING: 45' **PREPARATION: 10'** **SERVINGS: 5**

INGREDIENTS

- » 2 ripe avocados
- » 3 tablespoons coconut oil
- » 3 eggs
- » 2 cups almond flour
- » 1/2 cup cacao powder
- » 1 teaspoon baking soda
- » 1/2 teaspoon baking powder
- » 1 teaspoon vanilla extract
- » Stevia
- » Salt

DIRECTIONS

1. Warm-up oven to 350 F. Mix all fixings. Place into a loaf pan. Bake for 40-45 minutes. Serve.

NUTRITION:

Calories: 198, Carbs: 9g, Fat: 16g, Protein: 7g

33. SUNFLOWER BREAD

COOKING: 15' **PREPARATION: 120'** **SERVINGS: 15**

INGREDIENTS

- » 1 3/4 tsp fresh yeast
- » 1 1/4 cup water
- » 3 cups ground rye flour
- » 2 1/2 cups wheat flour
- » 7 oz rye sourdough starter
- » 1 tbsp salt
- » 3 tablespoon honey
- » 2/3 cup sunflower seeds
- » 1 tablespoon cumin

DIRECTIONS

1. Melt the yeast in a little water. Add all ingredients, mix well.

2. Let the dough rise within 1 to 2 hrs.

3. Shape the dough right into fifteen small rolls. Put it to the cooking sheet and also let them surge until doubled in dimension. Knead the dough after it has increased, and shape into a long roll.

4. Cut the dough into fifteen parts. Form right into rounded loaves.

5. Bake at 350 ° F within 10 minutes. Slice and serve.

NUTRITION:

Calories: 80, Carbs: 12g, Fat: 2g, Protein: 3g

34. COLLAGEN KETO BREAD KETO COLLAGEN BREAD

COOKING: 40'   PREPARATION: 20'   SERVINGS: 15

INGREDIENTS

- » 1/2 cup Unflavored Grass-Fed Collagen Protein
- » 6 tablespoons almond flour
- » 5 pastured eggs
- » 1 tbsp unflavored fluid coconut oil
- » 1 teaspoon aluminum-free baking powder
- » 1 teaspoon xanthan gum
- » Pinch of Himalayan pink salt
- » A squeeze of stevia

DIRECTIONS

1. Warm-up stove to 325 degrees F.
2. Grease the glass loaf pan with coconut oil. In a large bowl, break the egg whites, set aside.
3. In a little bowl, blend the dry components and set aside. In a little dish, whisk together the damp ingredients, egg yolks, and liquid coconut oil.
4. Include the dry and the damp components to the egg whites and blend till well integrated.
5. Bake for 40 minutes. Slice before serving.

NUTRITION:

Calories: 77, Protein: 7g, Carbs: 1g, Fiber: 1g, Sugar: 0g

35. KETO BREAKFAST PIZZA

COOKING: 15'   PREPARATION: 20'   SERVINGS: 2

INGREDIENTS

- » 2 cups grated cauliflower
- » 2 tablespoons coconut flour
- » 1/2 tsp salt
- » 4 eggs
- » 1 tbsp psyllium husk powder
- » Toppings: smoked salmon, avocado, natural herbs, spinach, olive oil

DIRECTIONS

1. Warm-up stove to 350 levels. Line a pizza tray with parchment.
2. In a mixing dish, add all items except toppings and mix up. Leave for 5 minutes.
3. Thoroughly put the breakfast pizza base onto the pan.
4. Cook for 15 minutes. Garnish with toppings. Serve.

NUTRITION:

Calories: 454, Total Fat: 31g, Total Carbs: 26g, Fiber: 17.2 g, Protein: 22g

36. CAULIFLOWER BREAD

COOKING: 35' **PREPARATION: 20'** **SERVINGS: 2**

INGREDIENTS

- » 2 cups grated cauliflower
- » 1-2 tablespoons coconut flour
- » 1/2 tsp salt
- » 4 eggs
- » 1/2 tsp garlic powder
- » 1/2 1 tbsp. psyllium husk
- » 3-4 pieces' bacon
- » 1/4 springtime onion
- » 1 avocado

DIRECTIONS

1. Warm-up oven to 350F.
2. Mix the two cups of grated cauliflower, salt, 2 eggs, 1 tbsp of coconut flour, psyllium, garlic powder, and 1 tablespoon flour.
3. Divide the cauliflower mix in 2. Place each cauliflower ball onto one of the lined cooking trays, shape the blend into even rectangular shapes. Cook in the stove within 15 minutes.
4. Bake with the bacon for an additional 10 minutes.
5. Boil water in a little pan, including the dash of apple cider vinegar plus salt.
6. Split two eggs into the boiling water to poach. Cook.
7. Transfer the cauliflower bread then serve with the poached eggs, crispy bacon, spring onion, and avocado.

NUTRITION:

Calories: 498, Total Fat: 38g, Carbohydrates: 14g, Protein: 27g

37. COCONUT FLOUR DONUTS

COOKING: 18' **PREPARATION: 15'** **SERVINGS: 8**

INGREDIENTS

- » 1/3 cup coconut flour
- » 1/3 cup Swerve Sweetener
- » 3 tbsp cacao powder
- » 1 tsp baking powder
- » 1/4 tsp salt
- » 4 big eggs
- » 1/4 cup butter thawed
- » 1/2 tsp vanilla essence
- » 6 tbsp brewed coffee

Glaze:
- » 1/4 cup powdered Swerve Sweetener
- » 1 tablespoon cocoa powder
- » 1 tbsp heavy cream
- » 1/4 tsp vanilla essence
- » 1 1/2 to 2 tbsp water

DIRECTIONS

1. Warm-up oven to 325F and grease the donut frying pan.

2. Mix the coconut flour, sweetener, cacao powder, baking powder, and salt. Then the eggs, melted butter, and vanilla essence. Stir in the cold coffee.

3. Separate the batter amongst the wells of the donut pan. Bake 16 to 20 minutes. Cooldown.

4. Glaze: In a medium shallow bowl, mix the powdered sugar and cocoa powder. Add the hefty cream and vanilla and whisk. Put water up until the glaze thins out. Serve.

NUTRITION:

Calories: 111, Carbs: 5g, Fat: 9g, Protein: 5g

38. TOFU MUSHROOMS

COOKING: 10' **PREPARATION: 5'** **SERVINGS: 3**

INGREDIENTS

- » 1 block tofu
- » 1 cup mushrooms
- » 4 tablespoons butter
- » 4 tablespoons Parmesan cheese
- » Salt
- » Ground black pepper

DIRECTIONS

1. Toss tofu cubes with melted butter, salt, and black pepper in a mixing bowl.
2. Sauté the tofu within 5 minutes. Stir in cheese and mushrooms.
3. Sauté for another 5 minutes. Serve.

NUTRITION:

Calories 211, Total Fat 18.5 g, Cholesterol 51 mg, Sodium 346 mg, Total Carbs 2 g, Protein 11.5 g

39. ONION TOFU

COOKING: 5' **PREPARATION: 8'** **SERVINGS: 3**

INGREDIENTS

- » 2 blocks tofu
- » 2 onions
- » 2 tablespoons butter
- » 1 cup cheddar cheese
- » Salt
- » Ground black pepper

DIRECTIONS

1. Rub the tofu with salt and pepper in a bowl.
2. Add melted butter and onions to a skillet to sauté within 3 minutes.
3. Toss in tofu and stir cook for 2 minutes. Stir in cheese and cover the skillet for 5 minutes on low heat. Serve.

NUTRITION:

Calories 184, Total Fat 12.7 g, Total Carbs 6.3 g, Sugar 2.7 g, Fiber 1.6 g, Protein 12.2 g

40. SPINACH RICH BALLET

COOKING: 30' **PREPARATION: 5'** **SERVINGS: 4**

INGREDIENTS

- » 1½ lbs. baby spinach
- » 8 teaspoons coconut cream
- » 14 oz. cauliflower
- » 2 tablespoons unsalted butter
- » Salt
- » Ground black pepper

DIRECTIONS

1. Warm-up oven at 360 degrees F.
2. Melt butter, then toss in spinach to sauté for 3 minutes.
3. Divide the spinach into four ramekins.
4. Divide cream, cauliflower, salt, and black pepper in the ramekins.
5. Bake within 25 minutes. Serve.

NUTRITION:

Calories 188, Total Fat 12.5 g, Cholesterol 53 mg, Sodium 1098 mg, Total Carbs 4.9 g, Protein 14.6 g

41. PEPPERONI EGG OMELET

COOKING: 20' **PREPARATION: 5'** **SERVINGS: 4**

INGREDIENTS

- » 15 pepperonis
- » 6 eggs
- » 2 tablespoons butter
- » 4 tablespoons coconut cream
- » Salt and ground black pepper

DIRECTIONS

1. Whisk eggs with pepperoni, cream, salt, and black pepper in a bowl.
2. Add ¼ of the butter to a warm-up pan.
3. Now pour ¼ of the batter in this melted butter and cook for 2 minutes each side. Serve.

NUTRITION:

Calories 141, Total Fat 11.3 g, Cholesterol 181 mg, Sodium 334 mg, Protein 8.9 g

42. NUT PORRIDGE

COOKING: 15' **PREPARATION: 10'** **SERVINGS: 4**

INGREDIENTS

- » 1 cup cashew nuts
- » 1 cup pecan
- » 2 tablespoons stevia
- » 4 teaspoons coconut oil
- » 2 cups of water

DIRECTIONS

1. Grind the cashews and peanuts in a processor.
2. Stir in stevia, oil, and water. Add the mixture to a saucepan and cook within 5 minutes on high. Adjust on low within 10 minutes. Serve.

NUTRITION:

Calories 260, Total Fat 22.9 g, Sodium 9 mg, Total Carbs 12.7 g, Sugar 1.8 g, Fiber 1.4 g, Protein 5.6 g

43. PARSLEY SOUFFLÉ

COOKING: 6' **PREPARATION: 5'** **SERVINGS: 1**

INGREDIENTS

- » 2 eggs
- » 1 red chili pepper
- » 2 tablespoons coconut cream
- » 1 tablespoon parsley
- » Salt

DIRECTIONS

1. Blend all the soufflé items to a food processor.
2. Put it in the soufflé dishes, then bake within 6 minutes at 390 degrees F. Serve.

NUTRITION:

Calories 108, Total Fat 9 g, Cholesterol 180 mg, Sodium 146 mg, Total Carbs 1.1 g, Protein 6 g

44. BOK CHOY SAMBA

COOKING: 15' **PREPARATION: 5'** **SERVINGS: 3**

INGREDIENTS

» 1 onion
» 4 bok choy
» 4 tablespoons coconut cream
» Salt
» Ground black pepper
» ½ cup Parmesan cheese

DIRECTIONS

1. Toss bok choy with salt and black pepper.
2. Add oil to a large pan and sauté onion within 5 minutes.
3. Stir in bok choy and cream. Stir for 6 minutes.
4. Toss in cheese and cover the skillet to cook on low within 3 minutes. Serve.

NUTRITION:

Calories 112, Total Fat 4.9 g , Cholesterol 10 mg, Sodium 355 mg, Total Carbs 1.9 g, Protein 3 g

45. EGGS WITH WATERCRESS

COOKING: 5' **PREPARATION: 10'** **SERVINGS: 6**

INGREDIENTS

» 6 organic eggs
» 1 medium ripe avocado
» 1/3 cup watercress
» ½ tablespoon lemon juice
» Salt

DIRECTIONS

1. Put water into the pot with the trivet inside. Spread the watercress in the trivet.

2. Cook for 3 minutes with high pressure. Drain the steamed watercress.

3. Toss the watercress with lemon juice, salt, avocado, and yolks in a bowl. Mix and mash.

4. Divide the egg yolk mixture at the center of all the egg whites. Serve.

NUTRITION:

Calories 132, Total Fat 10.9 g, Cholesterol 164 mg, Sodium 65 mg, Total Carbs 3.3 g, Protein 6.3 g

46. BANANA PORRIDGE

COOKING: 5'   **PREPARATION: 10'**   **SERVINGS: 2**

INGREDIENTS

- » ½ cup walnuts
- » 1 banana
- » ¾ cup hot water
- » 2 tablespoons coconut butter
- » ½ teaspoon cinnamon powder
- » 2 teaspoons maple syrup

DIRECTIONS

1. Pulse all the items using a blender, then transfer to a saucepan.
2. Warm-up over medium heat, 5 minutes, then transfers and serve.

NUTRITION:

Calories: 353, Fat: 28, Fiber: 3, Carbs: 21, Protein: 8

47. MUSHROOM SANDWICH

COOKING: 10'   **PREPARATION: 5'**   **SERVINGS: 1**

INGREDIENTS

- » 2 Portobello mushroom caps
- » 2 lettuce leaves
- » 2 avocado slices
- » ½ pound turkey meat, cooked
- » Olive oil

DIRECTIONS

1. Cook the turkey meat, and within 4 minutes, transfer and drain excess oil.

2. Warm-up pan with the olive oil, add mushroom caps, cook for 2 minutes on each side.

3. Remove then arrange 1 mushroom cap on a plate, add turkey, avocado slices, lettuce leaves, and serve.

NUTRITION:

Calories: 521, Fat: 25, Carbs: 3, Protein: 67

48. BELL PEPPER SANDWICH

COOKING: 10' **PREPARATION: 5'** **SERVINGS: 2**

INGREDIENTS

- » 2 cups bell peppers
- » ½ tablespoon avocado oil
- » 3 eggs
- » 15 oz turkey fillet
- » Olive oil

DIRECTIONS

1. Warm-up oil over medium-high heat, add bell peppers, stir and cook within 5 minutes
2. Warm-up another pans over medium heat, add the turkey meat, stir, cook within 3-4 minutes, transfer.
3. Mix the eggs, put to the pan with the bell peppers, cook for 7-8 minutes. Serve.

NUTRITION:

Calories: 580, Fat: 25, Fiber: 1, Carbs: 9, Protein: 75

49. MUSHROOM AND SALMON SLIDERS

COOKING: 15' **PREPARATION: 10'** **SERVINGS: 3**

INGREDIENTS

- » 3 Portobello mushroom caps
- » 10 oz turkey meat
- » 3 eggs
- » 4 ounces smoked salmon
- » Olive oil

DIRECTIONS

1. Warm-up a pan over medium-high heat, add the turkey, cook within 4 minutes, transfer.
2. Warm-up pan with the olive oil over medium heat, place egg rings in the pan, crack an egg in each, cook within 6 minutes, and transfer.
3. Warm-up the pan again, add mushroom caps, cook within 5 minutes, and transfer.
4. Top each mushroom cap with turkey slices, salmon, and eggs and serve.

NUTRITION:

Calories: 315, Fat: 15, Carbs: 1, Protein: 40

50. BEEF AND SQUASH SKILLET

COOKING: 20'   **PREPARATION: 10'**   **SERVINGS: 3**

INGREDIENTS

- » 15 ounces beef
- » 2 tablespoons ghee
- » 3 garlic cloves
- » 2 celery stalks
- » 1 yellow onion
- » Sea salt
- » Black pepper
- » ½ teaspoon coriander
- » 1 teaspoon cumin
- » 1 teaspoon garam masala
- » ½ butternut squash
- » 3 eggs
- » 1 small avocado
- » 15 ounces spinach

DIRECTIONS

1. Warm-up a pan with the ghee over medium heat, add onion, garlic, celery, a pinch of salt and pepper, cook within 3 minutes. Add beef, cumin, garam masala, and coriander, cook within 5 minutes more.
2. Add squash flesh and spinach, stir and make 3 holes in this mix.
3. Break an egg into the pan then bake at 375 degrees F, 15 minutes. Serve with avocado on top.

NUTRITION:

Calories: 594, Fat: 35, Fiber: 9, Carbs: 19, Protein: 54

51. TURKEY AND VEGGIES MIX

COOKING: 15'   **PREPARATION: 10'**   **SERVINGS: 4**

INGREDIENTS

- » 20 ounces of turkey meat
- » 4 tablespoons coconut oil
- » 1 small green bell pepper
- » ½ cup onion
- » 2 garlic cloves
- » 2 cups sweet potato
- » 1 avocado
- » 3 eggs
- » 2 cups spinach

DIRECTIONS

1. Warm-up a pan with the oil, add onion, stir and cook within 3 minutes.
2. After that, add the garlic and bell pepper, cook within 1 minute. Put the ground turkey, cook within 15 minutes more. Put the sweet potato, cook within 4 minutes. Put the spinach, cook within 2 minutes. Make 3 holes in the batter, break an egg in each, place pan under a preheated broiler, and cook within 3 minutes. Top with avocado slices and serve.

NUTRITION:

Calories: 619, Fat: 34, Fiber: 7, Carbs: 29, Protein: 49

52. PORK SKILLET

COOKING: 20'   **PREPARATION: 10'**   **SERVINGS: 4**

INGREDIENTS

- » 8 ounces mushrooms
- » 1-pound pork
- » 1 tablespoon olive oil
- » 2 zucchinis
- » ½ teaspoon garlic powder
- » ½ teaspoon basil
- » Sea salt
- » Black pepper
- » 2 tablespoons Dijon mustard

DIRECTIONS

1. Warm-up a pan with the oil over medium-high heat, add mushrooms, cook within 4 minutes.
2. Put zucchinis, salt, and black pepper cook within 4 minutes more.
3. Put pork, garlic powder, and basil, cook within 10 minutes.
4. Put the mustard, stir, and cook within 3 more minutes. Transfer and serve.

NUTRITION:

Calories: 226, Fat: 8, Fiber: 1, Carbs: 5, Protein: 3

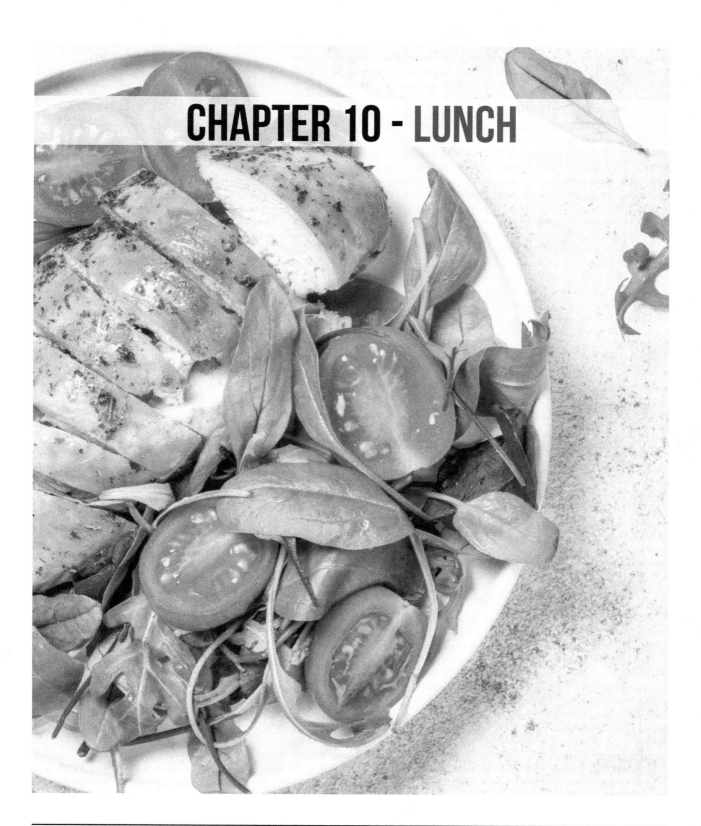

CHAPTER 10 - LUNCH

53. EASY KETO SMOKED SALMON LUNCH BOWL

COOKING: 0'   **PREPARATION: 15'**   **SERVINGS: 2**

INGREDIENTS

- » 12 ounces smoked salmon
- » 4 tablespoon mayonnaise
- » 2 ounces spinach
- » 1 tablespoon olive oil
- » 1 medium lime
- » Pepper
- » Salt

DIRECTIONS

1. Warm-up the butter to a pan over high heat.

2. Put the ground beef plus the pepper and salt. Cook.

3. Reduce heat to medium. Add the remaining butter and the green beans then cook within five minutes. Put pepper and salt, then transfer. Serve with a dollop of sour cream..

NUTRITION

Calories: 457, Net Carbs: 1.9g, Fats: 34.8g, Protein: 32.3g

54. EASY ONE-PAN GROUND BEEF AND GREEN BEANS

COOKING: 15'   **PREPARATION: 15'**   **SERVINGS: 2**

INGREDIENTS

- » 10 ounces ground beef
- » 9 ounces green beans
- » Pepper
- » Salt
- » 2 tablespoons sour cream
- » 3½ ounces butter

DIRECTIONS

1. Warm-up the butter to a pan over high heat.

2. Put the ground beef plus the pepper and salt. Cook.

3. Reduce heat to medium. Add the remaining butter and the green beans then cook within five minutes. Put pepper and salt, then transfer. Serve with a dollop of sour cream.

NUTRITION

Net Carbs: 6.65g, Calories: 787.5, Fats: 71.75g, Protein: 27.5g

55. EASY SPINACH AND BACON SALAD

COOKING: 15' **PREPARATION: 15'** **SERVINGS:4**

INGREDIENTS

» 8 ounces spinach
» 4 large hard-boiled eggs
» 6 ounces bacon
» 2 medium red onions
» 2 cups of mayonnaise
» Pepper
» Salt

DIRECTIONS

1. Cook the bacon, then chop into pieces, set aside.

2. Slice the hard-boiled eggs, and then rinse the spinach.

3. Combine the lettuce, mayonnaise, and bacon fat into a large cup, put pepper and salt.

4. Add the red onion, sliced eggs, and bacon into the salad, then toss. Serve.

NUTRITION

Fats: 45.9g, Calories: 509.15, Net Carbs: 2.5g, Protein: 19.75g

56. EASY KETO ITALIAN PLATE

COOKING:0' **PREPARATION: 15'** **SERVINGS: 2**

INGREDIENTS

» 7 ounces mozzarella cheese
» 7 ounces prosciutto
» 2 tomatoes
» 4 tablespoons olive oil
» 10 whole green olives
» Pepper
» Salt

DIRECTIONS

1. Arrange the tomato, olives, mozzarella, and prosciutto on a plate.

2. Season the tomato and cheese with pepper and salt. Serve with olive oil.

NUTRITION

Calories: 780.98, Net Carbs: 5.9g, Fats: 60.74g, Protein: 50.87g

57. FRESH BROCCOLI AND DILL KETO SALAD

COOKING: 7'   **PREPARATION: 15'**   **SERVINGS: 3**

INGREDIENTS

- » 16 ounces broccoli
- » 1/2 cup mayonnaise
- » 3/4 cup chopped dill
- » Salt
- » Pepper

DIRECTIONS

1. Boil salted water in a saucepan. Put the chopped broccoli in the pot and boil for 3-5 minutes. Drain and set aside. Once cooled, mix the rest of the fixing. Put pepper and salt, then serve.

NUTRITION

Calories: 303.33, Net Carbs: 6.2g, Fats: 28.1g, Protein: 4.03g

58. KETO SMOKED SALMON FILLED AVOCADOS

COOKING: 0'   **PREPARATION: 15'**   **SERVINGS: 1**

INGREDIENTS

- » 1 avocado
- » 3 ounces smoked salmon
- » 4 tablespoons sour cream
- » 1 tablespoon lemon juice
- » Pepper
- » Salt

DIRECTIONS

1. Cut the avocado into two. Place the sour cream in the hollow parts of the avocado with smoked salmon. Put pepper and salt, squeeze lemon juice over the top. Serve.

NUTRITION

Calories: 517, Net Carbs: 6.7g, Fats: 42.6g, Protein: 20.6g

59. LOW-CARB BROCCOLI LEMON PARMESAN SOUP

COOKING: 15'   **PREPARATION: 15'**   **SERVINGS: 4**

INGREDIENTS

- » 3 cups of water
- » 1 cup unsweetened almond milk
- » 32 ounces broccoli florets
- » 1 cup heavy whipping cream
- » 3/4 cup Parmesan cheese
- » Salt
- » Pepper
- » 2 tablespoons lemon juice

DIRECTIONS

1. Cook broccoli plus water over medium-high heat.

2. Take out 1 cup of the cooking liquid, and remove the rest.

3. Blend half the broccoli, reserved cooking oil, unsweetened almond milk, heavy cream, and salt plus pepper in a blender.

4. Put the blended items to the remaining broccoli, and stir with Parmesan cheese and lemon juice. Cook until heated through. Serve with Parmesan cheese on the top.

NUTRITION

Calories: 371, Net Carbs: 11.67g, Fats: 28.38g, Protein: 14.63g

60. PROSCIUTTO AND MOZZARELLA BOMB

COOKING: 10'   **PREPARATION: 15'**   **SERVINGS: 4**

INGREDIENTS

- » 4 ounces sliced prosciutto
- » 8 ounces mozzarella ball
- » Olive oil

DIRECTIONS

1. Layer half of the prosciutto vertically. Lay the remaining slices horizontally across the first set of slices. Place mozzarella ball, upside down, onto the crisscrossed prosciutto slices.

2. Wrap the mozzarella ball with the prosciutto slices. Warm-up the olive oil in a skillet, crisp the prosciutto, then serve.

NUTRITION

Calories: 253, Net Carbs: 1.08g, Fats: 19.35g, Protein: 18g

61. SUMMER TUNA AVOCADO SALAD

COOKING: 0' **PREPARATION: 15'** **SERVINGS: 2**

INGREDIENTS

- » 1 can tuna flake
- » 1 medium avocado
- » 1 medium English cucumber
- » ¼ cup cilantro
- » 1 tbsp lemon juice
- » 1 tbsp olive oil
- » Pepper
- » Salt

DIRECTIONS

1. Put the first 4 ingredients into a salad bowl. Sprinkle with the lemon and olive oil. Serve.

NUTRITION

Calories 303, Net Carbs: 5.2g, Fats: 22.6g, Protein: 16.7g

62. MUSHROOMS & GOAT CHEESE SALAD

COOKING: 10' **PREPARATION: 15'** **SERVINGS: 1**

INGREDIENTS

- » 1 tablespoon butter
- » 2 ounces cremini mushrooms
- » Pepper
- » Salt
- » 4 ounces spring mix
- » 1-ounce cooked bacon
- » 1-ounce goat cheese
- » 1 tablespoon olive oil
- » 1 tablespoon balsamic vinegar

DIRECTIONS

1. Sautee the mushrooms, put pepper and salt.

2. Place the salad greens in a bowl. Top with goat cheese and crumbled bacon.

3. Mix these in the salad once the mushrooms are done.

4. Whisk the olive oil in a small bowl and balsamic vinegar. Put the salad on top and serve.

NUTRITION

Calories: 243, Fat: 21gm, Carbs: 8g, Saturated Fat: 4g, Fiber: 1g

63. KETO BACON SUSHI

COOKING: 13'   **PREPARATION: 15'**   **SERVINGS: 4**

INGREDIENTS

- » 6 slices bacon
- » 1 avocado
- » 2 Persian cucumbers
- » 2 medium carrots
- » 4 oz. cream cheese

DIRECTIONS

1. Warm-up oven to 400F. Line a baking sheet. Place bacon halves in an even layer and bake, 11 to 13 minutes.

2. Meanwhile, slice cucumbers, avocado, and carrots into parts roughly the width of the bacon.

3. Spread an even layer of cream cheese in the cooled down bacon. Divide vegetables evenly and place it on one end. Roll up vegetables tightly. Garnish and serve.

NUTRITION

Carbohydrates: 11g, Protein: 28g, Fat: 30g

64. COLE SLAW KETO WRAP

COOKING: 0'   **PREPARATION: 15'**   **SERVINGS: 2**

INGREDIENTS

- » 3 c Red Cabbage
- » .5 c Green Onions
- » .75 c Mayo
- » 2 tsp Apple Cider Vinegar
- » 25 tsp Salt
- » 16 pcs Collard Green
- » 1-pound Ground Meat, cooked
- » .33 c Alfalfa Sprouts
- » Toothpicks

DIRECTIONS

1. Mix slaw items with a spoon in a large-sized bowl.

2. Place a collard green on a plate and scoop a tablespoon of coleslaw on the edge of the leaf. Top it with a scoop of meat and sprouts. Roll and tuck the sides.

3. Insert the toothpicks. Serve.

NUTRITION

Calories: 409, Net Carbs: 4g, Fiber: 2g, Fat: 42g, Protein: 2g

65. KETO CHICKEN CLUB LETTUCE WRAP

COOKING: 15'   **PREPARATION: 15'**   **SERVINGS: 1**

INGREDIENTS

- » 1 head iceberg lettuce
- » 1 tbsp. mayonnaise
- » 6 slices of organic chicken
- » Bacon
- » Tomato

DIRECTIONS

1. Layer 6-8 large leaves of lettuce in the center of the parchment paper, around 9-10 inches.

2. Spread the mayo in the center and lay with chicken, bacon, and tomato.

3. Roll the wrap halfway through, then roll tuck in the ends of the wrap.

4. Cut it in half. Serve.

INGREDIENTS

Net Carbs: 4g, Fiber: 2g,Fat: 78g, Protein: 28g, Calories: 837

66. KETO BROCCOLI SALAD

COOKING: 0'   **PREPARATION: 10'**   **SERVINGS: 4-6**

INGREDIENTS

For salad:
- » 2 broccoli
- » 2 red cabbage
- » 5 c sliced almonds
- » 1 green onions
- » 5 c raisins

For the orange almond dressing:
- » 33 c orange juice
- » 25 c almond butter
- » 2 tbsp coconut aminos
- » 1 shallot
- » Salt

DIRECTIONS

1. Pulse the salt, shallot, amino, nut butter, and orange juice using a blender.

2. Combine other fixing in a bowl. Toss it with dressing and serve.

NUTRITION

Net Carbs: 13g, Fiber: 0g, Fat: 94g, Protein: 22g, Calories: 1022

67. KETO SHEET PAN CHICKEN AND RAINBOW VEGGIES

COOKING: 25'   **PREPARATION: 15'**   **SERVINGS: 4**

INGREDIENTS

- » Nonstick spray
- » 1-pound Chicken Breasts
- » 1 tbsp Sesame Oil
- » 2 tbsp Soy Sauce
- » 2 tbsp Honey
- » 2 Red Pepper
- » 2 Yellow Pepper
- » 3 Carrots
- » ½ Broccoli
- » 2 Red Onions
- » 2 tbsp EVOO
- » Pepper & salt
- » .25 c Parsley

DIRECTIONS

1. Grease the baking sheet, warm-up the oven to a temperature of 400-degrees.

2. Put the chicken in the middle of the sheet. Separately, combine the oil and the soy sauce. Brush over the chicken.

3. Separate veggies across the plate. Sprinkle with oil and then toss. Put pepper & salt.

4. Set tray into the oven and cook within 25 minutes. Garnish using parsley. Serve.

INGREDIENTS

Net Carbs: 9g, Fiber: 0g, Fat: 30g, Protein: 30g, Calories: 437kcal

68. SKINNY BANG-BANG ZUCCHINI NOODLES

COOKING: 15'   **PREPARATION: 15'**   **SERVINGS: 4**

INGREDIENTS

For the noodles:
- » 4 medium zucchinis spiraled
- » 1 tbsp. olive oil

For the sauce:
- » 0.25 cup + 2 tablespoons Plain Greek Yogurt
- » 0.25 cup + 2 tablespoons Mayo
- » 0.25 cup + 2 tablespoons Thai Sweet Chili Sauce
- » 1.5 teaspoons Honey
- » 1.5 teaspoons Sriracha
- » 2 teaspoons Lime Juice

DIRECTIONS

1. Pour the oil into a large skillet at medium temperature. Stir in the spiraled zucchini noodles. Cook.

2. Remove then drain, and let it rest 10 minutes. Combine sauce items into a bowl.

3. Mix in the noodles to the sauce. Serve.

NUTRITION

Net carbs: 18g, Fiber: 0g, Fat: 1g, Protein: 9g, Calories: 161g

69. KETO CAESAR SALAD

COOKING: 0'   **PREPARATION: 15'**   **SERVINGS: 4**

INGREDIENTS

- » 1.5 cups Mayonnaise
- » 3 tablespoons Apple Cider Vinegar
- » 1 teaspoon Dijon Mustard
- » 4 Anchovy Fillets
- » 24 Romaine Heart Leaves
- » 4 oz Pork Rinds
- » Parmesan

DIRECTIONS

1. 1. Process the mayo with ACV, mustard, and anchovies into a blender. Prepare romaine leaves and pour the dressing. Top with pork rinds and serve.

INGREDIENTS

Net Carbs: 4g, Fiber: 3g, Fat: 86g, Protein: 47g, Calories: 993kcal

70. KETO BUFFALO CHICKEN EMPANADAS

COOKING: 30'   **PREPARATION: 20'**   **SERVINGS: 6**

INGREDIENTS

For the empanada dough:
- » 1 ½ cups mozzarella cheese
- » 3 oz cream cheese
- » 1 whisked egg
- » 2 cups almond flour

For the buffalo chicken filling:
- » 2 cups shredded chicken
- » 2 tablespoons Butter
- » 0.33 cup Hot Sauce

DIRECTIONS

1. Warm-up oven, 425-degrees.

2. Microwave the cheese & cream cheese within 1-minute. Stir the flour and egg into the dish.

3. With another bowl, combine the chicken with sauce and set aside.

4. Cover a flat surface with plastic wrap and sprinkle with almond flour.

5. Grease a rolling pin, press the dough flat.

6. Make the circle shapes out of this dough with a lid.

7. Portion out spoonful of filling into these dough circles.

8. Fold the other half over to close up into half-moon shapes.

9. Bake within 9 minutes. Serve.

NUTRITION

Net Carbs: 20g, Fiber: 0g, Fat: 96g, Protein: 74g, Calories: 1217kcal

71. PEPPERONI AND CHEDDAR STROMBOLI

COOKING: 20'   **PREPARATION: 15'**   **SERVINGS: 3**

INGREDIENTS

- » 1.25 cups Mozzarella Cheese
- » 0.25 cup Almond Flour
- » 3 tablespoons Coconut Flour
- » 1 teaspoon Italian Seasoning
- » 1 Egg
- » 6 oz Deli Ham
- » 2 oz Pepperoni
- » 4 oz Cheddar Cheese
- » 1 tbsp Butter
- » 6 cups Salad Greens

DIRECTIONS

1. Warm-up the oven, 400 degrees.
2. Melt the mozzarella. Mix flours & Italian seasoning in a separate bowl.
3. Dump in the melty cheese and mix with pepper and salt.
4. Stir in the egg and process the dough. Pour it onto that prepared baking tray.
5. Roll out the dough. Cut slits that mark out 4 equal rectangles.
6. Put the ham and cheese, then brush with butter and close up.
7. Bake within 17 minutes. Slice and serve.

INGREDIENTS

Net carbs: 20g, Fiber: 0g, Fat: 13g, Protein: 11g, Calories: 240kcal

72. TUNA CASSEROLE

COOKING: 10'   **PREPARATION: 15'**   **SERVINGS: 4**

INGREDIENTS

- » Tuna in oil, sixteen ounces
- » Butter two tablespoons
- » Salt
- » Black pepper
- » Chili powder, one teaspoon
- » Celery, six stalks
- » Green bell pepper, one
- » Yellow onion, one
- » Parmesan cheese, grated four ounces
- » Mayonnaise, one cup

DIRECTIONS

1. Warm-up oven to 400.
2. Fry the onion, bell pepper, and celery chops in the melted butter within five minutes.
3. Mix with the chili powder, parmesan cheese, tuna, and mayonnaise.
4. Grease a baking pan. Add the tuna mixture into the fried vegetables.
5. Bake within twenty minutes. Serve.

NUTRITION

Calories 953, Net Carbs: 5g, Fat: 83g, Protein: 43g

73. BRUSSELS SPROUT AND HAMBURGER GRATIN

COOKING: 20'　　　**PREPARATION: 15'**　　　**SERVINGS: 4**

INGREDIENTS

» Ground beef, one pound
» Bacon, eight ounces
» Brussel sprouts, fifteen ounces
» Salt
» Black pepper
» Thyme; one-half teaspoon
» Cheddar cheese, one cup
» Italian seasoning; one tablespoon
» Sour cream; four tablespoons
» Butter; two tablespoons

DIRECTIONS

1. Warm-up oven to 425.

2. Fry bacon and Brussel sprouts in butter within five minutes.

3. Stir in the sour cream and put into a greased baking pan.

4. Cook the ground beef and put salt and pepper, then add this mix to the baking pan.

5. Top with the herbs and the shredded cheese. Bake within twenty minutes. Serve.

NUTRITION

Calories: 770kcal, Net Carbs: 8g, Fat: 62g, Protein: 42g

74. CARPACCIO

COOKING: 5'　　　**PREPARATION: 15'**　　　**SERVINGS: 4**

INGREDIENTS

» 100 grams smoked prime rib
» 30 grams arugula
» 20 grams Parmesan cheese
» 10 grams pine nuts
» 7 grams of butter
» 3 tablespoons olive oil with orange
» 1 tablespoon lemon juice
» Pepper
» Salt

DIRECTIONS

1. Arrange the meat slices on a plate. Place the arugula on top of the meat.

2. Spread Parmesan cheese over the arugula.

3. Put the butter in a frying pan. Add the pine nuts, bake for a few minutes over medium heat and then sprinkle them over the carpaccio.

4. For the vinaigrette, mix the lemon juice into the olive oil, put pepper and salt, and drizzle over the carpaccio. Serve.

NUTRITION

Calories: 350 kcal, Protein: 31 g, Fat: 24 g, Fiber: 1 g, Carbohydrates: 2 g

75. KETO CROQUE MONSIEUR

COOKING: 7'   **PREPARATION: 15'**   **SERVINGS: 4**

INGREDIENTS

- » 2 eggs
- » 25 grams grated cheese
- » 25 grams ham
- » 40 ml of cream
- » 40 ml mascarpone
- » 30 grams of butter
- » Pepper
- » Salt
- » Basil leaves

NUTRITION

Calories: 350 kcal, Protein: 31 g, Fat: 24 g, Fiber: 1 g

— Carbohydrates: 2 g

DIRECTIONS

1. Beat eggs in a bowl, put salt and pepper.

2. Add the cream, mascarpone, and grated cheese and mix.

3. Melt the butter over medium heat. Adjust the heat to low.

4. Add half of the omelet mixture to the frying pan and then place the slice of ham. Put the rest of the omelet mixture over the ham. Fry within 2-3 minutes over low heat.

5. Then put the omelet back in the frying pan to fry for another 1-2 minutes.

6. Garnish with a few basil leaves. Serve.

76. KETO WRAPS WITH CREAM CHEESE AND SALMON

COOKING: 10'   **PREPARATION: 15'**   **SERVINGS: 4**

INGREDIENTS

- » 80 grams of cream cheese
- » 1 tablespoon dill
- » 30 grams smoked salmon
- » 1 egg
- » 15 grams of butter
- » Pinch cayenne pepper
- » Pepper
- » Salt

NUTRITION

Calories: 479 kcal, Protein: 16 g, Fats: 45 g — Net carbohydrates: 4 g

DIRECTIONS

1. Beat the egg well in a bowl.

2. Dissolve the butter over medium heat in a small frying pan. Put half of the beaten egg into the pan.

3. Carefully loosen the egg on the edges with a silicone spatula and turn the wafer-thin omelet, about 45 seconds each side. Remove.

4. Cut the dill into small pieces and put them in a bowl.

5. Add the cream cheese and the salmon, cut into small pieces. Mix.

6. Put a cayenne pepper and mix. Put salt and pepper.

7. Spread a layer on the wrap and roll it up. Cut the wrap in half and serve.

77. SAVORY KETO BROCCOLI CHEESE MUFFINS

COOKING: 10'   **PREPARATION: 15'**   **SERVINGS: 4**

INGREDIENTS

- » 4 eggs
- » 75 grams Parmesan cheese
- » 125 grams young cheese
- » 125 grams mozzarella
- » 75 grams of broccoli
- » 1.5 teaspoon baking powder
- » 0.25 teaspoon garlic powder
- » 0.25 teaspoon mustard

DIRECTIONS

1. Warm-up oven to 160° Celsius.

2. Boil water into a saucepan, put the broccoli pieces, for 1 minute. Drain.

3. Grate the Parmesan cheese and the young cheese. Cut the mozzarella into small pieces.

4. Beat the eggs, put the broccoli, cheese, and mustard.

5. Then add the garlic powder and baking powder and mix.

6. Add baking powder and garlic powder.

7. Fill a silicone muffin tray with the broccoli-cheese egg batter and bake within 10 minutes. Serve.

NUTRITION

Calories: 349 kcal, Protein: 28 g, Fats: 25 g, Fiber: 1 g, Carbohydrates: 3 g

78. KETO RUSK

COOKING: 9'   **PREPARATION: 15'**   **SERVINGS: 6**

INGREDIENTS

- » 35 grams of almond flour
- » 1 egg
- » 1 tablespoon butter
- » 0.5 teaspoon baking powder
- » 1/8 teaspoon salt

DIRECTIONS

1. Warm-up oven to 200° Celsius. Put all the fixing in a cup and mix.

2. Microwave within 90 seconds.

3. Cooldown and cut the dough into 5 equal slices and place it on a sheet with baking paper.

4. Bake for 5-6 minutes then serve.

NUTRITION

Calories: 53 kcal, Protein: 2 g, Fats: 4 g, Carbohydrates: 1 g

---

79. FLAXSEED HEMP FLOUR BUN

COOKING: 8' **PREPARATION: 15'** **SERVINGS: 4**

INGREDIENTS

» 1 teaspoon hemp flour
» 1 teaspoon linseed flour
» 1 teaspoon psyllium
» 1 teaspoon baking powder
» 1 egg
» 0.5 teaspoon butter

DIRECTIONS

1. Warm-up oven to 180°C. Put all dry items in a large cup, mix.

2. Add the egg and the butter then mix it again. Microwave within 1 minute.

3. Remove the sandwich and cut it into three slices. Bake those slices within 5 minutes. Serve.

NUTRITION

Calories: 182 kcal, Protein: 11g, Fats: 15g, Fiber: 12 g

80. KETO MUFFINS WITH ROQUEFORT

COOKING: 18' **PREPARATION: 15'** **SERVINGS: 4**

INGREDIENTS

» 150 grams zucchini
» 50 ml extra virgin olive oil
» Pepper
» 100 grams red pepper
» 75 grams Roquefort
» 100 grams mascarpone
» 6 eggs
» 1.5 teaspoon baking powder

DIRECTIONS

1. Warm-up oven to 175° Celsius.

2. Fry the zucchini and bell pepper within 5 minutes. Beat the eggs with the baking powder.

3. Mix the vegetables, the butter, mascarpone, and cheese and put over the muffin tins.

4. Bake within 15 minutes. Serve.

NUTRITION

Calories: 160 kcal, Protein: 6g, Fats: 14g, Fiber: 1g, Carbohydrates: 1g

81. KETO WRAP

COOKING: 5' **PREPARATION: 15'** **SERVINGS: 5**

INGREDIENTS

- » 1 egg
- » 0.5 teaspoon coconut fat
- » 0.5 teaspoon curry powder

DIRECTIONS

1. Warm-up coconut fat in a small frying pan over high heat.

2. Beat the egg plus the curry powder with salt in a bowl.

3. Put the batter into the frying pan. Bake this wafer-thin omelet within 10-20 seconds.

4. Turn the wrap over and bake for a few seconds. Serve.

NUTRITION

Calories: 128 kcal, Protein: 6g, Fats: 12g, Fiber: 0.3 g, Carbohydrates: 1 g

82. SAVORY KETO MUFFINS

COOKING: 20' **PREPARATION: 15'** **SERVINGS: 5**

INGREDIENTS

- » 4 eggs
- » 1 forest outing
- » 100 grams chorizo
- » 75 grams mascarpone
- » 100 grams grated cheese
- » Salt
- » Pepper

DIRECTIONS

1. Warm-up oven to 175° Celsius.

2. Beat the eggs with the mascarpone.

3. Add the spring onion, cheese, and chorizo to the egg batter. Put salt and pepper. Mix.

4. Bake within 9 - 14 minutes. Cooldown and serve.

NUTRITION

Calories: 315 kcal, Protein: 17g, Fats: 26g, Fiber: 1g, Carbohydrates: 0g

CHAPTER 11 - SNAKS

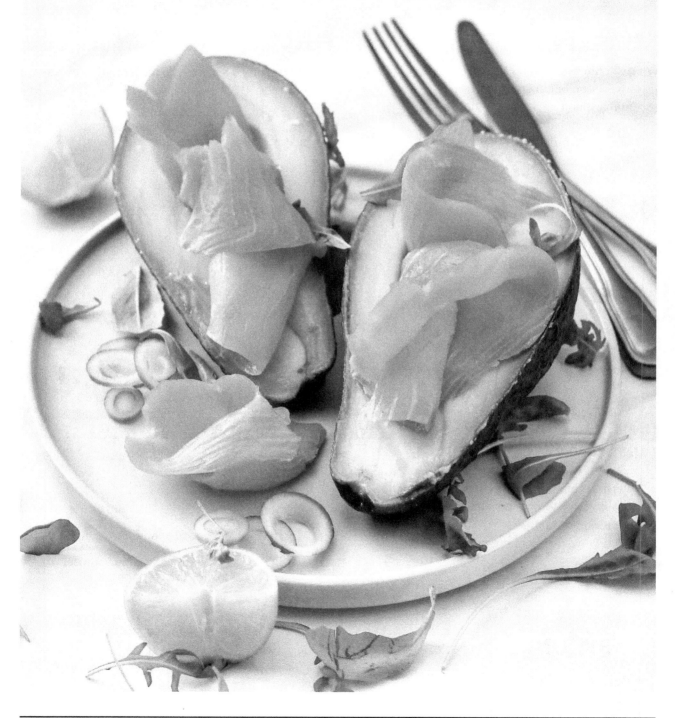

83. KETO RASPBERRY CAKE AND WHITE CHOCOLATE SAUCE

COOKING: 45'   **PREPARATION: 15'**   **SERVINGS: 4'**

INGREDIENTS

- » 5 ounces cacao butter
- » 4 teaspoons pure vanilla extract
- » 4 eggs
- » 3 cup raspberries
- » 2½ ounces grass-fed ghee
- » 1 teaspoon baking powder
- » 1 tablespoon apple cider vinegar
- » 1 cup green banana flour
- » ¾ cup coconut cream
- » ¾ cup granulated sweetener
- » 4 ounces cacao butter
- » 2 teaspoons pure vanilla extract
- » ¾ cup coconut cream
- » Salt

NUTRITION

Calories: 325 kcal, Total Fat: 12g, Total Carbs: 3g, Protein: 40g

DIRECTIONS

1. Mix the butter and the sweetener. Pour in the grass-fed ghee into the mix, blend.

2. Beat the eggs in a different bowl. Warm-up oven to 350 degrees F. Grease a baking pan.

3. Put the mixed eggs to the butter and sweetener mixture. Mix well.

4. Pour in the banana flour and mix. Then the vanilla extract, apple cider, coconut cream, baking powder, and mix again.

5. Spoon around the sliced raspberries. Then, sprinkle flour in the baking pan.

6. Put the mixture into the pan then bake within 45 minutes. Cool down.

For the sauce:

7. Mix cacao butter with 2 teaspoons pure vanilla extract. Add coconut cream and beat. Put salt and beat. Chop the remaining berries and throw them in the mix. Pour the mixture on the cake. Serve cold.

84. KETO CHOCOLATE CHIP COOKIES

COOKING: 10'   **PREPARATION: 15'**   **SERVINGS: 4**

INGREDIENTS

- » 7 spoons unsweetened coconut powder
- » 7 tablespoons Keto chocolate chips
- » 5 tablespoons butter
- » 2 flat tablespoon baking powder
- » 2 eggs
- » 2/3 confectioners swerve
- » 1 1/3 cups almond flour
- » A teaspoon vanilla extract

NUTRITION

Calories: 287 kcal, Total Fat: 19g, Total Carbs: 6.5g, Protein: 6.8g

DIRECTIONS

1. Warm-up oven to 325.

2. Melt half chocolate chips, then the butter. Mix.

3. Mix the eggs in chocolate and butter mixture.

4. Mix in the vanilla extract, coconut powder, confectioners swerve, and almond flour. Mix well.

5. Add chocolate chip cookies. Then, add baking powder, and mix until dough forms.

6. Spread out and cut out cookies, top with chocolate chips. Bake within 8 to 10 minutes. Serve.

85. KETO BEEF AND SAUSAGE BALLS

COOKING: 20'   **PREPARATION: 15'**   **SERVINGS: 3**

INGREDIENTS

For the meat:
- » 2 pounds ground beef
- » 2 pounds ground sausage
- » 2 eggs
- » ½ cup Keto mayonnaise
- » 1/3 cup ground pork rinds
- » ½ cup Parmesan cheese
- » Salt
- » Pepper
- » 2 tablespoons butter
- » 3 tablespoons oil

For the sauce:
- » 3 diced onions
- » 2 pounds mushrooms
- » 5 cloves garlic
- » 3 cups beef broth
- » 1 cup sour cream
- » 2 tablespoons mustard
- » Worcestershire sauce
- » Salt
- » Pepper
- » Parsley
- » 1 tablespoon Arrowroot powder

DIRECTIONS

1. Put meat, egg, and onions in a bowl, mix. Put beef, parmesan, egg, mayonnaise, sausage, pork rind in a bowl. Add salt and pepper. Warm-up oil in a skillet.

2. Mold the beef mixture into balls, fry within 7-10 minutes. Put aside.

3. Fry the diced onions, then the garlic and mushrooms, cook within 3 minutes. Then, add the broth. Mix in mustard, sour cream, and Worcestershire sauce. Boil within two minutes, then add in the meatballs. Add salt and pepper, simmer. Serve.

NUTRITION

Calories: 592 kcal, Total Fat: 53.9g, Total Carbs: 1.3g, Protein: 25.4g

86. KETO COCONUT FLAKE BALLS

COOKING: 0'   **PREPARATION: 15'**   **SERVINGS: 2**

INGREDIENTS

- » 1 Vanilla Shortbread Collagen Protein Bar
- » 1 tablespoon lemon
- » ¼ teaspoon ground ginger
- » ½ cup unsweetened coconut flakes
- » ¼ teaspoon ground turmeric

DIRECTIONS

1. Process protein bar, ginger, turmeric, and ¾ of the total flakes into a food processor.

2. Remove and add a spoon of water and roll till dough forms.

3. Roll into balls, and sprinkle the rest of the flakes on it. Serve.

NUTRITION

Calories: 204 kcal, Total Fat: 11g, Total Carbs: 4.2g, Protein: 1.5g

87. KETO CHOCOLATE GREEK YOGHURT COOKIES

COOKING: 30' **PREPARATION: 15'** **SERVINGS: 3**

INGREDIENTS

» 3 eggs
» 1/8 teaspoon tartar
» 5 tablespoons softened Greek yogurt

DIRECTIONS

1. Beat the egg whites, the tartar, and mix.

2. In the yolk, put in the Greek yogurt, and mix.

3. Combine both egg whites and yolk batter into a bowl.

4. Bake within 25-30 minutes, serve.

NUTRITION

Calories: 287 kcal, Total Fat: 19g, Total Carbs: 6.5g, Protein: 6.8g

88. KETO COCONUT FLAVORED ICE CREAM

COOKING: 0' **PREPARATION: 15'** **SERVINGS: 4**

INGREDIENTS

» 4 cups of coconut milk
» 2/3 cup xylitol
» ¼ teaspoon salt
» 2 teaspoons vanilla extract
» 1 teaspoon coconut extract

DIRECTIONS

1. Add the coconut milk in a bowl, with the sweetener, extracts, and salt. Mix.

2. Pour this mixture in the ice cube trays, and put it in the freezer. Serve.

NUTRITION

Calories: 244 kcal, Total Fat: 48g, Total Carbs: 6g, Protein: 15g

89. CHOCOLATE-COCONUT COOKIES

COOKING: 20'   **PREPARATION: 15'**   **SERVINGS: 4**

INGREDIENTS

- » 2 eggs
- » ½ cup of cocoa powder
- » ½ cup flour
- » ½ cup of coconut oil
- » ¼ cup grated coconut
- » Stevia

DIRECTIONS

1. Warm-up oven to 350 °F. Crack eggs and separate whites and yolks, mix separately.

2. Put salt to the yolks. Warm-up oil in a skillet, add cocoa, egg whites, and mix. Add in the salted yolks; then, add stevia. Add in coconut flour, and mix until dough forms.

3. On a flat surface, sprinkle grated coconut. Roll the dough around in the coconut, mix. Mold into cookies. Bake within 15 minutes, serve.

NUTRITION

Calories: 260 kcal, Total Fat: 26g, Total Carbs: 4.5g, Protein: 1g

90. KETO BUFFALO CHICKEN MEATBALLS

COOKING: 20'   **PREPARATION: 15'**   **SERVINGS: 3**

INGREDIENTS

- » 1-pound ground chicken
- » 1 large
- » 2/3 cup hot sauce
- » ½ cup almond flour
- » ½ teaspoon salt
- » ½ teaspoon pepper
- » ½ cup melted butter
- » 1 large onion
- » 1 teaspoon garlic

DIRECTIONS

1. Combine meat, egg, and onions in a bowl. Pour in almond flour, garlic, salt, and pepper in.

2. Warm-up oven to 350°F and grease a baking tray.

3. Mold the egg mixture into balls. Bake within 18-20 minutes.

4. Melt butter in the microwave for few seconds; mix it with hot sauce.

5. Put the sauce into meatballs. Serve.

NUTRITION

Calories: 360 kcal, Total Fat: 26g, Total Carbs: 4.5g, Protein: 1g

91. EGGPLANT AND CHICKPEA BITES

COOKING: 90' **PREPARATION: 15'** **SERVINGS: 6**

INGREDIENTS

» 3 large aubergines
» Spray oil
» 2 large cloves garlic
» 2 tbsp. coriander powder
» 2 tbsp. cumin seeds
» 400 g canned chickpeas
» 2 Tbsp. chickpea flour
» Zest and juice 1/2 lemon
» 1/2 lemon quartered
» 3 tbsp. tablespoon polenta

DIRECTIONS

1. Warm-up oven to 200°C. Grease the eggplant halves and place it on the meat side up on a baking sheet. Sprinkle with coriander and cumin seeds, and then place the cloves of garlic on the plate. Roast within 40 minutes, put aside.

2. Add chickpeas, chickpea flour, zest, and lemon juice. Crush roughly and mix well.

3. Form about twenty pellets and place them on a baking sheet. Fridge within 30 minutes.

4. Warm-up oven to 180°C. Remove the meatballs from the fridge and coat it in the polenta. Roast for 20 minutes. Serve with lemon wedges.

NUTRITION

Calories: 70, Carbs: 4g, Fat: 5g — Protein: 2g

92. BABA GANOUJ

COOKING: 20' **PREPARATION: 15'** **SERVINGS: 3**

INGREDIENTS

» 1 large aubergine
» 1 head of garlic
» 30 ml of olive oil
» Lemon juice

DIRECTIONS

1. Warm-up oven to 350 ° F.

2. Place the eggplant on the plate, skin side up. Roast, about 1 hour.

3. Place the garlic cloves in a square of aluminum foil. Fold the edges of the sheet. Roast with the eggplant, about 20 minutes. Let cool. Purée the pods with a garlic press.

4. Puree the flesh of the eggplant. Add the garlic puree, the oil, and the lemon juice.

5. Serve.

NUTRITION

Calories: 87, Carbs: 6g, Fat: 6g, Protein: 2g

93. SPICY CRAB DIP

COOKING: 20' **PREPARATION: 15'** **SERVINGS: 3**

INGREDIENTS

- » 8 oz cream cheese
- » 1 tbsp. onions
- » 1 tbsp. lemon juice
- » 2 tbsp. Worcestershire sauce
- » 1/8 tsp. t. black
- » Cayenne pepper
- » 2 tbsp. milk
- » 6 oz crabmeat

DIRECTIONS

1. Warm-up oven to 375 ° F.

2. Pour the cream cheese into a bowl. Add the onions, lemon juice, Worcestershire sauce, black pepper, and cayenne pepper. Mix. Stir in the milk and crab meat.

3. Cook uncovered within 15 minutes. Serve.

NUTRITION

Calories: 134, Carbs: 4g, Fat: 12g, Protein: 4g

94. PARMESAN CHEESE "POTATOES"

COOKING: 10' **PREPARATION: 15'** **SERVINGS: 3**

INGREDIENTS

- » 75 g Parmesan cheese
- » 1 tbsp Chia seeds
- » 2 tbsp whole flaxseeds
- » 2½ tbsp pumpkin seeds

DIRECTIONS

1. Warm-up oven to 180 ° C.

2. Combine both the cheese and seeds in a bowl.

3. Put small piles of the mixture on the baking paper, bake within 8 to 10 minutes

4. Remove and serve.

NUTRITION

Calories: 165, Carbs: 18g, Fat: 9g, Protein: 3g

95. CHILI CHEESE CHICKEN WITH CRISPY AND DELICIOUS CABBAGE SALAD

COOKING: 70'   **PREPARATION: 15'**   **SERVINGS: 5**

INGREDIENTS

Chili Cheese Chicken:
» 400 grams of chicken
» 200 grams tomatoes
» 100 grams of cream cheese
» 125 grams cheddar
» 40 grams jalapenos
» 60 grams of bacon

Crispy Cabbage Salad:
» 0.5 pcs casserole
» 200 grams Brussels sprouts
» 2 grams of almonds
» 3 tangerines
» 1 tablespoon olive oil
» 1 teaspoon apple cider vinegar
» 0.5 tsp salt
» 0.25 teaspoon pepper
» 1 tablespoon lemon

DIRECTIONS

1. Warm-up oven at 200 °. Put tomatoes half in the bottom of a baking dish. Put chicken fillets, half cream cheese on each chicken fillet, and sprinkle with cheddar. Spread jalapenos and bake within 25 minutes. Place bacon on a baking sheet with baking paper, and bake within 10 minutes.

For cabbage salad:

2. Blend the Brussels sprouts and cumin in a food processor.Make the dressing of juice from one tangerine, olive oil, apple cider vinegar, salt, pepper, and lemon juice. Put the cabbage in a dish and spread the dressing over. Chop almonds, cut the tangerine into slices, and place it on the salad. Sprinkle the bacon over the chicken dish. Serve.

NUTRITION

Calories: 515, Carbs: 35g, Fat: 23g, Protein: 42g

96. KETO PUMPKIN PIE SWEET AND SPICY

COOKING: 60'   **PREPARATION: 15'**   **SERVINGS: 5**

INGREDIENTS

Pie Bottom:
» 110 grams of almond flour
» 50 grams sucrine
» 0.5 tsp salt
» 1 scoop protein powder
» 1 paragraph eggs
» 80 grams of butter
» 15 grams of fiber

The Filling:
» 1 pcs Hokkaido
» 3 paragraph egg yolks
» 60 ml of coconut fat
» 1 teaspoon vanilla powder
» 15 grams of protein powder
» 1 teaspoon cinnamon
» 2 grams sucrine
» 0.5 tsp cardamom Black; 0.5 tsp cloves

DIRECTIONS

1. Warm-up oven to 175 °.

2. Combine all the dry fixing and add the wet ones. Mix and shape it into a dough lump. Put in a baking paper, then flatten the dough. Prick holes then bake within 8-10 minutes.

3. For filling:

4. Cut the meat of Hokkaido and cook within 15-20 minutes. Process it with the other fixing. Pour the stuffing into the baked pie and bake again within 25-30 minutes. Cool and serve.

NUTRITION

Calories: 229, Carbs: 4g, Fat: 22g, Protein: 8g

97. BLACKENED TILAPIA WITH ZUCCHINI NOODLES

COOKING: 10'　　　**PREPARATION: 15'**　　　**SERVINGS: 5**

INGREDIENTS

- » 2 zucchinis
- » ¾ teaspoon salt
- » 2 garlic cloves
- » 1 cup Pico de Gallo
- » 1 ½ pounds fish
- » 2 teaspoons olive oil
- » ½ teaspoon cumin
- » ¼ teaspoon garlic powder
- » ½ paprika
- » ½ teaspoon pepper

DIRECTIONS

1. Mix half salt, pepper, cumin, paprika, and garlic powder, rub to the fish thoroughly. Cook within 3 minutes each side and remove it. Cook zucchini and garlic, remaining salt within 2 minutes. Serve.

NUTRITION

Calories: 220, Carbs: 27g, Fat: 2g, Protein: 24g

98. BELL PEPPER NACHOS

COOKING: 10'　　　**PREPARATION: 15'**　　　**SERVINGS: 2**

INGREDIENTS

- » 2 bell peppers
- » 4 ounces beef ground
- » ¼ teaspoon cumin
- » ¼ cup guacamole
- » Salt
- » 1 cup cheese
- » ¼ teaspoon chili powder
- » 1 tablespoon vegetable oil
- » 2 tablespoons sour cream
- » ¼ cup Pico de Gallo

DIRECTIONS

1. Process protein bar, ginger, turmeric, and ¾ of the total flakes into a food processor.

2. Remove and add a spoon of water and roll till dough forms.

3. Roll into balls, and sprinkle the rest of the flakes on it. Serve.

NUTRITION

Calories: 475, Carbs: 19g, Fat: 24g, Protein: 50g

99. RADISH, CARROT & CILANTRO SALAD

COOKING: 0' **PREPARATION: 15'** **SERVINGS: 2**

INGREDIENTS

- » 1 ½ pounds carrots
- » ¼ cup cilantro
- » 1 ½ pound radish
- » ½ teaspoon salt
- » 6 onions
- » ¼ teaspoon black pepper
- » 3 tablespoons lemon juice
- » 3 tablespoons orange juice
- » 2 tablespoons olive oil

DIRECTIONS

1. Mix all the items until they merged properly. Chill and serve.

NUTRITION

Calories: 33, Carbs: 7g, Fat: 0g, Protein: 0g

100. ASPARAGUS-MUSHROOM FRITTATA

COOKING: 25' **PREPARATION: 15'** **SERVINGS: 2**

INGREDIENTS

- » 1 tablespoon olive oil
- » 1 garlic clove
- » ¼ cup onion
- » 2 cups button mushrooms
- » 1 asparagus
- » 1 tablespoon thyme
- » 6 eggs
- » ½ cup feta cheese
- » Salt
- » Black pepper

DIRECTIONS

1. Cook onions within 5 minutes. Put mushroom plus garlic then cook within 5 minutes. Mix thyme, salt, pepper, and asparagus and cook within 3 minutes. Beat eggs and cheese in a bowl and pour it in the pan and cook for 2 to 3 minutes. Bake within 10 minutes.

NUTRITION

Calories: 129, Carbs: 2g, Fat: 7g, Protein: 9g

101. SHRIMP AVOCADO SALAD

COOKING: 0'   **PREPARATION: 15'**   **SERVINGS: 1**

INGREDIENTS

- » 1/4cup onion
- » 1 tomato
- » 2 limes juice
- » 1 avocado
- » 1/4 tsp salt
- » Black pepper
- » 1 jalapeno
- » 1lb shrimp
- » 1 tbsp cilantro

DIRECTIONS

1. Mix onion, lime juice, salt, pepper, and let it stand 5 minutes. In another bowl, add chopped shrimp, avocado, tomato, jalapeno, and onion mixture. Put salt and pepper, toss and serve.

NUTRITION

Calories: 365, Carbs: 15g, Fat: 17g, Protein: 25g

102. SMOKY CAULIFLOWER BITES

COOKING: 25'   **PREPARATION: 15'**   **SERVINGS: 2**

INGREDIENTS

- » 1 cauliflower
- » 2 garlic cloves
- » 2 tbsp olive oil
- » 2 tbsp parsley
- » 1tsp paprika
- » 3/4tsp salt

DIRECTIONS

1. Mix cauliflower, olive oil, paprika, and salt. Warm-up oven at 450. Bake within 10 minutes. Put garlic and bake within 10 to 15 minutes. Serve with parsley.

NUTRITION

Calories: 69, Carbs: 8g, Fat: 3g, Protein: 1g

103. AVOCADO CRAB BOATS

COOKING: 2' **PREPARATION: 15'** **SERVINGS: 2**

INGREDIENTS

- » 12oz lump crab meat
- » 3tbsp lemon juice
- » 1/3cup Greek yogurt
- » 1/2tsp pepper
- » 1/2 onion
- » Salt
- » 2tbsp chives
- » 1cup cheddar cheese
- » 2 avocados

DIRECTIONS

1. Mix meat, yogurt, onion, chives, lemon juice, cayenne, and salt. Scoop the avocado flesh, fill the avocado bowl with meat mixture, and top with cheddar cheese. Microwave within 2 minutes and serve.

NUTRITION

Calories: 325, Carbs: 8g, Fat: 28g, Protein: 0g

104. COCONUT CURRY CAULIFLOWER SOUP

COOKING: 40' **PREPARATION: 15'** **SERVINGS: 2**

INGREDIENTS

- » 1tbsp olive oil
- » 2-3 tsp curry powder
- » 1 onion
- » 2tsp ground cumin
- » 3 garlic cloves
- » 1/2tsp turmeric powder
- » 1tsp ginger
- » 14oz coconut milk
- » 14oz tomatoes
- » 1 cup vegetable broth
- » 1 cauliflower
- » Salt
- » Pepper

DIRECTIONS

1. Mix olive oil and onion in a pot, sauté within 3 minutes. Put garlic, ginger, curry powder, cumin, and turmeric powder and sauté within 5 minutes. Put coconut milk, tomatoes, vegetable broth, and cauliflower. Cook on low within 20 minutes, blend the mixture through blender, and warm-up the soup within 5 minutes. Put salt and pepper. Serve.

NUTRITION

Calories: 112, Carbs: 0g, Fat: 0g — Protein: 0g

105. PARMESAN ASPARAGUS

COOKING: 15'　　　**PREPARATION: 15'**　　　**SERVINGS: 4**

INGREDIENTS

- » 4lb asparagus
- » Salt
- » 1/4lb butter
- » 2cups parmesan cheese shredded
- » 1/2tsp pepper

DIRECTIONS

1. Boil asparagus within 3 minutes. Drain and put aside. Preheat oven to 350. Arrange asparagus into the pan and pour butter, sprinkle pepper, salt, and parmesan cheese. Bake within 10 to 15 minutes. Serve.

NUTRITION

Calories: 83, Carbs: 5g, Fat: 5g, Protein: 6g

106. CREAM CHEESE PANCAKES

COOKING: 10'　　　**PREPARATION: 15'**　　　**SERVINGS: 12**

INGREDIENTS

- » 4oz cream cheese
- » Vanilla extract
- » 4 eggs
- » Butter

DIRECTIONS

1. Blend cream cheese and eggs in a blender, put aside. Grease skillet with butter. Cook the batter within 2 minutes. Serve with sprinkle cinnamon.

NUTRITION

Calories: 344, Carbs: 3g, Fat: 29g, Protein: 17g

107. SUGAR-FREE MEXICAN SPICED DARK CHOCOLATE

COOKING: 0' **PREPARATION: 15'** **SERVINGS: 1**

INGREDIENTS

- » 1/2cup cocoa powder
- » 1/4tsp cinnamon
- » 1/2tsp chili powder
- » 1/8tsp nutmeg
- » Black pepper
- » Salt
- » 1/4cup melted butter
- » 1/4tsp vanilla extract
- » 25 drops liquid stevia

DIRECTIONS

1. Mix cocoa powder, cinnamon, chili powder, nutmeg, black pepper, and salt. Put aside. Stir melted butter with vanilla extract and stevia and mix butter mixture with dry items. Put the mixture in chocolate molds. Chill and serve.

NUTRITION

Calories: 60, Carbs: 8g, Fat: 5g, Protein: 1g

108. TUNA IN CUCUMBER CUPS

COOKING: 0' **PREPARATION: 15'** **SERVINGS: 10**

INGREDIENTS

- » Mayonnaise, 1/3cup
- » Dill
- » Black pepper, 1tsp
- » Tuna, 1can
- » Cucumber, 1

DIRECTIONS

1. Mix the cucumber flesh with the remainder of the fixing and then fill the holes in the slices of cucumber. Garnish with fresh dill. Serve.

NUTRITION

Calories 22, Protein: 3g, Fat: 2g, Carbs: 2g

109. PARMESAN CRISPS

COOKING: 10' **PREPARATION: 15'** **SERVINGS: 2**

INGREDIENTS

- » Provolone cheese, 2
- » Jalapeno pepper
- » Parmesan cheese

DIRECTIONS

1. Warm-up oven to 425. Grease a baking sheet then set the eight tablespoons of parmesan cheese. Lay the slices of jalapeno over the parmesan cheese mounds. Put one square provolone over the eight parmesan mounds. Bake within nine minutes and serve.

NUTRITION

Calories 160, Protein: 15g, Fat: 9g, Carbs: 2g

110. ONION RINGS

COOKING: 15' **PREPARATION: 15'** **SERVINGS: 2**

INGREDIENTS

- » 2 Eggs
- » 1/2c Parmesan cheese
- » 1 tbsp Heavy whipping cream
- » 1/2c Coconut flour
- » 1/2c Pork rinds
- » 1 white Onion

DIRECTIONS

1. Warm-up oven to 425. Arrange the first bowl with the coconut flour, the second bowl with mixed whipping cream and beaten egg, and in the third bowl, with crushed pork rinds and grated parmesan cheese, mix. Dip the rings into the coconut flour, then into the egg-cream mixture, and lastly, into the mix of cheese and pork rinds. Bake within fifteen minutes. Serve.

NUTRITION

Calories: 205, Fat: 18g, Protein: 12g, Carbs: 4g

111. COLD CRAB DIP

COOKING: 0' **PREPARATION: 15'** **SERVINGS: 12**

INGREDIENTS

- » Lemon juice, 1tsp
- » Chives, 2tbsp
- » 1/2tsp Old Bay seasoning
- » Sour cream, 3tbsp
- » 8oz Crabmeat
- » 4oz Cream cheese

DIRECTIONS

1. Mix the cream cheese, lemon juice, seasoning, and sour cream. Fold the crab meat, then the chives, stirring. Serve.

NUTRITION

Calories: 42, Fat: 4g, Protein: 5g

112. BAKED COCONUT SHRIMP

COOKING: 20' **PREPARATION: 15'** **SERVINGS: 4**

INGREDIENTS

- » Medium shrimp, 1-pound
- » Black pepper, 1/2tsp
- » Coconut flakes, 2cups
- » Salt, 1/2tsp
- » Garlic powder, one quarter teaspoon
- » Eggs, three
- » Paprika, one quarter teaspoon
- » Coconut flour, 3tbsp

DIRECTIONS

1. Warm-up oven to 400. In the first bowl, put the beaten eggs, in the second bowl, put the coconut flakes, and in the last bowl, put a mix of the garlic powder, salt, paprika, pepper, and coconut flour. Dip each shrimp into the flour mixture first, then into the egg wash, and then roll them in the coconut flakes. Bake within ten minutes. Serve.

NUTRITION

Calories: 440, Protein: 3g, Fat: 32g, Carbs: 5g

113. SPICY DEVILED EGGS

COOKING: 0' **PREPARATION: 15'** **SERVINGS: 24**

INGREDIENTS

- » Sriracha sauce, 1tbsp
- » Chili powder, 1tbsp
- » Chives, minced, 1tbsp
- » Dijon mustard, 1tbsp
- » Mayonnaise, 1/3cup
- » Black pepper, 1tsp
- » 12 Eggs
- » Salt, 1tsp

DIRECTIONS

1. Mash the yolks into a paste. Mix in the salt, mayonnaise, chili powder, sriracha sauce, pepper, and the mustard. Refill the egg whites with this mixture. Serve with chopped chives on top.

NUTRITION

Calories: 55, Protein: 3g, Carbs: 1g, Fat: 5g

114. BACON-WRAPPED SCALLOPS

COOKING: 20' **PREPARATION: 15'** **SERVINGS: 4**

INGREDIENTS

- » Toothpicks, 16
- » Salt, 1/2tsp
- » Olive oil, 2tbsp
- » Black pepper, 1/2tsp
- » Sea scallops
- » Bacon

DIRECTIONS

1. Warm-up oven to 425. Grease a baking sheet.

2. Use 1/2 of a bacon slice to wrap around each scallop and stick in the toothpick.

3. Brush on the olive oil and put the salt and pepper. Bake within fifteen minutes. Serve.

NUTRITION

Calories 225, Protein: 13g, Fat: 16g, Carbs: 2g

115. BUFFALO CHICKEN JALAPENO POPPERS

COOKING: 30'   **PREPARATION: 15'**   **SERVINGS: 5**

INGREDIENTS

- » Ranch dressing
- » Green onions
- » 4 slices of bacon
- » 10 Jalapeno peppers
- » Garlic, 2tbsp
- » Cream cheese, 4oz
- » Chicken, 8oz
- » Buffalo wing sauce, one quarter cup
- » Onion powder, 1/2tsp
- » 1/2cup Blue cheese
- » Mozzarella cheese, one quarter cup
- » 1/2tsp Salt

DIRECTIONS

1. Warm-up oven to 350. Lay the half pieces of the jalapeno peppers on the cookie sheet.

2. Fry the onion powder, ground chicken, garlic, and salt within fifteen minutes.

3. Blend in the mozzarella cheese, wing sauce, and one-quarter cup of the crumbled blue cheese. Combine into the pepper halves, then top with bacon and blue cheese. Bake within thirty minutes then serve.

NUTRITION

Calories 250, Protein: 15g, Fat: 20g — Carbs: 4g

116. BAKED GARLIC PARMESAN WINGS

COOKING: 60'   **PREPARATION: 15'**   **SERVINGS: 6**

INGREDIENTS

- » Parsley, 1tbsp
- » Salt, 1tbsp
- » Onion powder, 1tsp
- » Chicken wings, 2-pounds
- » Butter, 1/2cup
- » Parmesan cheese, 1/2cup
- » Garlic powder, 2tsp
- » Baking powder, 2tsp
- » Black pepper, 1/2tsp

DIRECTIONS

1. Warm-up oven to 250. Sprinkle the pepper and salt on the wings and let them sit for ten minutes. Put baking powder over the wings, toss.

2. Bake the wings for thirty minutes. Adjust to 425 F and then bake again for thirty minutes.

3. Meanwhile, mix the minced garlic, parmesan cheese, onion powder, garlic powder, parsley, and melted butter. Toss wings in the sauce. Serve.

NUTRITION

Calories 459, Protein: 32g, Fat:40g, Carbs: 2g

115

117. SAUSAGE STUFFED MUSHROOMS

COOKING: 30'   **PREPARATION: 15'**   **SERVINGS: 20**

INGREDIENTS

- » Salt, 1/2tsp
- » Butter, 2tbsp
- » Sausage, 2
- » Garlic, 2tsp
- » Black pepper, 1/2tsp
- » Onion, one quarter cup
- » Baby Bella Mushrooms, twenty
- » Cheddar Cheese, 1cup

DIRECTIONS

1. Warm-up oven to 350. Fry sausage meat with butter, remove and put aside.

2. Cook the mushroom stalks, garlic, and diced onion into the pan with the leftover liquid within five minutes. Mix with the salt, cheddar cheese, pepper, and sausage. Fill all of the mushroom caps with this mixture. Bake within twenty minutes. Serve.

NUTRITION

Calories 60, Protein: 5g, Fat: 4g, Carbs: 2g

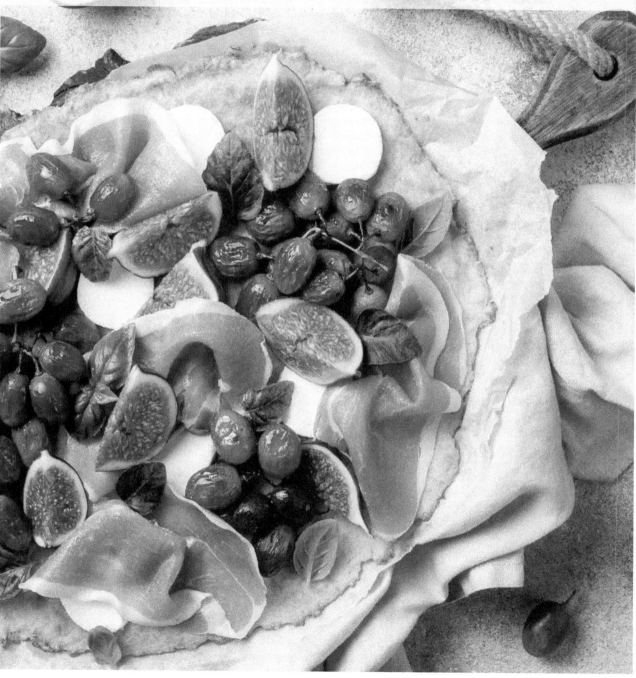

CHAPTER 11 - DINNER

118. GREEN CHICKEN CURRY

COOKING: 30'   **PREPARATION: 15'**   **SERVINGS: 4**

INGREDIENTS

- » 1-pound grass-fed chicken breasts
- » 1tbsp olive oil
- » 2tbsp green curry paste
- » 1 cup unsweetened coconut milk
- » 1cup chicken broth
- » 1 cup asparagus spears
- » 1 cup green beans
- » Salt
- » ground black pepper
- » ¼cup basil leaves

DIRECTIONS

1. Sauté the curry paste within 1–2 minutes. Add the chicken and cook within 8–10 minutes.

2. Add coconut milk and broth, boil. Cook again to low within 8–10 minutes.

3. Add the asparagus, green beans, salt, and black pepper, and cook within 4–5 minutes.

4. Serve.

NUTRITION

Calories 294, Net Carbs 4.3 g, Total Fat 16.2 g, Protein 28.6 g

119. CREAMY PORK STEW

COOKING: 85'   **PREPARATION: 15'**   **SERVINGS: 8**

INGREDIENTS

- » 3 tbsp unsalted butter
- » 2½ pounds boneless pork ribs
- » 1 yellow onion
- » 4 garlic cloves
- » 1½cups chicken broth
- » 2 cans sugar-free diced tomatoes
- » 2 tsp dried oregano
- » 1 tsp ground cumin
- » Salt
- » 2 tbsp lime juice
- » ½ cup sour cream

DIRECTIONS

1. Cook the pork, onions, and garlic within 4–5 minutes. Add the broth, tomatoes, oregano, cumin, and salt, and mix. Simmer to low. Combine in the sour cream plus lime juice and remove. Serve.

NUTRITION

Calories 304, Net Carbs 4.7 g, Total Fat 12.4 g, Protein 39.5 g

120. SALMON & SHRIMP STEW

COOKING: 25' **PREPARATION: 20'** **SERVINGS: 6**

INGREDIENTS

- » 2tbsp coconut oil
- » ½cup onion
- » 2 garlic cloves
- » 1 Serrano pepper
- » 1 tsp smoked paprika
- » 24 cups tomatoes
- » 4 cups chicken broth
- » 1-pound salmon fillets
- » 1-pound shrimp
- » 2 tbsp lime juice
- » Salt
- » Ground black pepper
- » 3 tablespoons parsley

DIRECTIONS

1. Sauté the onion within 5–6 minutes. Add the garlic, Serrano pepper, and paprika. Add the tomatoes and broth then boil. Simmer within 5 minutes. Add the salmon and simmer again, 3–4 minutes.

2. Put in the shrimp then cook within 4–5 minutes. Mix in lemon juice, salt plus black pepper, and remove. Serve with parsley.

NUTRITION

Calories 247, Net Carbs 3.9 g, Fiber 1.2 g, Sugar 2.1 g, Protein 32.7 g

121. CHICKEN CASSEROLE

COOKING: 70' **PREPARATION: 15'** **SERVINGS: 6**

INGREDIENTS

Chicken Layer:
- » 6 grass-fed chicken breasts
- » Salt
- » ground black pepper

Bacon Layer:
- » 5 bacon slices
- » ¼ cup yellow onion
- » ¼ cup jalapeño pepper
- » ½ cup mayonnaise
- » 1 package cream cheese
- » ½ cup Parmesan cheese
- » 1 cup cheddar cheese
- » Topping:
- » 1 package pork skins
- » ¼ cup butter
- » ½ cup Parmesan cheese

DIRECTIONS

1. Warm-up oven to 4250F.

2. Put the chicken breasts in the greased casserole then put salt and black pepper.

3. Bake within 30–40 minutes.

4. For the bacon layer:

5. Cook the bacon within 8–10 minutes. Transfer.

6. Sauté onion within 4–5 minutes. Remove, stir in bacon and remaining fixing.

7. Remove the casserole dish then put the bacon mixture.

8. Mix all topping fixing. Place the topping over the bacon mixture. Bake within 15 minutes. Serve.

NUTRITION

Calories 826, Net Carbs 2.5 g, Total Fat 62.9 g, Protein 60.6 g

122. CREAMY CHICKEN BAKE

COOKING: 70'   **PREPARATION: 15'**   **SERVINGS: 6**

INGREDIENTS

- 5 tbsp unsalted butter
- 2 onions
- 3 garlic cloves
- 1 tsp tarragon
- 8oz cream cheese
- 1 cup chicken broth
- 2 tbsp lemon juice
- ½ cup heavy cream
- 1½ teaspoons Herbs de Provence
- Salt
- ground black pepper
- 4 grass-fed chicken breasts

DIRECTIONS

1. Warm-up oven to 3500F.

2. Cook the onion, garlic, and tarragon within 4–5 minutes. Transfer.

3. Cook the cream cheese, ½ cup of broth, and lemon juice within 3–4 minutes.

4. Stir in the cream, herbs de Provence, salt, and black pepper, remove.

5. Pour remaining broth and chicken breast plus the cream mixture. Bake within 45–60 minutes. Serve.

NUTRITION

Calories 729, Net Carbs 5.6 g, Total Fat 52.8 g, Sugar 2 g, Protein 55.8 g

123. BEEF & VEGGIE CASSEROLE

COOKING: 55'   **PREPARATION: 20'**   **SERVINGS: 6**

INGREDIENTS

- 3 tbsp butter
- 1-pound grass-fed ground beef
- 1 yellow onion
- 2 garlic cloves
- 1 cup pumpkin
- 1 cup broccoli
- 2 cups cheddar cheese
- 1 tbsp Dijon mustard
- 6 organic eggs
- ½ cup heavy whipping cream
- Salt
- Ground black pepper

DIRECTIONS

1. Cook the beef within 8–10 minutes. Transfer.

2. Cook the onion and garlic within 10 minutes. Add the pumpkin and cook within 5–6 minutes.

3. Add the broccoli and cook within 3–4 minutes. Transfer to the cooked beef, combine.

4. Warm-up oven to 350°F.

5. Put 2/3 of cheese and mustard in the beef mixture, combine.

6. In another mixing bowl, add cream, eggs, salt, and black pepper, and beat.

7. In a baking dish, place the beef mixture and top with egg mixture, plus the remaining cheese.

8. Bake within 25 minutes. Serve.

NUTRITION

Calories 472, Net Carbs 5.5 g, Total Fat 34.6 g, Sodium 463 mg, Protein 32.6 g

124. BEEF WITH BELL PEPPERS

COOKING: 10'   **PREPARATION: 15'**   **SERVINGS: 4**

INGREDIENTS

- » 1 tbsp olive oil
- » 1-pound grass-fed flank steak
- » 1 red bell pepper
- » 1 green bell pepper
- » 1 tbsp ginger
- » 3 tbsp low-sodium soy sauce
- » 1½ tbsp balsamic vinegar
- » 2tsp Sriracha

DIRECTIONS

1. Sear the steak slices within 2 minutes. Cook bell peppers within 2–3 minutes.

2. Transfer the beef mixture. Boil the remaining fixing within 1 minute. Add the beef mixture and cook within 1–2 minutes. Serve.

NUTRITION

Calories 274, Net Carbs 3.8 g, Total Fat 13.1 g, Protein 32.9 g

125. BRAISED LAMB SHANKS

COOKING: 155'   **PREPARATION: 15'**   **SERVINGS: 4**

INGREDIENTS

- » 4 grass-fed lamb shanks
- » 2 tbsp butter
- » Salt
- » ground black pepper
- » 6 garlic cloves
- » 6 rosemary sprigs
- » 1 cup chicken broth

DIRECTIONS

1. Warm-up oven to 450°F.

2. Coat the shanks with butter and put salt plus pepper. Roast within 20 minutes.

3. Remove then reduce to 325°F.

4. Place the garlic cloves and rosemary over and around the lamb.

5. Roast within 2 hours. Put the broth into a roasting pan.

6. Increase to 400°F. Roast within 15 minutes more. Serve.

NUTRITION

Calories 1093, Net Carbs 2 g, Total Fat 44.2 g, Protein 161.4 g

126. SHRIMP & BELL PEPPER STIR-FRY

COOKING: 10'   **PREPARATION: 20'**   **SERVINGS: 6**

INGREDIENTS

- ½ cup low-sodium soy sauce
- 2 tablespoons balsamic vinegar
- 2 tablespoons Erythritol
- 1 tablespoon arrowroot starch
- 1 tablespoon ginger
- ½ teaspoon red pepper flakes
- 3 tablespoons olive oil
- ½ red bell pepper
- ½ yellow bell pepper
- ½ green bell pepper
- 1 onion
- 1 red chili
- 1½ pounds shrimp
- 2 scallion greens

DIRECTIONS

1. Mix soy sauce, vinegar, erythritol, arrowroot starch, ginger, and red pepper flakes. Set aside.
2. Stir-fry the bell peppers, onion, and red chili within 1–2 minutes.
3. In the center of the wok, place the shrimp and cook within 1–2 minutes.
4. Stir the shrimp with bell pepper mixture and cook within 2 minutes.
5. Stir in the sauce and cook within 2–3 minutes.
6. Stir in the scallion greens and remove. Serve hot.

NUTRITION

Calories 221, Net Carbs 6.5 g, Total Fat 9 g, Protein 27.6 g

127. VEGGIES & WALNUT LOAF

COOKING: 70'   **PREPARATION: 15'**   **SERVINGS: 10**

INGREDIENTS

- 1 tablespoon olive oil
- 2 yellow onions
- 2 garlic cloves
- 1 teaspoon dried rosemary
- 1 cup walnuts
- 2 carrots
- 1 celery stalk
- 1 green bell pepper
- 1 cup button mushrooms
- 5 organic eggs
- 1¼ cups almond flour
- Salt
- Ground black pepper

DIRECTIONS

1. Warm-up oven to 350°F. Sauté the onion within 4–5 minutes.
2. Add the garlic and rosemary and sauté within 1 minute.
3. Add the walnuts and vegetables within 3–4 minutes. Put aside
4. Beat the eggs, flour, sea salt, and black pepper.
5. Mix the egg mixture with vegetable mixture.
6. Bake within 50–60 minutes. Serve.

NUTRITION

Calories 242, Net Carbs 4.6 g, Total Fat 19.5 g, Protein 5.9 g

128. KETO SLOPPY JOES

COOKING: 70' **PREPARATION: 15'** **SERVINGS: 3**

INGREDIENTS

- » 1 ¼ cup almond flour
- » 5tbsp. ground psyllium husk powder
- » 1tsp. sea salt
- » 2tsp. baking powder
- » 2tsp. cider vinegar
- » 1 ¼ cups boiling water
- » 3 egg whites
- » 2tbsp. olive oil
- » 1 ½ lb. ground beef
- » 1 yellow onion
- » 4 garlic cloves
- » 14oz. crushed tomatoes
- » 1tbsp. chili powder
- » 1tbsp. Dijon powder
- » 1tbsp. red wine vinegar
- » 4tbsp. tomato paste
- » 2tsp. salt
- » ¼tsp ground black pepper
- » ½cup mayonnaise
- » 6oz. cheese

DIRECTIONS

1. Warm-up the oven to 350 degrees and then mix all the dry fixing.

2. Add some vinegar, egg whites, and boiled water. Whisk for 30 seconds.

3. Form the dough into 5 or 8 pieces of bread. Cook within 55 minutes.

4. Cook the onion and garlic. Add the ground beef and cook. Put the other fixing and cook. Simmer for 10 minutes in low. Serve.

NUTRITION

Calories: 215, Carbs: 19g, Fat: 10g, Protein: 30g

129. LOW CARB CRACK SLAW EGG ROLL IN A BOWL RECIPE

COOKING: 20' **PREPARATION: 15'** **SERVINGS: 2**

INGREDIENTS

- » 1lb. ground beef
- » 4 cups shredded coleslaw mix
- » 1tbsp. avocado oil
- » 1tsp. Sea salt
- » ¼tsp. black pepper
- » 4 cloves garlic
- » 3tbsp. ginger
- » ¼ cup coconut amines
- » 2 tsp. toasted sesame oil
- » ¼ cup green onions

DIRECTIONS

1. Warm-up avocado oil in a large pan, put in the garlic, and cook.

2. Add the ground beef and cook within 10 minutes, put salt and black pepper.

3. Lower the heat and add the coleslaw mix and the coconut amines. Stir to cook for 5 minutes.

4. Remove and put in the green onions and the toasted sesame oil. Serve.

NUTRITION

Calories: 116, Carbs: 2g, Fat: 13g, Protein: 8g

130. LOW CARB BEEF STIR FRY

COOKING: 20' **PREPARATION: 15** **SERVINGS: 4**

INGREDIENTS

- » ½ cup zucchini
- » ¼ cup organic broccoli florets
- » 1 baby book Choy
- » 2 tbsp. avocado oil
- » 2 tsp. coconut amines
- » 1 ginger
- » 8oz. skirt steak

DIRECTIONS

1. Sear the steak on high heat. Adjust to medium and put in the broccoli, ginger, ghee, and coconut amines. Add in the book Choy and cook for another minute.

2. Put the zucchini into the mix and cook. Serve.

NUTRITION

Calories: 275, Carbs: 12g, Fat: 5g, Protein: 40g

131. ONE PAN PESTO CHICKEN AND VEGGIES

COOKING: 25' **PREPARATION: 15'** **SERVINGS: 4**

INGREDIENTS

- » 2 tbsp. olive oil
- » 1 cup cherry diced tomatoes
- » ¼ cup basil pesto
- » 1/3 cup sun-dried tomatoes
- » 1-pound chicken thigh
- » 1-pound asparagus

DIRECTIONS

1. Warm-up a large skillet. Put two tablespoons of olive oil and sliced chicken on medium heat. Put salt and add ½ cup of the sun-dried tomatoes. Cook. Transfer the chicken and tomatoes.

2. Put the asparagus in the skillet and pour it in the pesto. Put the remaining sun-dried tomatoes. Cook within 5 to 10 minutes. Transfer.

3. Turn the chicken back in the skillet and pour it in pesto. Stir for 2 minutes. Serve with the asparagus.

NUTRITION

Calories: 340, Carbs: 9g, Fat: 24g, Protein: 23g

132. CRISPY PEANUT TOFU AND CAULIFLOWER RICE STIR-FRY

COOKING: 60'   **PREPARATION: 15'**   **SERVINGS: 4**

INGREDIENTS

- » 12oz. tofu
- » 1 tbsp. toasted sesame oil
- » 2 cloves minced garlic
- » 1 cauliflower head
- » Sauce:
- » 1 ½tbsp. Toasted sesame oil
- » ½tsp. chili garlic sauce
- » 2 ½tbsp. peanut butter
- » ¼ cup low sodium soy sauce
- » ½cup light brown sugar

DIRECTIONS

1. Warm-up oven to 400 degrees. Cube the tofu.
2. Bake for 25 minutes and cool.
3. Combine the sauce fixing. Put the tofu in the sauce and stir. Leave for 15 minutes.
4. Cook the veggies on a bit of sesame oil and soy sauce. Set it aside.
5. Grab the tofu and put it on the pan. Stir then set aside.
6. Steam the cauliflower rice for 5 to 8 minutes. Add some sauce and stir.
7. Add up the ingredients. Put the cauliflower rice with the veggies and tofu. Serve.

NUTRITION

Calories: 524, Carbs: 39g, Fat: 34g —

Protein: 25g

133. SIMPLE KETO FRIED CHICKEN

COOKING: 45'   **PREPARATION: 15'**   **SERVINGS: 4**

INGREDIENTS

- » 4 boneless chicken thighs
- » Frying oil
- » 2 eggs
- » 2tbsp. heavy whipping cream
- » Breading
- » 2/3cup grated parmesan cheese
- » 2/3cup blanched almond flour
- » 1tsp. salt
- » ½tsp. black pepper
- » ½tsp. cayenne
- » ½tsp. paprika

DIRECTIONS

1. Beat the eggs and heavy cream. Separately, mix all the breading fixing. Set aside.
2. Cut the chicken thigh into 3 even pieces.
3. Dip the chicken in the bread first before dipping it in the egg wash and then finally, dipping it in the breading again. Fry chicken within 5 minutes. Pat dry the chicken. Serve.

NUTRITION

Calories: 304, Carbs: 12g, Fat: 15g, Protein: 30g

134. KETO BUTTER CHICKEN

COOKING: 20' **PREPARATION: 15'** **SERVINGS: 4**

INGREDIENTS

- » 1.5lb. chicken breast
- » 1tbsp. coconut oil
- » 2tbsp. garam masala
- » 3tsp. grated ginger
- » 3tsp. garlic
- » 4oz. plain yogurt

Sauce:
- » 2tbsp. butter
- » 1tbsp ground coriander
- » ½cup heavy cream
- » ½tbsp. garam masala
- » 2tsp. ginger
- » 2tsp. minced garlic
- » 2tsp. cumin
- » 1tsp. chili powder
- » 1 onion
- » 14.5oz. crushed tomatoes
- » Salt

DIRECTIONS

1. Mix chicken pieces, 2 tablespoons garam masala, 1 teaspoon minced garlic, and 1 teaspoon grated ginger. Stir and add the yogurt. Chill for 30 minutes.

2. For the sauce, blend the ginger, garlic, onion, tomatoes, and spices. Put aside.

3. Cook the chicken pieces. Once cooked, pour in the sauce, and simmer for 5 minutes. Serve.

NUTRITION

Calories: 367, Carbs: 7g, Fat: 22g, Protein: 36g

135. KETO SHRIMP SCAMPI RECIPE

COOKING: 25' **PREPARATION: 15'** **SERVINGS: 2**

INGREDIENTS

- » 2 summer squash
- » 1-pound shrimp
- » 2tbsp. butter unsalted
- » 2tbsp. lemon juice
- » 2tbsp. parsley
- » ¼cup chicken broth
- » 1/8tsp. red chili flakes
- » 1 clove garlic
- » Salt
- » Pepper

DIRECTIONS

1. Put salt in the squash noodles on top. Set aside for 30 minutes.

2. Pat dry. Fry the garlic. Add some chicken broth, red chili flakes, and lemon juice.

3. Once it boils, add the shrimp, and cook. Lower the heat.

4. Add salt and pepper, put the summer squash noodles and parsley to the mix. Serve.

NUTRITION

Calories: 366, Carbs: 7g, Fat: 15g, Protein: 49g

136. KETO LASAGNA

COOKING: 60'   **PREPARATION: 15'**   **SERVINGS: 2**

INGREDIENTS

- » 8oz. block cream cheese
- » 3 eggs
- » Kosher salt
- » Ground black pepper
- » 2 cups mozzarella
- » ½cup parmesan
- » Pinch red pepper flakes
- » Parsley
- » Sauce:
- » ¾cup marinara
- » 1tbsp. tomato paste
- » 1lb. ground beef
- » ½cup parmesan
- » 1.5cup mozzarella
- » 1tbsp. extra virgin olive oil
- » 1tsp. dried oregano
- » 3 cloves garlic
- » ½cup onion
- » 16oz. ricotta

DIRECTIONS

1. Warm-up oven to 350 degrees.

2. Melt in the cream cheese, mozzarella, and parmesan. Put the eggs, salt, and pepper.

3. Bake for 15 to 20 minutes.

4. Cook the onion within 5 minutes, then the garlic. Put the tomato paste. Add the ground beef, put salt and pepper. Cook, then put aside.

5. Cook marinara sauce, put pepper, red pepper flakes, and ground pepper. Stir.

6. Take out the noodles and cut in half widthwise and then cut them again into 3 pieces.

7. Put 2 noodles at the bottom of the dish, then layer the parmesan and mozzarella shreds alternately.

8. Bake within 30 minutes. Garnish and serve.

NUTRITION

Calories: 508, Carbs: 8g, Fat: 39g, Protein: 33g

137. CREAMY TUSCAN GARLIC CHICKEN

COOKING: 30'   **PREPARATION: 15'**   **SERVINGS: 4**

INGREDIENTS

- » 1.5 pounds' chicken breast
- » ½cup chicken broth
- » ½cup parmesan cheese
- » ½cup sun-dried tomatoes
- » 1cup heavy cream
- » 1cup spinach
- » 2tbsp. olive oil
- » 1tsp. garlic powder
- » 1tsp. Italian seasoning

DIRECTIONS

1. Cook the chicken using olive oil, medium heat within 5 minutes, put aside.

2. Combine the heavy cream, garlic powder, Italian seasoning, parmesan cheese, and chicken broth. Add the sundried tomatoes and spinach and simmer. Add the chicken back and serve.

NUTRITION

Calories: 368, Carbs: 7g, Fat: 0g, Protein: 30g

138. ANCHO MACHO CHILI

COOKING: 90'   **PREPARATION: 24'**   **SERVINGS: 4**

INGREDIENTS

- » 2lbs. lean sirloin
- » 1 teaspoon salt
- » 0.25 teaspoon pepper
- » 1.5 tablespoons olive oil
- » Onion
- » Chili Powder
- » 7oz can tomato with green chilis
- » ½ cup chicken broth
- » 2 cloves garlic

DIRECTIONS

1. Warm-up oven to a temperature of 350F. Coat beef with pepper and salt.

2. Cook a third of the beef. Cook the onion for a few minutes. Put in the last four ingredients and simmer. Add in the beef with all its juices, and cook within two hours. Stir and serve.

NUTRITION

Net Carbs: 6g, Fat: 40g, Protein: 58g, Calories: 644kcal

139. CHICKEN SUPREME PIZZA

COOKING: 30'   **PREPARATION: 25'**   **SERVINGS: 4-8**

INGREDIENTS

- » 5oz cooked chicken breast
- » 1.5cups almond flour
- » 1 teaspoon Baking Powder
- » Salt half-teaspoon
- » 0.25 cup water
- » 1 Red Onion
- » 1 Red Pepper
- » Green Pepper
- » 1 cup Mozzarella Cheese

DIRECTIONS

1. Warm-up oven to a temperature of 400F.

2. Blend the flour both the salt and baking powder. Put the water and the oil added to the flour mixture to make the dough. Flatten the dough. Dump out the dough. Press it out, and coat the pan with oil.

3. Bake within 12 minutes. Remove then sprinkle with cheese and then add chicken, pepper, and onion. Bake again within 15 minutes, slice, and serve.

NUTRITION

Net Carbs: 4g, Fiber: 10g, Fat: 12g, Protein: 16g, Calories: 310kcal

140. BAKED JERKED CHICKEN

COOKING: 90'   **PREPARATION: 20'**   **SERVINGS: 4**

INGREDIENTS

- » 2 pounds' chicken thighs
- » 0.33 Olive Oil
- » Apple Cider Vinegar
- » 1 teaspoon salt
- » 1 teaspoon powdered onion
- » half-teaspoon garlic
- » half-teaspoon nutmeg
- » half-teaspoon pepper
- » half-teaspoon powdered ginger
- » half-teaspoon powdered cayenne
- » 0.25 teaspoon cinnamon
- » 0.25 teaspoon dried thyme

DIRECTIONS

1. Mix all fixings, excluding the chicken. Stir in the prepared chicken pieces. Stir well.

2. Marinade within 4 hours. Warm-up oven to a temperature of 375F.

3. Cook within 1.25 hours. Adjust to broil chicken within 4 minutes. Serve.

NUTRITION

Net Carbs: 4g, Fiber: 0g, Fat: 12g, Protein: 16g, Calories: 185kcal

141. CHICKEN SCHNITZEL

COOKING: 15'   **PREPARATION: 15'**   **SERVINGS: 3**

INGREDIENTS

- » 1-pound chicken breast
- » 0.5 cups almond flour
- » 1 egg
- » half-tablespoon powdered garlic
- » half-tablespoon powdered onion
- » Keto-Safe Oil

DIRECTIONS

1. Combine the garlic power flour and onion in a bowl. Separately, beat the egg.

2. With a mallet, pound out the chicken. Put the chicken in the egg mixture. Then roll well through the flour.

3. Take a deep-frying pan and warm-up the oil to medium-high temperature.

4. Add chicken in batches. Fry. Pat dry and serve.

NUTRITION

Net carbs: 32g, Fiber: 0g, Fat: 17g, Protein: 61g, Calories: 541kcl

142. BROCCOLI AND CHICKEN CASSEROLE

COOKING: 10'   **PREPARATION: 15'**   **SERVINGS: 4**

INGREDIENTS

- » 1 ½ lb. chicken breast
- » 8 oz softened cream cheese
- » 0.5 cups heavy cream
- » 1 teaspoon powdered garlic
- » 1 teaspoon powdered onion
- » half-teaspoon salt
- » half-teaspoon pepper
- » 2 cups, broccoli florets
- » 1 cup mozarella
- » 1 cup parmesan

DIRECTIONS

1. Warm-up oven to a temperature of 400F.

2. Combine the cream cheese to pepper and salt. Stir in the cubed chicken.

3. Put in the baking dish. Put the broccoli into the chicken-cheese mixture.

4. Top the dish with cheese, bake about 26 minutes and remove. Take off the foil and bake again for 10 minutes. Serve.

NUTRITION

Net carbs: 20g, Fiber: 0g, Fat: 25g, Protein: 21g, Calories: 391kcal

143. BAKED FISH WITH LEMON BUTTER

COOKING: 15'   **PREPARATION: 15'**   **SERVINGS: 2**

INGREDIENTS

- » 12 oz white fish fillets
- » 1 tablespoon olive oil
- » Pepper
- » Salt
- » 1 medium-sized broccoli
- » 2 tablespoons butter
- » 1 teaspoon garlic paste
- » 1 medium-sized lemon

DIRECTIONS

1. Warm-up the oven to a temperature of 430F.

2. Set the fish out onto the parchment paper, and put pepper and salt. Pour over olive oil and lemon slices. Bake within 15 minutes.

3. Steam the broccoli within five minutes. Put aside.

4. Warm-up, the butter, then stir in zest, garlic, remaining lemon slices, and broccoli. Cook for 2 minutes before serving.

NUTRITION

Net Carbs: 1g, Fiber: 0g, Fat: 15g, Protein: 34g, Calories: 276kcal

144. CHICKEN BROCCOLI ALFREDO

COOKING: 10' **PREPARATION: 15'** **SERVINGS: 4**

INGREDIENTS

- » 1 pound chicken breast
- » 0.5 cups spinach
- » 1 cup broccoli
- » 1 tablespoon butter
- » 0.5 cups heavy cream
- » 1 clove garlic
- » 2 tablespoons chopped onion
- » ½ tsp of salt
- » ½ tsp of pepper

DIRECTIONS

1. Boil broccoli within 10 minutes.

2. Melt the butter with onion and garlic, put the chicken. Sauté within 5 minutes.

3. Put the spinach and broccoli then stir in the cream with seasonings. Cook within 5 minutes and serve.

NUTRITION

Net carbs: 34g, Fiber: 0g, Fat: 19g, Protein: 34g, Calories: 523kcal

145. GRILLED CHEESY BUFFALO CHICKEN

COOKING: 10' **PREPARATION: 15'** **SERVINGS: 2**

INGREDIENTS

- » 10 oz chicken breast
- » Garlic 2 cloves
- » Mozzarella Cheese 0.25 cup
- » Butter 1 tablespoon
- » Hot Sauce 0.25 cup
- » Lemon Juice 1 tablespoon
- » Celery Salt 0.25 teaspoon
- » Pepper
- » Salt

DIRECTIONS

1. Mix the minced garlic, hot sauce, celery salt, melted butter, lemon juice, pepper, and salt then put the chicken into the mixture.

2. Fill each chicken breast with cheese. Roll up, then secure with a toothpick to close the pocket.

3. Grease the grill. Cook within 5 minutes, flipping and do another 5 minutes. Cooldown and serve.

NUTRITION

Net Carbs: 2g, Fiber: 1g, Fat: 5g, Protein: 24g, Calories: 150kcal

146. MIDDLE EASTERN SHAWARMA

INGREDIENTS

- » 1 pound lamb shoulder
- » 2 tablespoons yogurt
- » 1 tablespoon water
- » 1 teaspoon white vinegar
- » 2 teaspoons lemon juice
- » 1 teaspoon olive oil
- » 2 tablespoons chopped onion
- » 1 clove garlic
- » 0.25 teaspoon black pepper
- » 0.25 teaspoon cumin
- » 0.25 teaspoon nutmeg
- » 0.25 teaspoon cloves
- » 0.25 teaspoon mace
- » 0.25 teaspoon powdered cayenne

DIRECTIONS

1. In a bowl, whisk together egg, espresso powder, chocolate chips, Swerve, and cocoa powder.

2. Add mozzarella cheese and stir well.

3. Spray waffle maker with cooking spray.

4. Putes.

5. Cut chaffle sandwich in half and serve.

NUTRITION

Net Carbs: 1g, Fiber: 0g, Fat: 16g, Protein: 32g, Calories: 27kcal

147. TEX MEX CASSEROLE

INGREDIENTS

- » 1 cup Sour cream
- » 1 Scallion
- » 1 cup Guacamole
- » 1 cup Leafy greens
- » 2 pounds Ground beef
- » 3 tablespoons Tex Mex seasoning
- » 1 cup Monterey Jack cheese
- » 2 ounces Jalapenos pickled
- » 7 ounces Crushed Tomatoes
- » 2 ounces Butter

DIRECTIONS

1. Warm-up oven to 400. Cook the ground beef entirely in the melted butter. Add in the Tex Mex seasoning and the tomatoes and mix well.

2. Put the meat batter in a greased baking pan. Scatter the cheese, and the jalapenos on top, then bake within twenty-five minutes.

3. Chop up the scallion then mix it with the sour cream. Serve the meat mix with a spoon of the sour cream, a scoop of guacamole, and some leafy greens.

NUTRITION

Calories: 860kcal, Net carbs: 8g, Fat: 69g, Protein: 49g

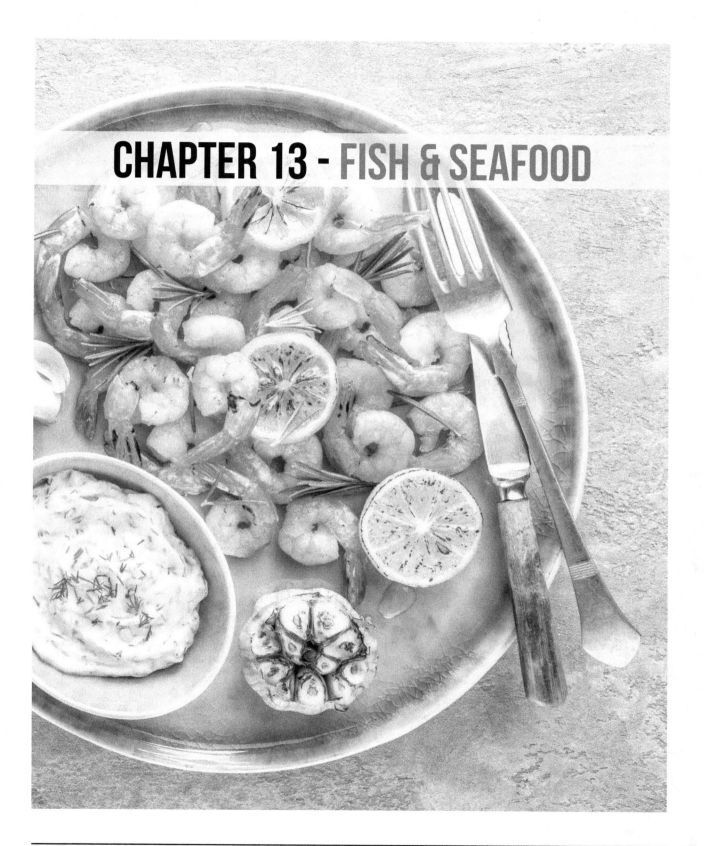

CHAPTER 13 - FISH & SEAFOOD

148. BAKED FISH FILLETS WITH VEGETABLES IN FOIL

COOKING: 40' **PREPARATION: 15'** **SERVINGS: 3**

INGREDIENTS

- » 1 lb. cod
- » 1 red bell pepper
- » 6 cherry tomatoes
- » 1 leek
- » ¼ onion
- » ½ zucchini
- » 1 clove garlic
- » 2 tbsp olives
- » 1 oz butter
- » 2 tbsp olive oil
- » ½ lemon sliced
- » Coriander leaves
- » Salt
- » Pepper

DIRECTIONS

1. Warm-up oven to 400°F. Transfer all the vegetables to a baking sheet lined with foil.

2. Cut the fish into bite-sized and add to the vegetables. Add salt and pepper, olive oil, and add pieces of butter. Bake for 35 – 40 minutes. Serve.

NUTRITION

Calories 339, Fat 19g, Protein 35g, Carbs 5g

149. FISH & CHIPS

COOKING: 30' **PREPARATION: 15'** **SERVINGS: 2**

INGREDIENTS

For chips:
- » ½ tbsp olive oil
- » 1 medium zucchini
- » Salt
- » Pepper
- » For fish:
- » ¾ lb. cod
- » Oil
- » ½ cup almond flour
- » ¼ tsp onion powder

For Sauce:
- » 2 tbsp dill pickle relish
- » ¼ tbsp curry powder
- » ½ cup mayonnaise
- » ½ tsp paprika powder
- » ½ cup parmesan cheese
- » 1 egg
- » Salt
- » Pepper

DIRECTIONS

1. Mix all the sauce fixing in a bowl. Set aside.

2. Warm-up oven to 400°F. Make thin zucchini rods, brush with oil, and spread on the baking sheet. Put salt and pepper then bake within 30 minutes.

3. Beat the egg in a bowl. On a separate plate, combine the parmesan cheese, almond flour, and the remaining spices.

4. Slice the fish into 1 inch by 1-inch pieces. Roll them on the flour mixture. Dip in the beaten egg and then in the flour again. Fry the fish for three minutes. Serve.

NUTRITION

Calories 463, Fat 26.2 g, Protein 49g, Carbs 6g

150. BAKED SALMON WITH ALMONDS AND CREAM SAUCE

COOKING: 20'   **PREPARATION: 10'**   **SERVINGS: 2**

INGREDIENTS

- » Almond Crumbs Creamy Sauce
- » 3 tbsp almonds
- » 2 tbsp almond milk
- » ½ cup cream cheese
- » Salt
- » Fish
- » 1 salmon fillet
- » 1 tsp coconut oil
- » 1 tbsp lemon zest
- » 1 tsp salt
- » White pepper

DIRECTIONS

1. Cut the salmon in half. Rub the salmon with the lemon zest, salt, and pepper. Marinade for 20 minutes.

2. Fry the fish on both sides. Top with almond crumbs and bake within 10 to 15 minutes.

3. Remove and put aside.

4. Place the baking dish on fire and add the cream cheese. Combine the fish baking juices and the cheese. Mix, then pour the sauce onto the fish. Serve.

NUTRITION

Calories 522, Fat 44g, Protein 28g — Carbs 2.4g

151. SHRIMP AND SAUSAGE BAKE

COOKING: 20'   **PREPARATION: 15'**   **SERVINGS: 4**

INGREDIENTS

- » 2 tbsp olive oil
- » 6 ounces chorizo sausage
- » ½ pound shrimp
- » ½ small sweet onion
- » 1 tsp garlic
- » ¼ cup Herbed Chicken Stock
- » Pinch red pepper flakes
- » 1 red bell pepper

DIRECTIONS

1. Sauté the sausage within 6 minutes. Add the shrimp and sauté within 4 minutes. Remove both and set aside. Cook the red pepper, onion, and garlic to the skillet within 4 minutes. Put the chicken stock along with the cooked sausage and shrimp. Simmer for 3 minutes.

2. Stir in the red pepper flake and serve.

NUTRITION

Calories 323, Fat 24g, Protein 20g, Carbs 6g

152. HERB BUTTER SCALLOPS

COOKING: 10'   **PREPARATION: 10'**   **SERVINGS: 4**

INGREDIENTS

- » 1-pound sea scallops
- » ground black pepper
- » 8 tbsp butter
- » 2 tsp garlic
- » 1 lemon juice
- » 2 tsp basil
- » 1 tsp thyme

DIRECTIONS

1. Pat dry the scallops then put pepper. Sear each side within 2 ½ minutes per side.

2. Remove then set aside. Sauté the garlic within 3 minutes. Stir in the lemon juice, basil, and thyme and return the scallops to the skillet, mix.

3. Serve.

NUTRITION

Calories 306, Fat 24g, Protein 19g, Carbs 4g

153. PAN-SEARED HALIBUT WITH CITRUS BUTTER SAUCE

COOKING: 15'   **PREPARATION: 10'**   **SERVINGS: 4**

INGREDIENTS

- » 4 halibut fillets
- » Sea salt
- » ground pepper
- » ¼ cup butter
- » 2 tbsp garlic
- » 1 shallot
- » 3 tablespoons dry white wine
- » 1 tbsp orange juice
- » 1 tbsp lemon juice
- » 2 tsp parsley
- » 2 tsp olive oil

DIRECTIONS

1. Pat dry the fish then put salt and pepper. Set aside.

2. Sauté the garlic and shallot within 3 minutes.

3. Whisk in the white wine, lemon juice, and orange juice and simmer within 2 minutes.

4. Remove the sauce and stir in the parsley; set aside.

5. Panfry the fish until within 10 minutes. Serve with sauce.

NUTRITION

Calories 319, Fat 26g, Protein 22g, Carbs 2g

154. BAKED COCONUT HADDOCK

COOKING: 12'　　　　**PREPARATION: 10'**　　　　**SERVINGS: 4**

INGREDIENTS

- » 4 (5 oz) boneless haddock fillets
- » Sea salt
- » Freshly ground pepper
- » 1 cup shredded unsweetened coconut
- » ½ cup ground hazelnuts
- » 2 tbsp coconut oil, melted

DIRECTIONS

1. Warm oven to 400°F.

2. Pat dry fillets and lightly season them with salt and pepper.

3. Stir together the shredded coconut and hazelnut in a small bowl.

4. Dredge the fish fillets in the coconut mixture so that both sides of each piece are thickly coated.

5. Put the fish on the baking sheet and lightly brush both sides of each piece with the coconut oil.

6. Bake the haddock until the topping is golden and the fish flakes easily with a fork, about 12 minutes total. Serve.

NUTRITION

Calories 299, Fat 24g, Protein 20g, Carbs 1g

CHAPTER 15 - MEAT RECIPES

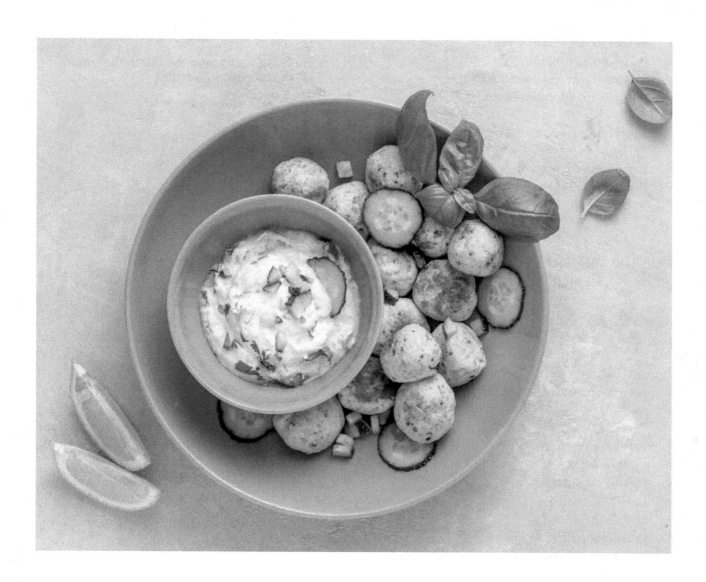

155. SPICY STEAK CURRY

COOKING: 40'   PREPARATION: 15'   SERVINGS: 6

INGREDIENTS

- » 1 cup plain yogurt
- » ½ teaspoon garlic paste
- » ½ teaspoon ginger paste
- » ½ teaspoon ground cloves
- » ½ teaspoon ground cumin
- » 2 teaspoons red pepper flakes
- » ¼ teaspoon ground turmeric
- » Salt
- » 2 pounds grass-fed round steak
- » ¼ cup olive oil
- » 1 medium yellow onion
- » 1½ tablespoons lemon juice
- » ¼ cup cilantro

DIRECTIONS

1. Mix yogurt, garlic paste, ginger paste, and spices. Add the steak pieces. Set aside.

2. Sauté the onion within 4-5 minutes. Add the steak pieces with marinade and mix.

3. Simmer within 25 minutes. Stir in the lemon juice and simmer 10 minutes.

4. Garnish with cilantro and serve.

NUTRITION

Calories: 440, Net Carbs: 4.8g, Carbohydrate: 5.5g, Fiber: 0.7g, Protein: 48.3g

156. BEEF STEW

COOKING: 100'   PREPARATION: 15'   SERVINGS: 4

INGREDIENTS

- » 1 1/3 pounds grass-fed chuck roast
- » Salt
- » ground black pepper
- » 2 tablespoons butter
- » 1 yellow onion
- » 2 garlic cloves
- » 1 cup beef broth
- » 1 bay leaf
- » ½ teaspoon dried thyme
- » ½ teaspoon dried rosemary
- » 1 carrot
- » 4 ounces celery stalks
- » 1 tablespoon lemon juice

DIRECTIONS

1. Put salt and black pepper in beef cubes.

2. Sear the beef cubes within 4-5 minutes. Add the onion and garlic, then adjust the heat to medium and cook within 4-5 minutes. Add the broth, bay leaf, and dried herbs and boil.

3. Simmer within 45 minutes. Stir in the carrot and celery and simmer within 30-45 minutes.

4. Stir in lemon juice, salt, and black pepper. Serve.

NUTRITION

Calories: 413, Net Carbs: 4.3g, Carbohydrate: 5.9g, Fiber: 1.6g, Protein: 52g

157. BEEF & CABBAGE STEW

COOKING: 70'   **PREPARATION: 15'**   **SERVINGS: 8**

INGREDIENTS

» 2 pounds grass-fed beef stew meat
» 1 1/3 cups hot chicken broth
» 2 yellow onions
» 2 bay leaves
» 1 teaspoon Greek seasoning
» Salt
» ground black pepper
» 3 celery stalks
» 1 package cabbage
» 1 can sugar-free tomato sauce
» 1 can sugar-free whole plum tomatoes

DIRECTIONS

1. Sear the beef within 4-5 minutes. Stir in the broth, onion, bay leaves, Greek seasoning, salt, and black pepper and boil. Adjust the heat to low and cook within 1¼ hours.

2. Stir in the celery and cabbage and cook within 30 minutes. Stir in the tomato sauce and chopped plum tomatoes and cook, uncovered within 15-20 minutes. Stir in the salt, discard bay leaves and serve.

NUTRITION

Calories: 247, Net Carbs: 4.9g, Carbohydrate: 7g, Fiber: 2.1g — Protein: 36.5g

158. BEEF & MUSHROOM CHILI

COOKING: 190'   **PREPARATION: 15'**   **SERVINGS: 8**

INGREDIENTS

» 2 pounds grass-fed ground beef
» 1 yellow onion
» ½ cup green bell pepper
» ½ cup carrot
» 4 ounces mushrooms
» 2 garlic cloves
» 1 can sugar-free tomato paste
» 2 tablespoons red chili powder
» 1 tablespoon ground cumin
» 1 teaspoon ground cinnamon
» 1 teaspoon red pepper flakes
» ½ teaspoon ground allspice
» Salt
» ground black pepper
» 4 cups of water
» ½ cup sour cream

DIRECTIONS

1. Cook the beef within 8-10 minutes. Stir in the remaining fixing except for sour cream and boil. Cook on low, covered, within 3 hours. Top with sour cream and serve.

NUTRITION

Calories: 246, Net Carbs: 5.9g, Carbohydrate: 8.2g, Fiber: 2.3g, Protein: 25.1g

159. STEAK WITH CHEESE SAUCE

COOKING: 17' **PREPARATION: 15'** **SERVINGS: 4**

INGREDIENTS

- » 18 ounces grass-fed filet mignon
- » Salt
- » ground black pepper
- » 2 tablespoons butter
- » ½ cup yellow onion
- » 5¼ ounces blue cheese
- » 1 cup heavy cream
- » 1 garlic clove
- » ground nutmeg

DIRECTIONS

1. Cook onion within 5-8 minutes. Add the blue cheese, heavy cream, garlic, nutmeg, salt, and black pepper and stir.

2. Cook for about 3-5 minutes.

3. Put salt and black pepper in filet mignon steaks. Cook the steaks within 4 minutes per side.

4. Transfer and set aside. Top with cheese sauce, then serve.

NUTRITION

Calories: 521, Net Carbs: 3g, Carbohydrate: 3.3g, Fiber: 0.3g, Protein: 44.7g

160. STEAK WITH BLUEBERRY SAUCE

COOKING: 20' **PREPARATION: 15'** **SERVINGS: 4**

INGREDIENTS

For Sauce:
- » 2 tablespoons butter
- » 2 tablespoons yellow onion
- » 2 garlic cloves
- » 1 teaspoon thyme
- » 1 1/3 cups beef broth
- » 2 tablespoons lemon juice
- » ¾ cup blueberries

For Steak:
- » 2 tablespoons butter
- » 4 grass-fed flank steaks
- » Salt
- » ground black pepper

DIRECTIONS

1. For the sauce: sauté the onion within 2-3 minutes.

2. Add the garlic and thyme and sauté within 1 minute. Stir in the broth and simmer within 10 minutes.

3. For the steak: put salt and black pepper. Cook steaks within 3-4 minutes per side.

4. Transfer and put aside. Add sauce in the skillet and stir. Stir in the lemon juice, blueberries, salt, and black pepper and cook within 1-2 minutes. Put blueberry sauce over the steaks. Serve.

NUTRITION

Calories: 467, Net Carbs: 4.6g, Fiber: 0.9g, Protein: 49.5g

161. GRILLED STEAK

COOKING: 12' **PREPARATION: 15'** **SERVINGS: 6**

INGREDIENTS

- » 1 teaspoon lemon zest
- » 1 garlic clove
- » 1 tablespoon red chili powder
- » 1 tablespoon paprika
- » 1 tablespoon ground coffee
- » Salt
- » ground black pepper
- » 2 grass-fed skirt steaks

DIRECTIONS

1. Mix all the ingredients except steaks. Marinate the steaks and keep aside within 30-40 minutes.

2. Grill the steaks within 5-6 minutes per side. Remove then cool before slicing. Serve.

NUTRITION

Calories: 473, Net Carbs: 0.7g, Carbohydrate: 1.6g, Fiber: 0.9g, Protein: 60.8g

162. ROASTED TENDERLOIN

COOKING: 50' **PREPARATION: 10'** **SERVINGS: 10**

INGREDIENTS

- » 1 grass-fed beef tenderloin roast
- » 4 garlic cloves
- » 1 tablespoon rosemary
- » Salt
- » ground black pepper
- » 1 tablespoon olive oil

DIRECTIONS

1. Warm-up oven to 425 degrees F.

2. Place beef meat into the prepared roasting pan. Massage with garlic, rosemary, salt, and black pepper and oil. Roast the beef within 45-50 minutes.

3. Remove, cool, slice, and serve.

NUTRITION

Calories: 295, Net Carbs: 0.4g, Fiber: 0.2g, Protein: 39.5g, Fat: 13.9g

163. GARLICKY PRIME RIB ROAST

COOKING: 95'   **PREPARATION: 15'**   **SERVINGS: 15**

INGREDIENTS

- » 10 garlic cloves
- » 2 teaspoons dried thyme
- » 2 tablespoons olive oil
- » Salt
- » ground black pepper
- » 1 grass-fed prime rib roast

NUTRITION

Calories: 499, Net Carbs: 0.6g, Carbohydrate: 0.7g, Fiber: 0.1g, Protein: 61.5g, Fat: 25.9g

DIRECTIONS

1. Mix the garlic, thyme, oil, salt, and black pepper. Marinate the rib roast with garlic mixture within 1 hour.

2. Warm-up oven to 500 degrees F.

3. Roast within 20 minutes. Lower to 325 degrees F and roast within 65-75 minutes.

4. Remove then cooldown within 10-15 minutes, slice, and serve.

164. MEATBALLS CURRY

COOKING: 25'   **PREPARATION: 15'**   **SERVINGS: 6**

INGREDIENTS

For Meatballs:
- » 1-pound lean ground pork
- » 2 organic eggs
- » 3 tablespoons yellow onion
- » ¼ cup fresh parsley leaves
- » ¼ teaspoon fresh ginger
- » 2 garlic cloves
- » 1 jalapeño pepper
- » 1 teaspoon Erythritol
- » 1 tablespoon red curry paste
- » 3 tablespoons olive oil

For Curry:
- » 1 yellow onion
- » Salt
- » 2 garlic cloves
- » ¼ teaspoon ginger
- » 2 tablespoons red curry paste
- » 1 can unsweetened coconut milk
- » Ground black pepper
- » ¼ cup fresh parsley

DIRECTIONS

For meatballs:

1. Mix all the ingredients except oil. Make small-sized balls from the mixture.

2. Cook meatballs within 3-5 minutes. Transfer and put aside.

For curry:

3. Sauté onion, and salt within 4-5 minutes. Add the garlic and ginger. Add the curry paste, and sauté within 1-2 minutes. Add coconut milk, and meatballs then simmer.

4. Simmer again within 10-12 minutes. Put salt and black pepper. Remove then serve with fresh parsley.

NUTRITION

Calories: 444, Net Carbs: 6.4g, Carbohydrate: 8.6g, Fiber: 2.2g, Protein: 17g

165. BEEF TACO BAKE

PREPARATION: 15' **SERVINGS: 6**

INGREDIENTS

For Crust:
» 3 organic eggs
» 4 ounces cream cheese
» ½ teaspoon taco seasoning
» 1/3 cup heavy cream
» 8 ounces cheddar cheese

For Topping:
» 1-pound grass-fed ground beef
» 4 ounces green chilies
» ¼ cup sugar-free tomato sauce
» 3 teaspoons taco seasoning
» 8 ounces cheddar cheese

NUTRITION

Calories: 569, Net Carbs: 3.8g, Carbohydrate: 4g, Fiber: 0.2g, Protein: 38.7g

DIRECTIONS

1. Warm-up oven to 375 degrees F.

For the crust:

2. Beat the eggs, and cream cheese, taco seasoning, and heavy cream. Place cheddar cheese in the baking dish. Spread cream cheese mixture over cheese.

3. Bake within 25-30 minutes. Remove then set aside within 5 minutes.

For topping:

4. Cook the beef within 8-10 minutes. Stir in the green chilies, tomato sauce, and taco seasoning and transfer. Place the beef mixture over the crust and sprinkle with cheese. Bake within 18-20 minutes. Remove then slice and serve.

166. MEATBALLS IN CHEESE SAUCE

COOKING: 25' **PREPARATION: 20'** **SERVINGS: 5**

INGREDIENTS

For Meatballs:
» 1-pound ground pork
» 1 organic egg
» 2 ounces Parmesan cheese
» ½ tablespoon dried basil
» 1 teaspoon garlic powder
» ½ teaspoon onion powder
» Salt
» ground black pepper
» 3 tablespoons olive oil

For Sauce:
» 1 can sugar-free tomatoes
» 2 tablespoons butter
» 7 ounces spinach
» 2 tablespoons parsley
» 5 ounces mozzarella cheese
» Sground black pepper ; Salt

DIRECTIONS

1. Mix all the fixing except oil in a large bowl. Make small-sized balls from the mixture.

2. Cook the meatballs within 3-5 minutes. Add the tomatoes. Simmer within 15 minutes.

3. Stir fry the spinach within 1-2 minutes in butter. Put salt and black pepper.

4. Remove then put the cooked spinach, parsley, and mozzarella cheese into meatballs and stir.

5. Cook within 1-2 minutes. Remove and serve.

NUTRITION

Calories: 398, Net Carbs: 4.7g, Carbohydrate: 6.6g, Fiber: 1.9g, Protein: 38.6g, Fat: 24.8g

167. CHOCOLATE CHILI

COOKING: 135' **PREPARATION: 15'** **SERVINGS: 8**

INGREDIENTS

- » 2 tablespoons olive oil
- » 1 small onion
- » 1 green bell pepper
- » 4 garlic cloves
- » 1 jalapeño pepper
- » 1 teaspoon dried thyme
- » 2 tablespoons red chili powder
- » 1 tablespoon ground cumin
- » 2 pounds lean ground pork
- » 2 cups fresh tomatoes
- » 4 ounces sugar-free tomato paste
- » 1½ tablespoons cacao powder
- » 2 cups chicken broth
- » 1 cup of water
- » Salt
- » ground black pepper
- » ¼ cup cheddar cheese

DIRECTIONS

1. Sauté the onion and bell pepper within 5-7 minutes.

2. Add the garlic, jalapeño pepper, thyme, and spices and sauté within 1 minute.

3. Add the pork and cook within 4-5 minutes. Stir in the tomatoes, tomato paste, and cacao powder and cook within 2 minutes.

4. Add the broth and water, boil. Simmer, covered within 2 hours. Stir in the salt and black pepper. Remove then top with cheddar cheese and serve.

NUTRITION

Calories: 326, Net Carbs: 6.5g, Carbohydrate: 9.1g, Fiber: 2.6g, Protein: 23.3g, Fat: 22.9g

168. PORK STEW

COOKING: 45' **PREPARATION: 15'** **SERVINGS: 6**

INGREDIENTS

- » 2 tablespoons olive oil
- » 2 pounds pork tenderloin
- » 1 tablespoon garlic
- » 2 teaspoons paprika
- » ¾ cup chicken broth
- » 1 cup sugar-free tomato sauce
- » ½ tablespoon Erythritol
- » 1 teaspoon dried oregano
- » 2 dried bay leaves
- » 2 tablespoons lemon juice
- » Salt
- » ground black pepper

DIRECTIONS

1. Cook the pork within 3-4 minutes. Add the garlic and cook within 1 minute.

2. Stir in the remaining fixing and boil. Simmer, covered within 30-40 minutes

3. Remove then discard the bay leaves. Serve.

NUTRITION

Calories: 277, Net Carbs: 2.5g, Carbohydrate: 3.6g, Fiber: 1.1g, Protein: 41g — Fat: 10.4g

169. PORK & CHILES STEW

INGREDIENTS

- » 3 tablespoons unsalted butter
- » 2½ pounds boneless pork ribs
- » 1 large yellow onion
- » 4 garlic cloves
- » 1½ cups chicken broth
- » 2 cans sugar-free tomatoes
- » 1 cup canned roasted poblano chilies
- » 2 teaspoons dried oregano
- » 1 teaspoon ground cumin
- » Salt
- » ¼ cup cilantro
- » 2 tablespoons lime juice

DIRECTIONS

1. Cook the pork, onions, and garlic within 5 minutes.

2. Add the broth, tomatoes, poblano chilies, oregano, cumin, and salt and boil.

3. Simmer, covered within 2 hours. Mix with the fresh cilantro and lime juice and remove it. Serve.

NUTRITION

Calories: 288, Net Carbs:6g, Carbohydrate: 8.8g, Fiber: 2.8g, Protein: 39.6g

CHAPTER 15 - DESSERTS

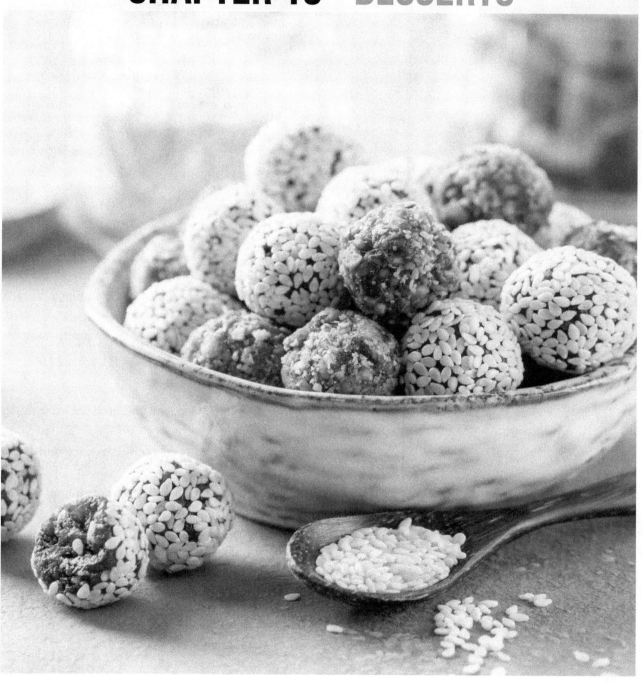

170. KETO CHEESECAKES

COOKING: 10' **PREPARATION: 15'** **SERVINGS: 9**

INGREDIENTS

- » 2 tablespoons butter
- » 1 tablespoon caramel syrup; sugar-free
- » 3 tablespoons coffee
- » 8 ounces cream cheese
- » 1/3 cup swerve
- » 3 eggs

For the frosting:

- » 8 ounces mascarpone cheese
- » 3 tablespoons caramel syrup
- » 2 tablespoons swerve
- » 3 tablespoons butter

DIRECTIONS

1. Pulse cream cheese with eggs, 2 tablespoons butter, coffee, 1 tablespoon caramel syrup, and 1/3 cup twist in a processor. Scoop into a cupcakes pan and bake within 15 minutes. Chill for 3 hours.

2. Combine 3 tablespoons butter, 3 tablespoons caramel syrup, 2 tablespoons swerve, and mascarpone cheese. Top over cheesecakes and serve.

NUTRITION

Calories: 254, Fat: 23, Fiber: 0, Carbs: 1, Protein: 5

171. EASY KETO DESSERT

COOKING: 35' **PREPARATION: 15'** **SERVINGS: 4**

INGREDIENTS

- » 1/3 cup cocoa powder
- » 1/3 cup erythritol
- » 1 egg
- » 1/4 cup almond flour
- » 1/4 cup walnuts
- » 1/2 teaspoon baking powder
- » 7 tablespoons ghee
- » 1/2 teaspoon vanilla extract
- » 1 tablespoon of peanut butter
- » Salt

DIRECTIONS

1. Warm-up 6 tablespoons ghee and the erythritol, cook for 5 minutes.

2. Transfer, mix with salt, vanilla extract, and cocoa powder. Put egg, beat.

3. Add baking powder, walnuts, and almond flour; stir and pour into a skillet.

4. Mix 1 tablespoon ghee with peanut butter, warm-up in the microwave a second.

5. Drizzle over brownies mix in the skillet and bake for 30 minutes.

6. Slice and serve.

NUTRITION

Calories: 223, Fat: 32, Fiber: 1, Carbs: 3 —
Protein: 6

172. KETO BROWNIES

COOKING: 20' **PREPARATION: 15'** **SERVINGS: 9**

INGREDIENTS

- » 6 ounces of coconut oil
- » 4 ounces cream cheese
- » 5 tablespoons swerve
- » 6 eggs
- » 2 teaspoons vanilla
- » 3 ounces of cocoa powder
- » 1/2 teaspoon baking powder

DIRECTIONS

1. Blend eggs with coconut oil, cocoa powder, baking powder, vanilla, cream cheese, and swerve using a mixer.

2. Put into a lined baking dish, at 350 degrees F, and bake for 20 minutes.

3. Chill and serve.

NUTRITION

Calories: 178, Fat: 14, Fiber: 2, Carbs: 3, Protein: 5

173. RASPBERRY AND COCONUT

COOKING: 5' **PREPARATION: 15'** **SERVINGS: 12**

INGREDIENTS

- » 1/4 cup swerve
- » 1/2 cup coconut oil
- » 1/2 cup raspberries; dried
- » 1/2 cup coconut
- » 1/2 cup coconut butter

DIRECTIONS

1. Blend dried berries using a processor.

2. Warm-up the butter over medium heat.

3. Add oil, coconut, and swerve; cook for 5 minutes.

4. Pour half into a baking pan. Add raspberry powder.

5. Put the rest of the butter mixture, chill and serve.

NUTRITION

Calories: 234, Fat: 22, Fiber: 2, Carbs: 4, Protein: 2

174. CHOCOLATE PUDDING DELIGHT

COOKING: 10'   **PREPARATION: 60**   **SERVINGS: 2**

INGREDIENTS

- » 1/2 teaspoon stevia powder
- » 2 tablespoons cocoa powder
- » 2 tablespoons water
- » 1 tablespoon gelatin
- » 1 cup of coconut milk
- » 2 tablespoons maple syrup

DIRECTIONS

1. Warm-up the coconut milk over medium heat; add stevia and cocoa powder and mix.

2. Mix gelatin with water; then add to the pan.

3. Mix, add maple syrup, chill for 45 minutes. Serve.

NUTRITION

Calories: 140, Fat: 2, Fiber: 2, Carbs: 4, Protein: 4

175. SPECIAL KETO PUDDING

COOKING: 4H 15'   **PREPARATION: 10'**   **SERVINGS: 2**

INGREDIENTS

- » 1 cup of coconut milk
- » 4 teaspoons gelatin
- » 1/4 teaspoon ginger
- » 1/4 teaspoon liquid stevia
- » A pinch of nutmeg
- » A pinch of cardamom

DIRECTIONS

1. In a bowl, mix 1/4 cup milk with gelatin.

2. Put the remaining coconut milk in a pot and warm-up.

3. Add gelatin mix, cold, and chill for 4 hours.

4. Transfer to a food processor, add stevia, cardamom, nutmeg, and ginger and blend.

5. Serve cold.

NUTRITION

Calories: 150, Fat: 1, Fiber: 0, Carbs: 2, Protein: 6

176. PEANUT BUTTER FUDGE

COOKING: 135'   **PREPARATION: 10'**   **SERVINGS: 12**

INGREDIENTS

- » 1 cup peanut butter
- » 1 cup of coconut oil
- » 1/4 cup almond milk
- » 2 teaspoons vanilla stevia
- » A pinch of salt

Topping:
- » 2 tablespoons swerve
- » 1/4 cup cocoa powder
- » 2 tablespoons melted coconut oil

DIRECTIONS

1. Mix peanut butter with 1 cup coconut oil; microwave until it melts.

2. Add a pinch of salt, almond milk, and stevia; mix and pour into a lined loaf pan.

3. Chill for 2 hours and slice.

4. Mix 2 tablespoons melted coconut with cocoa powder and swerve.

5. Drizzle the sauce on top and serve.

NUTRITION

Calories: 265, Fat: 23, Fiber: 2, Carbs: 4, Protein: 6

177. COCONUT PEAR CREAM

COOKING: 4H   **PREPARATION: 5'**   **SERVINGS: 4**

INGREDIENTS

- » 1 tablespoon lime juice
- » 4 tablespoons coconut cream
- » 4 pears
- » 1 ½ cups date sugar

DIRECTIONS

1. Mix all the fixings and cook on low for 4 hours.

2. Blend using an immersion blender, and serve.

NUTRITION

Calories: 208, Fat 4, Fiber: 8, Carbs: 45, Protein: 15

178. LEMONY COCONUT CREAM

COOKING: 3H　　　**PREPARATION: 5'**　　　**SERVINGS: 4**

INGREDIENTS

- » 4 cups of coconut milk
- » 1 cup of coconut sugar
- » 1 lemon juice
- » 2 tablespoons ground cinnamon
- » ½ cup coconut

DIRECTIONS

1. Mix all the fixings, cook on low for 3 hours, and serve cold.

NUTRITION

Calories: 793, Fat: 60, Fiber: 8, Carbs: 70, Protein: 6

179. BLACKBERRY STEW

COOKING: 4H　　　**PREPARATION: 5'**　　　**SERVINGS: 4**

INGREDIENTS

- » 4 cups blackberries
- » 2 tablespoons coconut oil
- » 1/3 cup rose water
- » 2/3 cup coconut sugar

DIRECTIONS

1. Mix all the fixings, and cook on low for 4 hours.
2. Serve cold.

NUTRITION

Calories: 246, Fat: 7, Fiber: 7, Carbs: 47, Protein: 2

180. PEACH JAM

COOKING: 6H　　　**PREPARATION: 5'**　　　**SERVINGS: 8**

INGREDIENTS

- » 3 pounds peaches
- » 1 cup of water
- » 1 teaspoon vanilla extract
- » 1 cup date sugar

DIRECTIONS

1. Mix all the fixings, and cook on low for 6 hours.
2. Stir the jam, and serve.

NUTRITION

Calories: 117, Fat: 0, Fiber: 0, Carbs: 30, Protein: 0

181. STRAWBERRY BOWLS

COOKING: 3H　　　**PREPARATION: 5'**　　　**SERVINGS: 4**

INGREDIENTS

- » 2 pounds of strawberries
- » ½ cup honey
- » 2 tablespoons lemon zest
- » 1 cup of coconut water

DIRECTIONS

1. Combine all the ingredients, cook on low for 3 hours, and serve cold.

NUTRITION

Calories: 215, Fat: 0, Fiber: 5, Carbs: 55, Protein: 2

182. PINEAPPLE STEW

COOKING: 3H **PREPARATION: 5'** **SERVINGS: 4**

INGREDIENTS

- » 1/2 fresh pineapple
- » 2 cups apple juice
- » ¼ cup of coconut sugar

DIRECTIONS

1. Combine all the ingredients, cook on low for 3 hours, and serve.

NUTRITION

Calories: 165, Fat: 0, Fiber: 2, Carbs: 42, Protein: 0

183. RHUBARB COMPOTE

COOKING: 4H **PREPARATION: 5'** **SERVINGS: 6**

INGREDIENTS

- » 1-pound rhubarb
- » 1 cup of water
- » 4 tablespoons honey
- » 1 teaspoon vanilla extract

DIRECTIONS

1. Mix all the fixings, and cook on low for 4 hours, and serve.

NUTRITION

Calories: 60, Fat: 0, Fiber: 1, Carbs: 15, Protein: 0

184. BANANA BOWLS

COOKING: 2H   **PREPARATION: 5'**   **SERVINGS: 4**

INGREDIENTS

» 1 tablespoon coconut sugar
» 4 bananas
» ½ cup of coconut oil

DIRECTIONS

1. Mix all the fixings, and cook on low for 2 hours.
2. Serve.

NUTRITION

Calories: 346, Fat: 27, Fiber: 3, Carbs: 28, Protein: 1

185. GRAPES COMPOTE

COOKING: 2H   **PREPARATION: 10'**   **SERVINGS: 4**

INGREDIENTS

» 1 ½ cups grape juice
» 1-pound green grapes
» 2 tablespoons coconut sugar

DIRECTIONS

1. Mix all the fixings, and cook on low for 2 hours.
2. Serve.

NUTRITION

Calories: 131, Fat: 0, Fiber: 1, Carbs: 33, Protein: 1

186. APRICOT PUDDING

COOKING: 4H   PREPARATION: 5'   SERVINGS: 6

INGREDIENTS

- » 3 eggs
- » 2 cups apricots
- » 1 cup of coconut milk
- » 1/2 teaspoon baking soda
- » 2 tablespoons lemon juice
- » 1 ¼ cups coconut flour
- » 2 tablespoons coconut sugar
- » 1/3 cup coconut oil
- » 1 teaspoon vanilla extract
- » Olive oil

DIRECTIONS

1. 1. Combine all the other ingredients, put into the slow cooker, cook on low for 4 hours, and serve cold.

NUTRITION

Calories: 298, Fat: 27, Fiber: 3, Carbs: 12, Protein: 4

187. BLUEBERRIES AND CREAM

COOKING: 3H   PREPARATION: 5'   SERVINGS: 4

INGREDIENTS

- » 4 cups blueberries
- » 1 ½ cups coconut cream
- » ½ cup of coconut sugar

DIRECTIONS

1. Mix all the fixings, and cook on low for 3 hours.
2. Blend in an immersion blender, and serve cold.

NUTRITION

Calories: 384, Fat: 22, Fiber: 5, Carbs: 51, Protein: 3

188. PUMPKIN CREAM

COOKING: 2H   **PREPARATION: 10'**   **SERVINGS: 2**

INGREDIENTS

- » 1 cup pumpkin puree
- » ½ cup almond milk
- » 1 teaspoon ground cinnamon
- » 2 tablespoons coconut sugar
- » 1 teaspoon vanilla extract

DIRECTIONS

1. Mix all the fixings, and cook on low for 2 hours.
2. Serve.

NUTRITION

Calories 211, Fat: 14, Fiber: 5, Carbs: 20, Protein: 2

189. MAPLE PUMPKIN DESSERT

COOKING: 3H   **PREPARATION: 5'**   **SERVINGS: 6**

INGREDIENTS

- » 1 ½ teaspoon ground cinnamon
- » ½ teaspoon baking soda
- » 2 tablespoons lemon juice
- » 1/3 cup pure maple syrup
- » 1 cup pumpkin puree
- » 3 cups of coconut milk
- » 1 teaspoon grated ginger
- » 2 teaspoons vanilla extract
- » 1 cup walnuts

DIRECTIONS

1. Mix all the fixings, and cook on low for 3 hours.
2. Serve.

NUTRITION

Calories: 472, Fat: 41, Fiber: 5, Carbs: 24, Protein: 8

190. COCONUT PINEAPPLE BOWLS

COOKING: 3H   **PREPARATION: 5'**   **SERVINGS: 2**

INGREDIENTS

- » 1 cup pineapple chunks
- » 2 tablespoons coconut flakes
- » 1 cup of coconut milk
- » 1 tablespoon ground cinnamon

DIRECTIONS

1. Mix all the fixing, and cook on low for 3 hours.
2. Serve.

NUTRITION

Calories: 343, Fat: 30, Fiber: 6, Carbs: 21, Protein: 3

191. CINNAMON CRUNCH CEREAL

COOKING: 20'   **PREPARATION: 10'**   **SERVINGS: 5**

INGREDIENTS

- » For the Cereal
- » Almond Flour (1 cup)
- » Cinnamon (2 teaspoons)
- » Coconut (0.5 cup)
- » Erythritol (0.33 cup)
- » Butter (6 tablespoons)
- » For sugar topping
- » 1 tbsp erythritol sweetener
- » ½ tsp ground cinnamon

DIRECTIONS

1. Warm-up to a temperature of 300F.
2. Put the flour, coconut, sweetener, and cinnamon in a processor. Pulse.
3. Put the butter pieces and pulse.
4. Put the mixture in the pan and cover it with another sheet of parchment. Flatten out the ingredients. Bake for 20-30 minutes.
5. Combine the topping. Sprinkle over the cereal.
6. Cooldown and serve.

NUTRITION

Net carbs: 6g, Fiber: 5g, Fat: 20g, Protein: 9g, kcal: 236

192. ALMOND PAPAYA MIX

COOKING: 2H **PREPARATION: 10'** **SERVINGS: 8**

INGREDIENTS

» 1 cup of coconut milk
» 1 cup papaya
» 2 tablespoons almonds

DIRECTIONS

1. Mix all the fixing, and cook on low for 2 hours.
2. Serve cold.

NUTRITION

Calories: 85, Fat: 7, Fiber: 1, Carbs: 3, Protein: 1

193. CINNAMON ROLLS

COOKING: 20' **PREPARATION: 10'** **SERVINGS: 8**

INGREDIENTS

» Mozzarella (1.5 cups)
» Almond Flour (0.75 cups)
» Cream Cheese (2 tablespoons)
» Egg (1)
» ½ tsp baking powder

Filling

» 2tbsp water
» 2 tbsp Sweetener
» 2 tsp cinnamon
» Frosting
» 2 tbsp cream cheese
» 1 tbsp Greek yogurt
» Vanilla Extract (2 drops)

DIRECTIONS

1. Warm-up the oven to heat at 360F.
2. Dissolve the shredded mozzarella and cream cheese in a microwave. Remove.
3. Stir in the egg.
4. Mix in the flour and baking powder. Make a ball of smooth dough, divided into 4.
5. Form long rolls, flatten thin.
6. For the cinnamon filling:
7. Boil water, then put in the sweetener and cinnamon.
8. Put the cinnamon paste over the flattened dough rolls.
9. Roll into a bun and cut sideways in half.
10. Place the buns on a nonstick pie dish.
11. Bake within 18 minutes.
12. Prepare the frosting by thoroughly mixing yogurt, sweetener, and cream cheese. Serve.

NUTRITION

Net carbs: 10g, Fiber: 0g, Fat: 9g, Protein: 4g, kcal: 243

194. CHOCOLATE ICE CREAM

COOKING: 15' **PREPARATION: 10'** **SERVINGS: 8**

INGREDIENTS

- » 2 cups heavy whipping cream
- » 4 egg yolks
- » 10 packet no-calorie sweetener
- » Dry Cocoa Powder (0.25 cup, unsweetened)
- » Chocolate Sweetener (2 tablespoons)
- » Vanilla Extract (1 teaspoon)

DIRECTIONS

1. Warm-up the cream to heat over low.

2. Stir in the egg yolks on low heat within 7 minutes.

3. Remove and combine in the sweetener, chocolate powder, syrup, and vanilla.

4. Add the mixture to the ice cream maker. Freeze and serve.

NUTRITION

Net carbs: 2g, Fiber: 0g, Fat: 11g, Protein: 7g, kcal: 150

195. STRAWBERRY ICE CREAM

COOKING: 0' **PREPARATION: 10'** **SERVINGS: 3**

INGREDIENTS

- » 1 cup strawberries
- » 1 ½ vanilla whey protein powder
- » Almond Butter (1 tablespoon)
- » Coconut Oil (2 tablespoons)
- » Heavy cream (0.5 cups)
- » Sweetener (2 tablespoons)

DIRECTIONS

1. Pulse all the fixing in a blender, chill and serve.

NUTRITION

Net carbs: 36g, Fiber: 0g, Fat: 11g, Protein: 5g, kcal: 253

196. LAVA CAKE

COOKING: 10' **PREPARATION: 10'** **SERVINGS: 2**

INGREDIENTS

- » Cocoa Powder (4 tablespoons, unsweetened)
- » Baking Powder (a half-teaspoon)
- » Egg (1)
- » Heavy cream (2 tablespoons)
- » Stevia (3 tablespoons)
- » Vanilla Extract (1 teaspoon)
- » Salt

DIRECTIONS

1. Warm-up the oven to heat at 350F.
2. Combine the stevia and cocoa powder, mix with eggs.
3. Stir in baking powder, cream, and vanilla. Add salt.
4. Dump out the batter evenly into cups and bake for 10 minutes. Serve.

NUTRITION

Net carbs: 66g, Fiber: 0g, Fat: 41g, Protein: 5g, kcal: 660

197. LEMON MOUSSE

COOKING: 5H 15' **PREPARATION: 0'** **SERVINGS: 4**

INGREDIENTS

- » Heavy cream (1 cup)
- » Jell-O with Lemon Flavor (1 pack)
- » Lemon Juice (1 tablespoon)
- » Erythritol (1 teaspoon)
- » Sweetener

DIRECTIONS

1. Whisk the cream until points start to form. Prepare the Jell-O and chill within 12 minutes.
2. Combine the Jell-O and cream mixture within 3 minutes. Flavor it with sweetener and lemon juice.
3. Chill up to 5 hours and serve

NUTRITION

Net carbs: 3g, Fiber: 0g, Fat: 27g, Protein: 5g, Calories: 249

198. CHOCOLATE ALMOND BUTTER FAT BOMBS

COOKING: 5'　　　**PREPARATION: 60'**　　　**SERVINGS: 4**

INGREDIENTS

- » 2 oz unsweetened chocolate
- » Butter (4 tablespoons)
- » Almond Butter (0.33 cup)
- » Peanut Butter (1 tablespoon)
- » Coconut Oil (1 tablespoon)
- » Stevia (1 teaspoon)

DIRECTIONS

1. Melt the chocolate, put into a silicone mold. Chill for 15 minutes.

2. Put everything into a mixer. Put stevia then process.

3. Pour mixture into the silicone mold.

4. Chill for 45 minutes, serve.

NUTRITION

Net carbs: 12g, Fiber: 0g, Fat: 60g, Protein: 10g, kcal: 98

199. WHITE CHOCOLATE

COOKING: 5'　　　**PREPARATION: 15'**　　　**SERVINGS: 10**

INGREDIENTS

- » 8 oz raw cacao butter
- » ½ cup erythritol
- » Vanilla Protein Powder (0.25 cup)
- » Vanilla Extract (2 teaspoons)
- » Salt (0.25 teaspoon)

DIRECTIONS

1. Melt the cacao butter on low heat; whisk in Swerve.

2. Cooldown within 15 minutes, then put it into a blender.

3. Stir in the remaining items and process in the blender.

4. Pour the mixture onto the chocolate bar molds.

5. Chill, serve.

NUTRITION

Net carbs: 2g, Fiber: 0g, Fat: 52g, Protein: 5g, kcal: 498

200. COCONUT PEANUT BUTTER BALLS

COOKING: 135'   **PREPARATION: 15'**   **SERVINGS: 8**

INGREDIENTS

- » 2 tablespoons olive oil
- » 1 small onion
- » 1 green bell pepper
- » 4 garlic cloves
- » 1 jalapeño pepper
- » 1 teaspoon dried thyme
- » 2 tablespoons red chili powder
- » 1 tablespoon ground cumin
- » 2 pounds lean ground pork
- »

DIRECTIONS

1. Sauté the onion and bell pepper within 5-7 minutes.

2. Add the garlic, jalapeño pepper, thyme, and spices and sauté within 1 minute.

3. Add the pork and cook within 4-5 minutes. Stir in the tomatoes, tomato paste, and cacao powder and cook within 2 minutes.

4. Add the broth and water, boil. Simmer, covered within 2 hours. Stir in the salt and black pepper. Remove then top with cheddar cheese and serve.

NUTRITION

Calories: 326, Net Carbs: 6.5g, Carbohydrate: 9.1g, Fiber: 2.6g, Protein: 23.3g, Fat: 22.9g

CHAPTER 16 - 30 DAYS MEAL PLAN

Day	Breakfast	Lunch	Snack	Dinner	Dessert
1	Cheese Crepes	Easy Keto Smoked Salmon Lunch Bowl	Keto Raspberry Cake & White Chocolate Sauce	Green Chicken Curry	Keto Cheesecakes
2	Ricotta Pancakes	Easy one-pan ground beef & green beans	Keto Chocolate Chips Cookies	Creamy Pork Stew	Keto Easy Dessert
3	Yogurt Waffles	Easy Spinach & Bacon Salad	Keto beef & Sausage balls	Salmon & Shrimp Stew	Keto Brownies
4	Broccoli Muffins	Easy Keto Italian Plate	Keto Coconut Flake Balls	Chicken Casserole	Raspberry & Coconut
5	Pumpkin Bread	Fresh broccoli & Dill Keto Salad	Keto Chocolate Greek Yoghurt Cookies	Creamy Chicken Bake	Chocolate Pudding Delight
6	Eggs in Avocado cups	Keto Smoked Salmon filled Avocados	Keto coconut flavored ice cream	Beef & Veggie Casserole	Special Keto Pudding
7	Cheddar Scramble	Low-carb Broccoli Lemon Parmesan Soup	Chocolate-coconut Cookies	Beef with Bell Peppers	Peanut Butter Fudge
8	Bacon Omelet	Prosciutto & Mozzarella Bomb	Keto Buffalo Chicken Meatballs	Braised Lamb Shanks	Coconut Pear Cream
9	Green Veggies Quiche	Summer Tuna Avocado Salad	Eggplant & Chickpea Bites	Shrimp & Bell Pepper Stir-Fry	Blackberry Stew

10	Chicken & Asparagus Frittata	Mushrooms & Goat Cheese Salad	Baba Ganouj	Veggies & Walnut Loaf	Peach Jam
11	Southwest Scrambled Egg Bites	Keto Bacon Sushi	Spicy Crab dip	Keto Sloppy Joes	Strawberry Bowls
12	Bacon Egg Bites	Cole Slaw Keto Wrap	Potatoes" of Parmesan Cheese	Low Carb Crack Slaw Egg Roll in a Bowl Recipe	Pineapple Stew
13	Omelet Bites	Keto Chicken Club Lettuce Wrap	Chili cheese Chicken with crispy & delicious cabbage salad	Low Carb Beef Stir Fry	Rhubarb Compote
14	Cheddar & Bacon Egg Bites	Keto Broccoli Salad	Keto Pumpkin Pie sweet & spicy	One Pan Pesto Chicken & Veggies	Banana Bowls
15	Avocado Pico Egg Bites	Keto Sheet Pan Chicken & Rainbow Veggies	Blackened Tilapia with Zucchini Noodles	Crispy Peanut Tofu & Cauliflower Rice Stir-Fry	Grapes Compote
16	Salmon Scramble	Skinny Bang-Bang Zucchini Noodles	Bell Pepper Nachos	Simple Keto Fried Chicken	Apricot Pudding
17	Mexican Scrambled Eggs	Keto Caesar Salad	Radish, Carrot & Cilantro Salad	Keto Butter Chicken	Blueberries & Cream
18	Caprese Omelet	Keto Buffalo Chicken Empanadas	Asparagus-Mushroom Frittata	Keto Shrimp Scampi Recipe	Pumpkin Cream
19	Sausage Omelet	Pepperoni & Cheddar Stromboli	Shrimp Avocado Salad	Keto Lasagna	Maple Pumpkin Dessert

169

20	Brown Hash with Zucchini	Tuna Casserole	Smoky Cauliflower Bites	Creamy Tuscan Garlic Chicken	Coconut Pineapple Bowls
21	Crunchy Radish & Zucchini Hash Browns	Brussels Sprout & Hamburger Gratin	Avocado Crab Boats	Ancho Macho Chili	Cinnamon Crunch Cereals
22	Fennel Quiche	Carpaccio	Coconut Curry Cauliflower Soup	Chicken Supreme Pizza	Cinnamon Rolls
23	Turkey Hash	Keto Croque Monsieur	Parmesan Asparagus	Baked Jerked Chicken	Chocolate Ice cream
24	Crustless Veggie Quiche	Keto wraps with Cream Cheese & Salmon	Cream Cheese Pancakes	Chicken Schnitzel	Strawberry ice cream
25	Keto Zucchini Bread	Savory Keto Broccoli Cheese Muffins	Sugar-free Mexican Spiced Dark Chocolate	Broccoli & Chicken Casserole	Lava Cake
26	Keto Almond Bread Recipe	Keto Rusk	Tuna in Cucumber Cups	Baked Fish with Lemon Butter	Lemon Mousse
27	Quick Keto Toast	Flaxseed hemp Flour Bun	Parmesan Crisp	Chicken Broccoli Alfredo	Chocolate Almond Butter Fat Bombs
28	Keto Loaf of Bread	Keto Muffins with Roquefort	Onion Rings	Grilled Cheesy Buffalo Chicken	White chocolate
29	Blueberry Loaf	Keto Wrap	Cold Crab Dip	Middle Eastern Shawarma	Coconut Peanut Butter Balls
30	Simple Loaf of Bread	Savory Keto Muffins	Baked Coconut Shrimp	Tex Mex Casserole	No-bake Cheesecake

CHAPTER 17 - BEST PHYSICAL EXERCISES FOR WOMEN

How you take care of your body and how you stay active will dictate your quality of life and how good you will look. If you do not take care of your body, you might be fifty years old and look like you are sixty-five years old. But if you do good things for your body, you might be sixty-five years old and look like you are fifty years old. Age is just a number. And even if you haven't been active in a long time, or ever, it is never too late to start on some activity plan to increase your life quality.

Once a woman crosses that fifty-year mark, she begins losing one percent of her muscle each year. But muscle tone and fiber do not need to be lost with aging. With a proper workout, you can continue to build new muscle and maintain what you already have until you are in your nineties.

Regular physical exercise will help you to avoid developing that middle-age spread around the abdomen or to lose it if you already have it. Exercise will help you maintain a proper weight for your height and build, which will help you avoid many, if not all, of the age-related, obesity-related diseases such as cardiovascular diseases and diabetes.

TYPES OF EXERCISES

These exercises will build up your heart and lungs, which are, after all, very important muscles in your body.

Strength training — We are not talking about bodybuilding, but if you want to go for it. It will include working out with resistance bands or lifting weights. Either activity will help to build muscle.

One thing to note here, especially if you have not been active in a while, is not to begin a vigorous activity level the same day you begin the Keto diet. When your body is getting used to the diet and going through ketosis, you will not feel like indulging in a lot of extra activity, and your workout routine will be doomed to failure. This journey is all about making you the best you can, so don't sabotage yourself in the first few weeks.

Stretching — this exercise is so important for older women. It will also help you improve your balance because you might find yourself standing or reaching new and different ways.

Quad stretch — This is a simple exercise that can be done at home. Hold onto a chair or your partner for balance assistance if you need it. Then with the opposite hand, lift the foot on that side behind you. Pull upward gently; you can feel the beginning of a stretch in the front of your leg. As people get older, they may lean forward for balance, and this muscle, the quad, can become shorter and less efficient over time. Hold this position steady for at least thirty seconds and repeat on the other side.

Hamstring stretch — This activity can be done on the sofa, the bed, or the floor. Lay one leg in front of you and point your toes to the ceiling. Slowly fold your body over until you feel a stretching in the back of your leg and hold it for thirty seconds.

Calf stretch — Place your hands on the wall and step back with one foot. Put your back foot flat on the floor, and the front knee should be slightly bent. Then lean forward toward the wall until you feel a stretch in your calf muscle. Hold it for thirty seconds and repeat on the other leg.

Balancing — Balancing activities are so important for older adults to reduce the risk of falls. Tai Chi and Yoga are both excellent activities for assisting with better balance. You can find DVDs, routines online, or classes taught by certified instructors. J Keep in mind that flexibility activities also help with the effects of arthritis. While you will want to explore the different types of yoga before deciding on the best for you, here is a yoga pose that anyone can do at home and wake the whole body in the morning.

Mountain Pose — Stand straight with your feet together. Pull in your stomach muscles as tight as you can and let your shoulders relax. Keep your legs strong but do not lock your knees. Breathe deeply and regularly in and out for ten breaths.

Strength Training — This activity is especially essential for keeping your muscles strong and healthy for your life phase. You can do many strength training activities without weights or add some light hand weights for an extra challenge.

Punching — This will strengthen your arms and shoulders and get your blood moving at the same time. Stand straight with your feet apart slightly wider than your shoulders.

Keep your stomach firm. Punch straight out with one fist and then the other for at least twenty repetitions.

Squat — This activity is excellent for strengthening the bottom and the thighs. It will help you sit down — not fall down — and rise from a seated position with ease and grace. Stand on your feet as far apart as your hips are wide to provide a stable stance. Push your bottom backward as you bend your knees. Your knees should never go out front further than your toes, and try to keep your weight over your heels. If you feel more secure, this activity can be done in front of a chair if you lose your balance and inadvertently sit down.

Cardiovascular/Aerobic — The purpose here is to engage in some activity that gets your heart pumping faster and your lungs expanding further. Swimming, walking, running, cycling, aerobics classes, and dancing are great activities for getting the circulation going again. Just remember to begin slowly and pay attention to your body. In other words, if something hurts, stop. But make sure it is really hurt. There is a difference between "Wow, I'm really out of shape, because I haven't walked anywhere in a while" and "My knee hurts when I do that." And any time you are ever in doubt, seek medical attention.

Seated Activities — The body will deteriorate if not used, so you need to engage in physical activities, but you really can't stand up for long enough to do anything meaningful. You can sit down and do many activities designed to get you back into a regular movement routine.

MAKE THE BELLY FLAT EXERCISES

All women over 50 want to clear their belly flats and achieved a new younger slim tummy. Here is a stepwise description of the most effective abdominal exercise:

RAISING THE SUPINE LEG

This exercise can be done daily. It acts on strengthening the lower abdominal muscles and also the hip flexors. Follow these steps:

Lie on a flat surface, then keep your arms on the sides and maintain them on the flat surface. Your legs should be straight and close together.

Raise your legs slowly. You can start with 3 to around 6 inches from the ground. As you do this, your heels should be close together. Increase the distance you raise your legs each day.

Flatten the lower back and tighten your abdominal muscle. It will help you hold your legs in the raised position for some time.

Vary the height, you raised your legs and held them in the new position.

You can hold your legs for as long as your body withstands.

To the beginners, initiate the exercise by holding the legs in the raised position for 30 seconds. But, if you can do 120 seconds, consider yourself doing ok.

V-UP SIT-UP

It is no joke exercise. It should be performed by those who are used to belly workouts. It targets to strengthen both the upper and the lower abdominal muscles. You can also use it to build the hip flexors. Follow these steps: Lie on a flat surface in a supine position. Your arms should be extended behind the head while the legs should be straightened.

As you perform this exercise, ensure your elbows and knees remain straight throughout the exercise.

Use your abdominal muscles to bring your arms and legs close together by bending your waist. The legs and arms should be raised simultaneously to a vertical position so that you assume a V shape.

Lower your legs and arms to the supine position. Repeat the procedure.

Relax and inhale each time you lower the limbs and exhale as you lift them to the vertical position.

BENT LEG SIT UP

This exercise can be carried out by almost everyone who is physically fit. It targets to strengthen the upper and lower abdominal muscles and also the hip flexors. It requires at least two people to be performed effectively. Follow these steps:

Lie on a flat surface. Clasp your hand behind your head.

Hold your knees at an angle of 45 degrees. To keep your feet on the floor, let your trainer/assistant hold your feet to the floor.

Use your abdominal muscles to bend your waist so that your elbows touch the knees.

Slowly take your upper body to the initial position. Repeat the exercise without pausing to work out the abdominal muscles.

Regulate your breathing such that you inhale when lowering your upper body and exhale when raising your body.

Here is an exercise that does not require the use of any tools. It has been known for its effectiveness in strengthening the abdominal muscles and hip flexors. It can be complete by people of all ages. Follow these steps:

Assume the push-up position. Your arms should be in line with your chest, while your feet should be positioned extended outward. At this position, you are resting on the balls of your feet and hands.

Lift one leg to your chest and take it back slowly. Your other leg should be kept in its original position. It would be best if you only used your abdominal muscle in lifting your leg; therefore, your hips should not rotate.

REPEAT THE PROCEDURE WITH THE OTHER LEG.

As you get used to it, you can increase the procedure's speed so that you may perform as many times as possible.

NAUTILUS ABDOMINAL CHAIR

In this exercise, a nautilus chair is used. The exercise is simple and can be used by beginners. It is very effective in strengthening all the abdominal muscles. Follow these steps:

Sit on the Nautilus chair. Place your feet underneath the ankle pads to lock them up against movement. The best way to perform this exercise is to sit upright so that the Nautilus chair's upper pads correspond to your shoulders. It would be best if you pressed on them using your chest.

Hold your arms on your chest. Close them up and let them remain in this position throughout the exercise.

Bend your waist and use your chest to push down the upper pads as far as you can. It will force you to flex your trunk. Your upper body will move forward and down, creating tension on your abdominal muscles.

Hold on to this position for about 5 seconds. Slowly allow yourself to get back to the initial position.

Repeat the exercise at least five times.

CHAPTER 18 - TROUBLESHOOTING AND FAQ

It should be noted that having doubts about the Keto diet's effectiveness or asking numerous questions about it is entirely normal. This guide will troubleshoot several regularly asked questions for you:

WHY IS IT IMPORTANT TO STICK TO THE KETOGENIC MEAL PLAN?

The Ketogenic diet is important because:

It reduces your blood's insulin and sugar level.

It lowers your body's blood pressure.

It improves your LDL Cholesterol levels.

It is a therapy for brain disorders.

It lowers your body's triglycerides.

It assists you in shedding weight.

It reduces your appetite.

Suppose you are looking to boost your blood sugar and insulin levels or lose appetite, lose weight, lower your triglycerides, remedying brain disorders, lower your blood pressure, or become healthier. In that case, you have all the reasons to stick to the Keto diet.

HOW LONG WOULD IT TAKE FOR THE KETOGENIC DIET TO BE EFFECTIVE?

The fact is that the amount of time it would take you to enter Ketosis is not the same amount of time someone else could need to get into Ketosis. Additionally, many people find it hard for their bodies to enter Ketosis. Let us take a look at how long it could take you to enter Ketosis.

For you to benefit from the diet, your body needs to get into Ketosis first. Ketosis is a state that your body adapts to when it starts burning fats into molecules referred to as ketones. Ketones are your body's primary energy source once your body stops burning carbohydrates to produce glucose, usually the primary energy source on the regular diet.

It would require you between 2 to 5 days to get into Ketosis if you are an average consumer of carbohydrates. It is approximate if you consume 50 to 60 grams of carbohydrates in a day. The duration of time could be altered depending on several factors, including; the body's metabolism, age, physical activity level, protein, carbohydrates, and fat intake.

Other people take longer to get into Ketosis because they most probably ingest carbohydrates without knowing.

IS IT POSSIBLE TO GAIN WEIGHT WHILE ON THE KETOGENIC DIET?

Although the Ketogenic diet is responsible for a healthy way of losing weight, the diet could gain weight. By talking about the Ketogenic diet, we are talking about the increased consumption of fats. You could gain weight on a diet without your knowledge.

WHAT IS THE DIRTY KETOGENIC DIET?

As stated numerous times, the regular Ketogenic diet advocates for about 70% of fats, 20% of protein, and finally 10% of carbohydrates. The 'dirty Ketogenic diet' follows these same rules. Their difference is that it does not focus on where these fats, proteins, or carbohydrates come from. It could mean instead of eating foods rich in a good fast, you could opt to eat a bunless double cheeseburger. Unlike the Ketogenic diet, which follows and advocates for healthy oils like coconut oil, the dirty Ketogenic diet allows you to consume pork rinds.

HOW WILL I KNOW IF MY BODY IS IN KETOSIS?

Numerous signs would indicate that your body is in Ketosis. For instance, if you happen to wake up with a fruity metallic taste in your mouth after adopting the diet, it is evidence to indicate that your body is already manufacturing ketones and that you are already in Ketosis. It is also possible to experience mental sharpness if your body manufactures elevated levels of ketones.

However, the only way to be sure that your body is in Ketosis is to test your body's ketones levels medically. You could opt to visit your local physician or your local doctor, who will then run a few tests on you to determine if your body is in Ketosis. Or, you could opt to self-test and test your urine using the urine test, blood using the blood test, or your breath using the Breathalyzer and determine your body's ketones levels.

WHAT COULD PUT ME OUT OF KETOSIS, AND HOW CAN I QUICKLY GET MYSELF BACK INTO KETOSIS?

Getting your body out of Ketosis is very easy. It is because your body could get out of Ketosis immediately after a meal, even if that meal contains small traces of carbohydrates, and your body could revert to burning carbohydrates for energy for a few hours. It is why it is advisable to stick to the Ketogenic diet with discipline. However, this is all normal, and you do not have to press the panic button already. It is because your body is designed to burn carbohydrates for energy, and it will automatically revert to burning carbohydrates if some are available in your meal.

It is important to note that ingesting artificial ketones has not been fully clinically tested; thus, it is not recommended to get your body back into Ketosis. There are ways that you could do to assist your body to get back into Ketosis, and these include; integrating periods of fasting or consuming certain types of fats that are Keto-friendly, like MCTs.

I AM A PHYSICALLY ACTIVE PERSON; CAN I STILL PRACTICE THE KETOGENIC DIET?

It is effortless to assume that your lack of ingesting carbohydrates could interfere with your body's production of energy, which could, in return, affect your performance, given that you are an active person. This assumption is not correct. It is because research conducted on the Ketogenic diet has proven that the ketones produced by your body can boost your performance.

WHAT IS A KETOGENIC ADAPTATION, AND WHAT DOES IT FEEL LIKE?

The term 'Ketogenic Adaptation' refers to the transition of your body from primarily burning carbohydrates to produce glucose to burning fats to produce ketone bodies to be used instead of glucose. It will take a few days for your body, after adapting to the Ketogenic diet, to completely burn all the glucose in your body before shifting its attention to burning fats to produce ketone bodies.

During the Ketogenic Adaptation period, it is a possibility that you will experience symptoms of carbohydrates withdrawal at the beginning. Still, once your body has adjusted to using fats to produce ketone bodies for energy, you will find your cravings for carbohydrates reducing.

IS ALCOHOL APPROPRIATE WHILE ON THE KETOGENIC DIET?

Alcohol is rich in carbs. The Ketogenic diet advocates for a meal that is high in fats, moderate in protein, and very low in carbohydrates. Alcohol is defying that order and ratio.

You are probably not a lover of both hard liquor and wines, but you are a big fan of beer. Well, beer is made up of barley, yeast, water, and hops, meaning that beer is not Keto friendly. From its content, beer should be avoided at all costs. It is because beer is made from the breaking down of barley into sugary maltose; yeast acts on and ends up creating an elevated amount of sugar compared to wines and hard liquor. However, there is one beer you could opt to use, which is gluten-free and low in carbs, the Omission Ultimate Light Golden Ale.

WHAT CHINESE FOOD YOU COULD EAT WHEN ON THE KETOGENIC DIET?

If you are a Chinese food lover and are on the Ketogenic diet, this book has you covered. The first step to ensure that you have a great Keto friendly Chinese food is to plan your visit to a Chinese restaurant. It is essential to decide how much carbohydrates you are planning on consuming. In this case, you are on the Ketogenic diet, which means you will have to keep your carbohydrates consumption in line with the diet requirements. If the restaurant has provided its recipe online, you could opt to check it and be sure that the restaurant is offering a Keto friendly diet. You could also call and ask, or you could even message the restaurant.

CONCLUSION

REACHING YOUR GOAL

The saying remains true — you will realize that what you put into your body will dictate how you feel. While on the Keto diet, you are building up energy stores for your body to utilize. That means that you should be feeling a necessary boost in your energy levels and the ability to pass each moment of each day without struggling. You can say goodbye to the sluggish feeling that often accompanies other diet plans. When you are on Keto, you should only be experiencing the benefits of additional energy and unlimited potential. Your diet isn't going to always feel like a diet. After some time, you will realize that you enjoy eating a Keto menu very much. Because your body will be switching the way it metabolizes, it will also change what it craves. Don't be surprised if you end up hungering fats and proteins as you progress on the Keto diet — this is what your body will eventually want.

TRACKING PROGRESS

Using a compare and contrast method is always great for monitoring progress. Remember how you felt before starting the Keto diet. If you haven't started already, you can use this time to document your current state of being. Make sure to record your mindset and the cravings that you have. When you have these figures to compare your progress to, you will use this as a motivating tool. Remember to allow yourself the feeling of pride as you make it through each day of being on the Keto diet. Commit yourself and the diet. That will present its own set of trials to face, but they will not be so complicated that you lose your way. Believe in your ability to see this through.

YOU ARE WHAT YOU EAT

Think about how you used to feel while eating your sugary and carb-loaded cravings. Your immediate response will likely suggest that you felt great but think about the bigger picture. Did you gain more energy from eating these things? Eating junk food only serves your immediate cravings. When you think about it, this junk food indeed doesn't have a place in your life.

Choose to feel satisfied when you can know for sure that you are treating your body correctly. You should be able to handle the joy that comes from the fact that you are giving your body fuel that it can utilize. While eating your Keto-friendly food might not show you the same immediate rush that eating your favorite junk food does, it will benefit you much more in the long run. You will be able to notice its advantages long after you digest the food, which is essential. A simple change in perspective is what you need to realize that your happiness isn't directly tied to the cravings that you satisfy. Your satisfaction needs to stem from a deeper place.

YOUR LIFE WILL IMPROVE

There comes the point while being on the Keto diet that you make a shift from trying to succeeding. That will happen at various points for people, but when it happens to you, embrace it. Instead of concentrating on the fact that you are following a diet, you can begin to shift your focus to your receiving benefits. You need to ensure that you appreciate your life!

YOUR BODY WILL CHANGE

One of the exciting benefits that you will begin enjoying is the way that your appearance will change. Your skin should have a healthy glow to it, appearing youthful. As the aging process takes place, feeling ashamed of your skin can become a prominent issue that impacts your self-esteem significantly. Aging is a process that no one is exempt from, but the Keto diet can help you do it more gracefully. When you notice that your skin is improving, you can commit to taking better care of it.

Your efforts should not only inspire those around you, but they should also serve as a way to motivate yourself. Acknowledge your progress and recognize the challenges that you had to face while arriving there. You will wonder what you even used to eat before. That is why Keto tends to be a permanent solution. Even those who agree to try it for a few months end up sticking with it for much longer. Just keep it up unless it no longer feels right. If you are getting all of your benefits plus the satisfaction of being full of eating clean foods, you will likely continue feeling great while on Keto.

THANK YOU

Finally, if you enjoyed this book, then I'd like to ask you for a favor, would you be kind enough to leave a review for this book on Amazon? It'd be greatly appreciated!

It would be crucial to help me with this project that I care about a lot. I believe that regardless of the book and the mission that matters. Everybody deserves a healthier and more just life. Maybe people are not aware of it.

Maybe we can help.

With Love,

Jillian Collins

CPSIA information can be obtained
at www.ICGtesting.com
Printed in the USA
LVHW101149141220
674127LV00006B/193